Biomarkers in Neurodegenerative Diseases

Biomarkers in Neurodegenerative Diseases

Editor

Arnab Ghosh

MDPI • Basel • Beijing • Wuhan • Barcelona • Belgrade • Manchester • Tokyo • Cluj • Tianjin

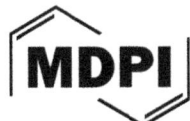

Editor
Arnab Ghosh
Cleveland State University
USA

Editorial Office
MDPI
St. Alban-Anlage 66
4052 Basel, Switzerland

This is a reprint of articles from the Special Issue published online in the open access journal *Biomedicines* (ISSN 2227-9059) (available at: https://www.mdpi.com/journal/biomedicines/special_issues/biomarkers_neurodegenerative).

For citation purposes, cite each article independently as indicated on the article page online and as indicated below:

LastName, A.A.; LastName, B.B.; LastName, C.C. Article Title. *Journal Name* **Year**, *Volume Number*, Page Range.

ISBN 978-3-0365-5729-8 (Hbk)
ISBN 978-3-0365-5730-4 (PDF)

© 2022 by the authors. Articles in this book are Open Access and distributed under the Creative Commons Attribution (CC BY) license, which allows users to download, copy and build upon published articles, as long as the author and publisher are properly credited, which ensures maximum dissemination and a wider impact of our publications.

The book as a whole is distributed by MDPI under the terms and conditions of the Creative Commons license CC BY-NC-ND.

Contents

Arnab Ghosh
Biomarkers in Neurodegenerative Diseases
Reprinted from: *Biomedicines* **2022**, *10*, 215, doi:10.3390/biomedicines10020215 1

Enes Akyuz, Chiara Villa, Merve Beker and Birsen Elibol
Unraveling the Role of Inwardly Rectifying Potassium Channels in the Hippocampus of an
$A\beta_{(1-42)}$-Infused Rat Model of Alzheimer's Disease
Reprinted from: *Biomedicines* **2020**, *8*, 58, doi:10.3390/biomedicines8030058 5

Almuth F. Kessler, Jonas Feldheim, Dominik Schmitt, Julia J. Feldheim,
Camelia M. Monoranu, Ralf-Ingo Ernestus, Mario Löhr and Carsten Hagemann
Monopolar Spindle 1 Kinase (MPS1/TTK) mRNA Expression is Associated with Earlier
Development of Clinical Symptoms, Tumor Aggressiveness and Survival of Glioma Patients
Reprinted from: *Biomedicines* **2020**, *8*, 192, doi:10.3390/biomedicines8070192 15

Alessandro Fulgenzi, Daniele Vietti and Maria Elena Ferrero
EDTA Chelation Therapy in the Treatment of Neurodegenerative Diseases: An Update
Reprinted from: *Biomedicines* **2020**, *8*, 269, doi:10.3390/biomedicines8080269 29

Riaz Ahmad, Amjad Khan, Hyeon Jin Lee, Inayat Ur Rehman, Ibrahim Khan,
Sayed Ibrar Alam and Myeong Ok Kim
Lupeol, a Plant-Derived Triterpenoid, Protects Mice Brains against $A\beta$-Induced Oxidative Stress
and Neurodegeneration
Reprinted from: *Biomedicines* **2020**, *8*, 380, doi:10.3390/biomedicines8100380 43

Adrian Florian Bălașa, Cristina Chircov and Alexandru Mihai Grumezescu
Body Fluid Biomarkers for Alzheimer's Disease—An Up-To-Date Overview
Reprinted from: *Biomedicines* **2020**, *8*, 421, doi:10.3390/biomedicines8100421 57

Laura Bordoni, Irene Petracci, Jean Calleja-Agius, Joan G. Lalor and Rosita Gabbianelli
NURR1 Alterations in Perinatal Stress: A First Step towards Late-Onset Diseases? A
Narrative Review
Reprinted from: *Biomedicines* **2020**, *8*, 584, doi:10.3390/biomedicines8120584 79

Chung-Yao Chien, Szu-Wei Hsu, Tsung-Lin Lee, Pi-Shan Sung and Chou-Ching Lin
Using Artificial Neural Network to Discriminate Parkinson's Disease from Other Parkinsonisms
by Focusing on Putamen of Dopamine Transporter SPECT Images
Reprinted from: *Biomedicines* , , 12, doi:10.3390/biomedicines9010012 95

Seungil Paik, Rishi K. Somvanshi, Helen A. Oliveira, Shenglong Zou and Ujendra Kumar
Somatostatin Ameliorates β-Amyloid-Induced Cytotoxicity via the Regulation of CRMP2
Phosphorylation and Calcium Homeostasis in SH-SY5Y Cells
Reprinted from: *Biomedicines* **2021**, *9*, 27, doi:10.3390/biomedicines9010027 107

Sayed Ibrar Alam, Min Gi Jo, Tae Ju Park, Rahat Ullah, Sareer Ahmad, Shafiq Ur Rehman
and Myeong Ok Kim
Quinpirole-Mediated Regulation of Dopamine D2 Receptors Inhibits Glial Cell-Induced
Neuroinflammation in Cortex and Striatum after Brain Injury
Reprinted from: *Biomedicines* **2021**, *9*, 47, doi:10.3390/biomedicines9010047 125

Carlotta Giorgi, Esmaa Bouhamida, Alberto Danese, Maurizio Previati, Paolo Pinton and Simone Patergnani
Relevance of Autophagy and Mitophagy Dynamics and Markers in Neurodegenerative Diseases
Reprinted from: *Biomedicines* **2021**, 9, 149, doi:10.3390/biomedicines9020149 . . . . **143**

Jacopo Meldolesi
News about the Role of Fluid and Imaging Biomarkers in Neurodegenerative Diseases
Reprinted from: *Biomedicines* **2021**, 9, 252, doi:10.3390/biomedicines9030252 . . . . **169**

Editorial

Biomarkers in Neurodegenerative Diseases

Arnab Ghosh

Center for Gene Regulation in Health and Disease, Department of Biological, Geological and Environmental Sciences, Cleveland State University, Cleveland, OH 44115, USA; a.ghosh100@csuohio.edu

An increasing number of people are affected by various neurodegenerative diseases each year, impacting the quality of life of millions of people worldwide. However, considerable knowledge gaps in the mechanistic understanding of these diseases present a challenge to address this threat to human life successfully. Recent endeavors in basic research, clinical trials, and other research areas have provided vital insights to discover novel biomarkers for improved diagnosis and better treatment options for patients suffering from such diseases. Articles published as part of the Special Issue "Biomarkers in Neurodegenerative Diseases" highlight the recent advances in this field and emerging strategies to counter such diseases in the future.

Three research articles published in the Special Issue focused on molecular mechanisms involving Alzheimer's disease (AD). First, Paik et al. used human SH-SY5Y neuroblastoma cells to show the neuroprotective role of Somatostatin-14 (SST). The possible mechanism involves the ability of SST to regulate the intracellular calcium levels and Collapsin Response Mediator Protein 2 (CRMP2) phosphorylation [1]. Second, Akyuz and coworkers measured the expression of neuronal inwardly rectifying potassium (Kir) channels in an $A\beta(1-42)$-infused rat model of AD [2]. These findings open up newer possibilities to discover novel biomarkers or therapeutic targets against AD in the future. Finally, Ahmad et al. showed that lupeol (a plant-based triterpenoid compound) could improve memory function in the AD mouse model. Lupeol's antioxidant and anti-inflammatory properties were proposed to be responsible for this observation [3]. Naturally occurring biologically active compounds present a promising target to evaluate as a potential therapy against many pathological conditions, including neurodegenerative diseases.

Kessler and others show a correlation between dysregulation of Monopolar Spindle 1 Kinase (MPS1) and tumor aggressiveness in glioblastoma multiforme (GBM) patients [4]. The researchers performed qPCR on frozen tumor tissue samples of GBM patients and compared them with non-pathological tissue samples. However, a more extensive study involving an increased number of patients is necessary to test whether MPS1 mRNA levels can be a reliable indicator of tumor aggressiveness in cancer patients across different subgroups.

One key aspect of neurologic disorders includes complications arising from traumatic brain injuries (TBIs). In this regard, Alam et al. investigated the role of quinpirole in dopamine D2 receptor (D2R) activation using a mouse model simulating TBI [5]. This study implicated quinpirole in D2R regulation and suggested a mechanism via the Akt/GSK3-β signaling pathway, leading to brain function recovery by reducing inflammatory responses. This observation opens up additional prospects to improve brain functions in patients suffering neurologic ailments due to TBI. Nevertheless, further studies are necessary to test the hypothesis definitively.

Fulgenzi et al. provide an excellent update in the investigation of chelation therapy involving EDTA as a potential treatment for neurologic disorders. They studied more than 300 patients from a broad age group to monitor their toxic metal burdens before and after receiving EDTA as part of the therapy [6]. Information obtained from the study provides excellent guidance for more detailed analyses involving larger patient groups to investigate the efficacy of chelation therapy in the future.

One of the critical challenges for better treatment outcomes is correctly identifying the causes behind indicators of different neurologic conditions. Chien and coworkers used an artificial neural network to distinguish between dopamine transporter single-photon emission computed tomography (DAT-SPECT) images obtained from patients with Parkinson's disease or parkinsonism resulting from other illnesses with high (more than 80%) accuracy [7].

Apart from these original research papers, the Special Issue also contains an excellent collection of review articles highlighting recent progress, challenges, and future directions in the field. For example, the review articles published by Jacopo Meldolesi and Bălașa et al. are excellent resources summarizing the significant advances made in fluid and imaging biomarkers for the early detection of neurodegenerative disorders in recent times [8,9]. The authors also make a great effort to outline the deficiencies of our present knowledge in the field and potential ways to address these shortcomings. Giorgi et al. focused on recent advancements in understanding the mechanisms of autophagy and mitophagy processes and their relevance to neurodegenerative diseases [10]. Knowledge obtained from studying these cellular processes could lead to better therapeutic strategies against such conditions in the future. Finally, Bordoni and colleagues summarized the significance of dysregulation of a transcription factor called Nuclear Receptor Related 1 (NURR1) protein for perinatal stress [11]. Such stress is known to substantially increase the possibility of chronic diseases (such as neurologic conditions) later in life.

I hope that these excellent research works and review articles published as part of the Special Issue will provide an invaluable reference for further research to counter the menaces posed by neurologic disorders in the future.

Funding: This research received no external funding.

Institutional Review Board Statement: Not applicable.

Informed Consent Statement: Not applicable.

Data Availability Statement: Not applicable.

Acknowledgments: I would like to thank the authors who decided to publish their valuable work and the journal editors for their enormous efforts to make the Special Issue a success.

Conflicts of Interest: The author declares no conflict of interest.

References

1. Paik, S.; Somvanshi, R.K.; Oliveira, H.A.; Zou, S.; Kumar, U. Somatostatin Ameliorates β-Amyloid-Induced Cytotoxicity via the Regulation of CRMP2 Phosphorylation and Calcium Homeostasis in SH-SY5Y Cells. *Biomedicines* **2021**, *9*, 27. [CrossRef] [PubMed]
2. Akyuz, E.; Villa, C.; Beker, M.; Elibol, B. Unraveling the Role of Inwardly Rectifying Potassium Channels in the Hippocampus of an Aβ(1–42)-Infused Rat Model of Alzheimer's Disease. *Biomedicines* **2020**, *8*, 58. [CrossRef] [PubMed]
3. Ahmad, R.; Khan, A.; Lee, H.J.; Ur Rehman, I.; Khan, I.; Alam, S.I.; Kim, M.O. Lupeol, a Plant-Derived Triterpenoid, Protects Mice Brains against Aβ-Induced Oxidative Stress and Neurodegeneration. *Biomedicines* **2020**, *8*, 380. [CrossRef] [PubMed]
4. Kessler, A.F.; Feldheim, J.; Schmitt, D.; Feldheim, J.J.; Monoranu, C.M.; Ernestus, R.-I.; Löhr, M.; Hagemann, C. Monopolar Spindle 1 Kinase (MPS1/TTK) mRNA Expression is Associated with Earlier Development of Clinical Symptoms, Tumor Aggressiveness and Survival of Glioma Patients. *Biomedicines* **2020**, *8*, 192. [CrossRef] [PubMed]
5. Alam, S.I.; Jo, M.G.; Park, T.J.; Ullah, R.; Ahmad, S.; Rehman, S.U.; Kim, M.O. Quinpirole-Mediated Regulation of Dopamine D2 Receptors Inhibits Glial Cell-Induced Neuroinflammation in Cortex and Striatum after Brain Injury. *Biomedicines* **2021**, *9*, 47. [CrossRef] [PubMed]
6. Fulgenzi, A.; Vietti, D.; Ferrero, M.E. EDTA Chelation Therapy in the Treatment of Neurodegenerative Diseases: An Update. *Biomedicines* **2020**, *8*, 269. [CrossRef] [PubMed]
7. Chien, C.-Y.; Hsu, S.-W.; Lee, T.-L.; Sung, P.-S.; Lin, C.-C. Using Artificial Neural Network to Discriminate Parkinson's Disease from Other Parkinsonisms by Focusing on Putamen of Dopamine Transporter SPECT Images. *Biomedicines* **2021**, *9*, 12. [CrossRef] [PubMed]
8. Meldolesi, J. News about the Role of Fluid and Imaging Biomarkers in Neurodegenerative Diseases. *Biomedicines* **2021**, *9*, 252. [CrossRef] [PubMed]

9. Bălașa, A.F.; Chircov, C.; Grumezescu, A.M. Body Fluid Biomarkers for Alzheimer's Disease—An Up-To-Date Overview. *Biomedicines* **2020**, *8*, 421. [CrossRef] [PubMed]
10. Giorgi, C.; Bouhamida, E.; Danese, A.; Previati, M.; Pinton, P.; Patergnani, S. Relevance of Autophagy and Mitophagy Dynamics and Markers in Neurodegenerative Diseases. *Biomedicines* **2021**, *9*, 149. [CrossRef] [PubMed]
11. Bordoni, L.; Petracci, I.; Calleja-Agius, J.; Lalor, J.G.; Gabbianelli, R. NURR1 Alterations in Perinatal Stress: A First Step towards Late-Onset Diseases? A Narrative Review. *Biomedicines* **2020**, *8*, 584. [CrossRef] [PubMed]

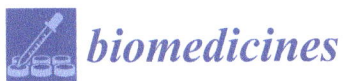

Article

Unraveling the Role of Inwardly Rectifying Potassium Channels in the Hippocampus of an Aβ$_{(1-42)}$-Infused Rat Model of Alzheimer's Disease

Enes Akyuz [1,*], Chiara Villa [2,*], Merve Beker [3] and Birsen Elibol [3]

1. Department of Biophysics, Faculty of Medicine, Yozgat Bozok University, Yozgat 66100, Turkey
2. School of Medicine and Surgery, University of Milano-Bicocca, 20900 Monza, Italy
3. Department of Medical Biology, Faculty of Medicine, Bezmialem Vakif University, Istanbul 34093, Turkey; mbeker@bezmialem.edu.tr (M.B.); bcan@bezmialem.edu.tr (B.E.)
* Correspondence: enesakyuz25@gmail.com (E.A.); chiara.villa@unimib.it (C.V.)

Received: 7 February 2020; Accepted: 12 March 2020; Published: 13 March 2020

Abstract: Alzheimer's disease (AD) is a progressive neurodegenerative disorder with a complex etiology and characterized by cognitive deficits and memory loss. The pathogenesis of AD is not yet completely elucidated, and no curative treatment is currently available. Inwardly rectifying potassium (Kir) channels are important for playing a key role in maintaining the resting membrane potential and controlling cell excitability, being largely expressed in both excitable and non-excitable tissues, including neurons. Accordingly, the aim of the study is to investigate the role of neuronal Kir channels in AD pathophysiology. The mRNA and protein levels of neuronal Kir2.1, Kir3.1, and Kir6.2 were evaluated by real-time PCR and Western blot analysis from the hippocampus of an amyloid-β(Aβ)$_{(1-42)}$-infused rat model of AD. Extracellular deposition of Aβ was confirmed by both histological Congo red staining and immunofluorescence analysis. Significant decreased mRNA and protein levels of Kir2.1 and Kir6.2 channels were observed in the rat model of AD, whereas no differences were found in Kir3.1 channel levels as compared with controls. Our results provide in vivo evidence that Aβ can modulate the expression of these channels, which may represent novel potential therapeutic targets in the treatment of AD.

Keywords: Alzheimer's disease; amyloid beta; hippocampus; Kir channels; K$^+$ channels

---

1. Introduction

Alzheimer's disease (AD; MIM#104300) is a chronic irreversible neurodegenerative disorder and represents the most common form of dementia in elderly individuals [1]. AD is clinically characterized by a progressive memory deterioration, thinking difficulty, confusion, and changes in personality, behavior, and language, resulting in autonomy loss that finally requires full-time medical care [2]. The neuropathological hallmarks of AD include the presence of extracellular senile plaques constituted by the amyloid-β (Aβ) peptide and intracellular neurofibrillary tangles (NFTs) composed of hyper-phosphorylated paired helical filaments of the microtubule-associated protein tau (MAPT) [3]. Among Aβ species, Aβ$_{(1-42)}$, which is generated from Aβ precursor protein (APP) sequentially cleaved by β-secretase and γ-secretase, is considered more toxic than Aβ$_{(1-40)}$ because of its strong tendency to aggregate [4]. The Aβ deposition in the brain triggers a series of neurodegenerative processes, including synaptic toxicity, microglia-mediated inflammation, mitochondrial dysfunction, and oxidative stress, which in turn lead to cell death [5]. Furthermore, Aβ pathogenesis reduces the synthesis of acetylcholine (ACh) and negatively affects the acetylcholinesterase (AChE) activity [6]. Despite its prevalence, the AD pathogenesis is not completely understood, and, currently, there are no effective treatments to slow or halt the progression of its symptoms [7].

Emerging evidence points out a key role of ion channels in the progress and development of a variety of neurological disorders, including epilepsy [8,9], autism spectrum disorders [10], multiple sclerosis [11], and AD [12]. Among them, the inwardly rectifying potassium (K^+) channels (Kir) are essential for maintaining the resting membrane potential and controlling the cell excitability by the regulation intracellular and extracellular flow of K^+ ions in different types of cells, including neurons. To date, seven subfamilies (Kir1-Kir7) have been identified according to their sequence similarity and function properties [13]. An important involvement of Kir2.x, Kir3.x, and Kir6.x channels in the pathogenesis of AD has been supported by both in vitro and in vivo models [11]. Evidence showed an impaired activity or an altered expression of these channels, probably modulated by Aβ [12,14]. Given the limitations of investigating AD in human subjects, current studies mostly rely on animal models in order to understand the underlying molecular mechanisms of this disorder. Some experimental in vivo models mimicking the major neuropathological hallmarks in AD have already been developed for studying Kir channels in the disease pathogenesis [12,15], but no data are available regarding an $Aβ_{(1-42)}$-infused rat model of AD.

Herein, we aim to better elucidate the role of Kir2.1, Kir3.1, and Kir6.2 channels in AD pathophysiology by analyzing their mRNA and protein levels in the hippocampus of an $Aβ_{(1-42)}$-infused rat model of AD. This represents a valuable tool that recapitulates some key features of human AD, including Aβ plaque, cholinergic dysfunction, neuron loss, ventricular enlargement, and behavior deficiencies.

2. Materials and Methods

2.1. Animals

Adult female Sprague–Dawley rats (6-month-old; n = 14) were housed in a quiet, temperature and humidity-controlled room (21 ± 2 °C; 62% ± 7% relative humidity; 12-h cycles dark/light). Rats were fed ad libitum with a standard dry rat diet and tap water. All procedures were carried out in strict accordance with the recommendations in the Guide for the Care and Use of Laboratory Animals adopted by the National Institutes of Health (NIH, Bethesda, MD, USA) and the Declaration of Helsinki. Experimental protocol of this study was approved by the local scientific ethical committee of Bezmialem Vakif University, Istanbul, Turkey (2015/229). All efforts were made to minimize animal suffering.

2.2. $Aβ_{(1-42)}$-Infused Rat Model

A solvent of 35% acetonitrile plus 0.1% trifluoroacetic acid was used to reconstitute the $Aβ_{(1-42)}$ peptide (SCP0038, Sigma-Aldrich, St. Louis, MO, USA) and soluble peptide suspensions were incubated at 37 °C for 72 h with gentle shaking for fibril formation. The rats were injected intra-cerebroventricularly (ICV) with oligomeric $Aβ_{(1-42)}$ to induce AD. Briefly, after seven days of acclimation, rats were anesthetized with an intraperitoneal injection of a ketamine and xylazine mixture (100 and 10 mg/kg body weight, respectively) and then placed in a stereotaxic apparatus. A stainless steel cannula was stereotaxically implanted into the right hippocampus of rats (coordinates from bregma: −3.60 mm anteroposterior; −2.00 mm lateral; −4.00 mm vertical) and fixed to the skull with dental cement. A mini-osmotic pump (Alzet 2002, Durect, Cupertino, CA, USA) was attached and implanted subcutaneously near the scapula for a continual infusion.

2.3. Experimental Design

Rats that underwent ICV infusion were randomly divided into two groups (n = 7 per group): (i) sham control that received injections of 0.9% NaCl saline solution, and (ii) $Aβ_{(1-42)}$-infused group injected with $Aβ_{(1-42)}$ oligomers at the rate of 300 pmol/day for 14 days. Rats were sacrificed with decapitation after a 14-day infusion. The brains were quickly removed, and their both right and left hippocampi were dissected and then stored at −80 °C until molecular analysis.

2.4. Histological Congo Red Staining

Coronal sections from the hippocampus were prepared at 20 μm thickness using a cryostat and fixed in ice-chilled 4% paraformaldehyde (PFA). For labeling Aβ deposits, slices were stained with 1% Congo red solution (Sigma-Aldrich, St. Louis, MO, USA) in 80% of absolute ethanol and 1% of NaOH. After being washed, sections were counterstained with cresyl violet, dehydrated in absolute ethanol, and then cleared in xylene. Specimens were mounted on slides and evaluated under a light microscope (Nikon Microscopy, Tokyo, Japan). For quantification, images were analyzed by color segmentation plugin–ImageJ software (NIH, Bethesda, MD, USA). The entire area of deposits was considered.

2.5. Immunofluorescence Analysis

The PFA-fixed slices were blocked with 10% normal goat serum for 1 h. Sections were immunostained with the application of 1:100 dilution of primary anti-Aβ rabbit polyclonal antibody (8243, Cell Signaling Technology, Danvers, MA, USA) followed by goat anti-rabbit Alexa Fluor® 488 conjugated secondary antibody (A11034, Thermo Fisher Scientific, Waltham, MA, USA) at 1:200 dilution. Nuclei were marked blue with 40,6-diamidino-2-phenylindole (DAPI). The sections were mounted on slides and evaluated under a fluorescence microscope (Axio, Zeiss, Germany).

2.6. cDNA Synthesis and Real-Time PCR

Total RNA was isolated from homogenized hippocampal tissue with TRIzol and PureLink RNA mini kit (Thermo Fisher Scientific, Waltham, MA, USA), according to the manufacturer's instructions. One microgram of the total extract amount of RNA was treated with DNase I and reverse-transcribed using High Capacity cDNA Reverse Transcription Kit according to the manufacturer's suggested protocol (Applied Biosystems, Foster City, CA, USA). The first-strand cDNA was used as a template for real-time PCR (RT–PCR) using rat specific primers for *Kcnj2* (Kir2.1), *Kcnj3* (Kir3.1), and *Kcnj11* (Kir6.2), as reported in Table 1. RT–PCR reaction was performed with the SYBR Green PCR kit (iTaq™ Universal SYBR® Green, Biorad, Hercules, CA, USA) using a CFX96 real-time system sequence detector (Biorad, Hercules, CA, USA). Data, normalized to the housekeeping control gene (*Gapdh*), are expressed as fold change values respect to the sham control group according to the $2^{-\Delta\Delta Ct}$ algorithm, as previously described [16].

Table 1. List of primers for RT–PCR.

Genes	Forward Primer (5′–3′)	Reverse Primer (5′–3′)
Kcnj2	GCAAACTCTGCTTGATGTGG	TCATACAAAGGGCTGTCTTCG
Kcnj3	CTGACCGCTTCACATAGC	CTCCAGACTGGGATAGAC
Kcnj11	CCTACACCAGGTGGACATCC	CAGGCTGCGGTCCTCATCAA

2.7. Western blotting (WB)

Total protein extracts were obtained by lysing 0.25 g hippocampal tissue with 1 X RIPA lysis buffer (50 mM Tris-HCl pH 7.4, 150 mM NaCl, 1% Triton X-100, 0.1 % SDS) added with 1 mM DTT, 1 mM EDTA and EGTA, and 1.5% protease inhibitor cocktail and phosphatase inhibitor cocktail. Total protein concentration was measured using the Pierce BCA Protein Assay Kit (Thermo Fisher Scientific, Waltham, MA, USA) by a Multiskan™ GO Microplate spectrophotometer. Equal amounts of proteins were boiled for 5 min and separated by SDS–PAGE followed by transfer to PVDF membrane. Then, the membranes were blocked with 5% milk solution prepared in TBST (Tris-buffered saline, 0.1% Tween 20) buffer and incubated with one of the following primary antibodies against Kir2.1 (rabbit polyclonal, 1:200, Abcam, Cambridge, UK [ab65796]), Kir3.1 (mouse monoclonal, 1:200, Alomone Labs, Jerusalem, Israel [APC-005]), Kir6.2 (rabbit polyclonal, 1:200, Alomone Labs, Jerusalem, Israel [APC-020]), or β-actin (mouse monoclonal, 1:5000, Thermo Fisher Scientific, Waltham, MA, USA [AC-15]). Membranes were washed three times in TBST and then incubated with ECL anti-mouse or anti-rabbit horseradish peroxidase-conjugated IgG secondary antibodies (1:5000, GE Healthcare Life Sciences, Amersham, UK). The protein bands were developed with luminol-based substrate (Advansta, San Jose, CA, USA) and chemiluminescent signal was digitally acquired by CCD camera with Fusion FX7 (Vilber Lourmat, France) system. Densitometric analysis of Western blot bands was performed using the "gel analyzer" function of ImageJ software (NIH, Bethesda, MD, USA).

2.8. Statistical Analysis

Data are generally given as mean values ± standard error of the mean (SEM). Pairwise comparisons were performed by Mann–Whitney U-test. The version 18 of Statistical Package for Social Science (SPSS 18, IBM Corporation, Chicago, IL, USA) was used for statistical analysis of the data. Differences were considered significant at * $p < 0.05$ and ** $p < 0.01$.

3. Results

3.1. Injection of Aβ$_{(1-42)}$ Oligomers Mimicked Alzheimer's Disease in Rats

As a result of Aβ$_{(1-42)}$ infusion for 14 days, both Congo red histological staining and immunofluorescence analysis confirmed the extracellular presence of oligomeric and aggregated forms of Aβ in the hippocampus of rat model as compared with the sham control (2.73-fold change over sham controls, * $p < 0.05$, Figure 1; 2.21-fold change over sham control, * $p < 0.05$, Figure 2, respectively).

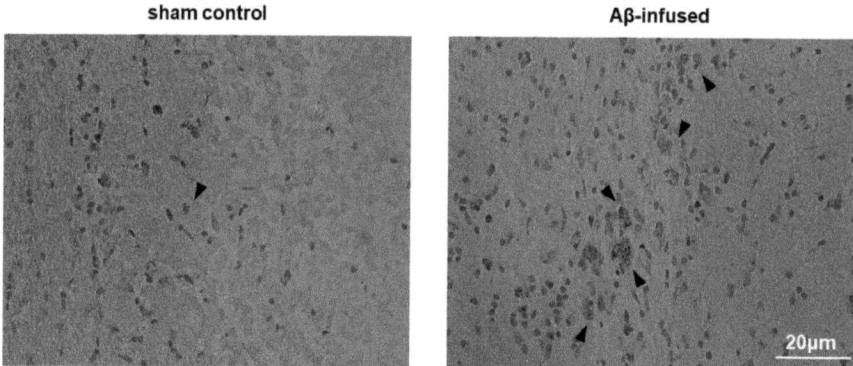

Figure 1. Representative images of hippocampus sections stained with Congo red in sham control and Aβ$_{(1-42)}$-infused rat model. Extracellular Aβ deposits were visualized in brownish color and indicated by arrows; the nuclei were counterstained with cresyl violet (purple). Pictures were taken at the magnification of ×20. Scale bar: 20 μm.

3.2. Aβ$_{(1-42)}$-Infused Rats Exhibited Low mRNA Levels of Neuronal Kir2.1 and Kir6.2 Channels

With the purpose of investigating a possible role of neuronal Kir channels in AD pathogenesis, we firstly analyzed mRNA levels of Kir2.1, Kir3.1, and Kir6.2 channels in both ipsilateral and contralateral hippocampi from rats by RT–PCR.

Significantly decreased mRNA levels of Kir2.1 (*Kcnj2*) and Kir6.2 (*Kcnj11*) channels were observed in both ipsilateral and contralateral hemispheres of Aβ$_{(1-42)}$-infused rats as compared with sham controls (Figure 3A: 4.85-fold change and 3.15-fold change over controls, ** $p < 0.01$; Figure 3C: 5.30-fold change and 3.00-fold change over controls, ** $p < 0.01$ and * $p < 0.05$, respectively). However, no significant differences were found in mRNA levels of the Kir3.1 (*Kcnj3*) channel in both hemispheres (Figure 3B, $p > 0.05$).

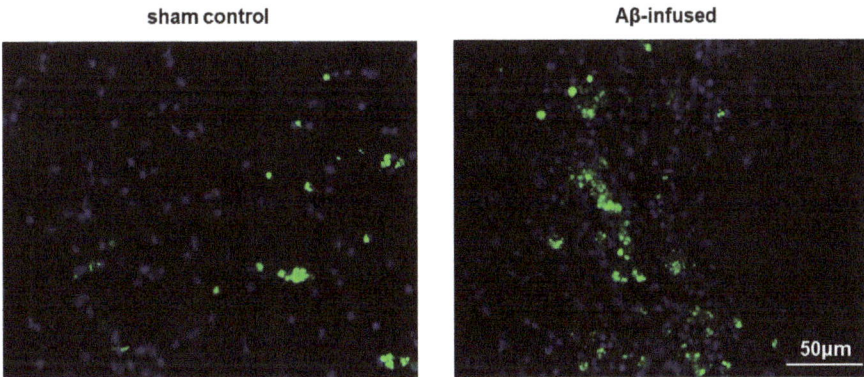

Figure 2. Representative images of hippocampus section stained with anti-Aβ antibody (green fluorescence) in sham control and Aβ$_{(1-42)}$-infused rat model. Cell nuclei were counterstained with DAPI (blue fluorescence). Scale bar: 50 µm.

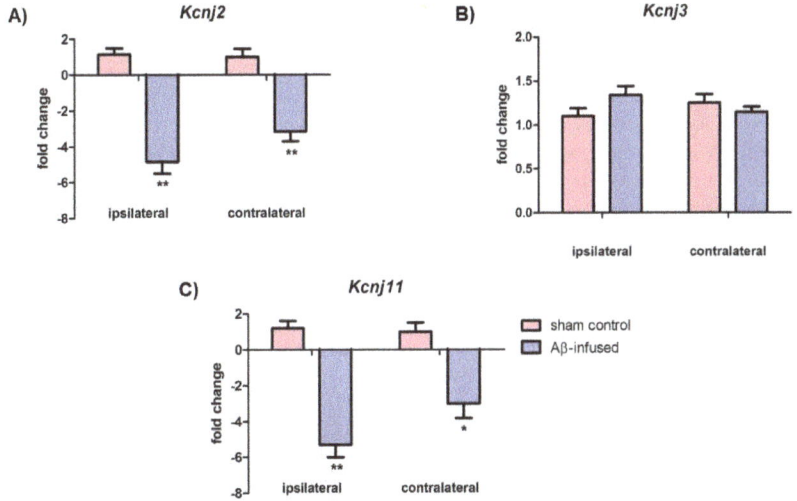

Figure 3. Relative mRNA levels of (**A**) *Kcnj2* (Kir2.1), (**B**) *Kcnj3* (Kir3.1), and (**C**) *Kcnj11* (Kir6.2) in ipsilateral and contralateral hippocampi from both sham control and Aβ$_{(1-42)}$-infused rat model. Data are expressed as fold change of mRNA levels normalized to the housekeeping control gene (*Gapdh*) and represent the mean ± SEM obtained in 3 independent experiments, n = 7 for each group, * $p < 0.05$, ** $p < 0.01$.

3.3. Low mRNA Levels of Kir2.1 and Kir6.2 Channels Correlate with Decreased Protein Levels in Aβ$_{(1-42)}$-Infused Rat Model

In order to assess if changes in mRNA levels of Kir channels result in different protein levels, total protein extract from both ipsilateral and contralateral hippocampus tissues were analyzed via WB analysis by using specific anti-Kir antibodies and the relative protein abundance was quantified by densitometric measurements.

Significantly decreased Kir2.1 protein levels were detected only in the ipsilateral hemisphere of Aβ$_{(1-42)}$-infused rats as compared with sham controls (Figure 4A: 0.41 ± 0.50 vs. 0.72 ± 0.25, ** $p < 0.01$). Decreased Kir6.2 protein levels were observed in both ipsilateral and contralateral hippocampus tissues of Aβ$_{(1-42)}$-infused rats as compared with sham controls (Figure 4C: 0.61 ± 0.35 vs. 0.82 ± 0.52, *

$p < 0.05$, and 0.52 ± 0.25 vs. 0.71 ± 0.40, * $p < 0.05$, respectively). On the other hand, no significant differences in Kir3.1 protein levels were found in Kir3.1 protein levels in both hemispheres (Figure 4B, $p > 0.05$), confirming previous mRNA data (Figure 3B).

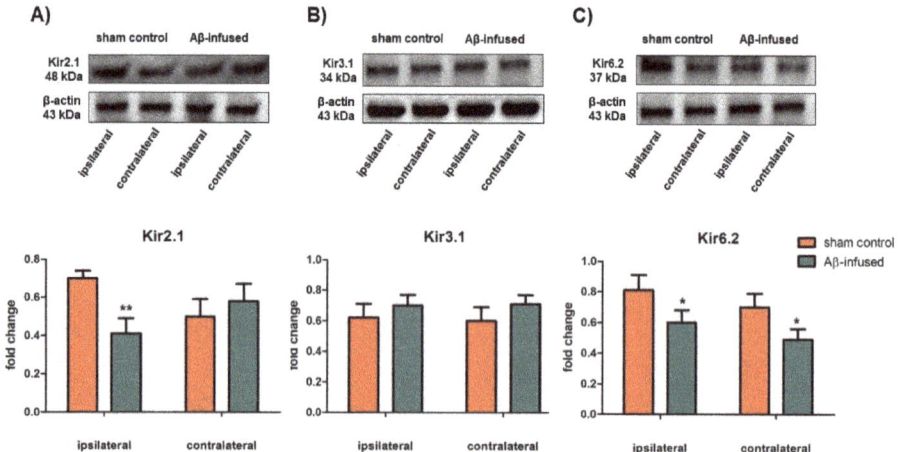

Figure 4. Protein expression levels of Kir2.1 (**A**), Kir3.1 (**B**), and Kir6.2 (**C**) channels in ipsilateral and contralateral hippocampi from both sham control and Aβ$_{(1-42)}$-infused rat model. Upper panel: representative images of WB analysis on total protein extracts. β-actin was used as endogenous control for equal protein load. Lower panel: densitometric analysis of Kir2.1 (**A**), Kir3.1 (**B**), and Kir6.2 (**C**) protein levels. Data are expressed as fold change ratio on sham control and normalized to the β-actin protein levels. Bars represent the mean ± SEM obtained in 3 independent experiments, $n = 7$ for each group, * $p < 0.05$, ** $p < 0.01$.

4. Discussion

Functional and expression alterations of K$^+$ channels cause disruptions in neuronal balance and membrane excitability, contributing to the development and progress of several neurological diseases, including AD [8–12]. Among them, Kir channels have the ability to mediate the inward flow of K$^+$ ions at hyperpolarizing membrane voltages more readily than the outward flow of K$^+$ at depolarizing voltages [13]. They are involved in a number of essential physiological processes, such as the regulation of hormone secretion, generation of electrical impulses, and control of vascular smooth muscle tone. It is known that a variety of severe human disorders are directly related to a dysfunction of Kir channel proteins [17]. Moreover, intracellular Na$^+$ and K$^+$ levels were found to be increased in brain regions of AD patients, pointing out a cellular ion imbalance in AD pathophysiology [18]. So, given their function in maintaining the resting membrane potential and K$^+$ homeostasis of most cells [13], we aim to highlight the role of neural Kir channels in AD by analyzing their mRNA and protein levels in the hippocampus of Aβ$_{(1-42)}$-infused rat model of the disease.

The classical Kir2 subfamily exhibits a strong inward rectifying property and it is the major responsible for the I_{K1} current. Kir2.1 channels hyperpolarize the cells in response to an increase in the external K$^+$ concentration [19]. Our data showed a decrease in both mRNA and protein levels of Kir2.1, suggesting a reduced Kir current in the hippocampus of AD model rats. We can speculate that Aβ peptide may decrease the expression of this channel, affecting the hippocampal activity balance underlying memory and learning processes damaged in AD [14]. However, other authors reported no differences in Kir2.1 mRNA expression in the hippocampus of rats with cholinergic impairment, probably because of the use of different models [15].

In addition to Kir2.1, a decrease in both transcript and protein levels of Kir6.2 channel has also been observed. In contrast with I_{K1} channels, Kir6 (also known as adenosine triphosphate (ATP)-sensitive

K^+, K_{ATP}) subfamily are weakly inwardly rectifying and are inhibited by intracellular ATP levels [13]. They correlate the metabolic status of neurons to their excitability by detecting changes of intracellular phosphate potential (e.g., ATP/ADP ratio) [20]. Functional channels consist of four pore-forming Kir6 subunits (Kir6.1 and Kir6.2) and four sulfonylurea receptor (SUR) subunits (SUR1, SUR2 A, and SUR2 B). In neurons, the K_{ATP} channels are mainly constituted by the coassembly of Kir6.2/SUR1 subunits [13]. They are also involved in the generation of the glucose-sensitive K^+ current in neurons, indicating that the increase in neuronal excitation observed when the concentration of external glucose raises is due to the closure of K_{ATP} channels [21]. It is well-known that the Kir6 subfamily is involved in AD pathogenesis and phenotype [12]. The first evidence has been addressed by a study in which increased transcript levels of Kir6.1 were observed in the hippocampus of cholinergic impaired rats, whereas mRNA expression of Kir6.2 was significantly increased in the cortex [15]. Consistent with these findings, high Kir6.2 protein levels were also found in both hippocampal reactive astrocytes from a triple transgenic mouse model of AD (3 xTg-AD) [22]. On the other hand, we found a decrease in both mRNA and protein levels of Kir6.2 in the hippocampus of A$\beta_{(1-42)}$-infused rats. These contrasting results may be due to the use of different AD models. Interestingly, the transgenic overexpression of the Kir6.2 channel in the forebrain protects mice from neuronal damage and hypoxic–ischemic injury seen in stroke [23]. Moreover, it has been shown that Kir6.2 knock-out mice showed severe deficits in long-term memory processes and learning [24,25]. Therefore, we can hypothesize that the impairment of memory occurring in AD may be related to a downregulation of the Kir6.2 subunit.

Concerning Kir3.1 channels, no statistical differences were found. Also named as G-protein-coupled Kir (GIRK) channels, they are activated by some neurotransmitters (e.g., acetylcholine GABA, dopamine) through the stimulation of their G protein coupled receptors (GPCRs), resulting in a reduced action potential firing and a cell membrane hyperpolarization. GIRK channels are detected in the extra-synaptic membrane of CA1 hippocampal pyramidal neurons and play a role in the production of slow inhibitory post-synaptic potential [13]. However, our data did not show any significant differences in either transcript or protein levels of Kir3.1 channel in both hemispheres of hippocampus from the A$\beta_{(1-42)}$-infused rat model, in line with an already reported study [15]. We can speculate that this evidence may be due to two contrasting effects of Aβ on these channels in a more complex neuronal network. Indeed, it has been reported that this peptide led to a GIRK3 channel upregulation, which resulted in K^+ efflux from neurons triggering, thus, the Aβ-mediated apoptotic pathway [26]. On the contrary, other authors reported an opposite effect of Aβ in which it modulated GIRK3 expression by downregulating these channels [14].

In summary, our data support the evidence that Aβ can modulate the expression of neuronal Kir channels in the AD pathogenesis. The fact that we reported some results that are contrasting with the previous ones may be related to the use of different in vivo models that recapitulate distinct features of the disorder. Indeed, due to the lack of complete understanding of AD etiology, the development of adequate animal models resembling all stages of disease progression, as well as the merging convergent pathways of neurodegeneration, still represents a need for AD research. However, the complementary use of several models will help to understand molecular mechanisms underlying the disease and to develop novel strategies based on the modulation of Kir channels or their accessory subunits for AD prevention and therapy.

5. Conclusions

Overall, our data corroborate the working hypothesis that Kir channels play a causative role in AD pathogenesis, as suggested by their altered mRNA and protein levels found in the A$\beta_{(1-42)}$-infused rat model. However, it cannot be excluded a complex mechanism of Aβ, which makes such reported alterations the result of an impaired metabolic pathway involving related channels or other proteins. We are aware that our study has several limitations, including the confirmation that differences observed in protein amounts are translated into an altered channel function activity by patch-clamp recordings and the lack of tests assessing learning and memory deficits. Moreover, it should be noted that, although cerebral infusion of Aβ in rats can recapitulate some hallmarks of human AD, it cannot properly reproduce the progressive neurodegeneration occurring during the disease, so further studies in different models are necessary to cover all aspects of the disease.

Author Contributions: Conceptualization, E.A.; methodology, E.A. and B.E.; formal analysis, E.A., C.V., M.B. and B.E.; investigation, E.A., C.V., M.B. and B.E.; data curation, E.A., C.V., M.B. and B.E.; writing—original draft preparation, E.A., C.V., M.B. and B.E.; writing—review and editing, E.A., C.V., M.B. and B.E.; supervision, E.A., C.V. and B.E.; project administration, E.A. All authors have read and agreed to the published version of the manuscript.

Funding: This study was supported by the grant from Bezmialem Vakif University Scientific Research Found (BVU-BAP) (12.2014/2 and 9.2015/26).

Conflicts of Interest: The authors declare no conflict of interest. The funders had no role in the design of the study; in the collection, analyses, or interpretation of data; in the writing of the manuscript; or in the decision to publish the results.

References

1. Crous-Bou, M.; Minguillón, C.; Gramunt, N.; Molinuevo, J.L. Alzheimer's disease prevention: From risk factors to early intervention. *Alzheimers Res. Ther.* **2017**, *9*, 71. [CrossRef]
2. Anand, R.; Gill, K.D.; Mahdi, A.A. Therapeutics of Alzheimer's disease: Past, present and future. *Neuropharmacology* **2014**, *76 (Pt. A)*, 27–50. [CrossRef]
3. Sanabria-Castro, A.; Alvarado-Echeverria, I.; Monge-Bonilla, C. Molecular Pathogenesis of Alzheimer's Disease: An Update. *Ann. Neurosci.* **2017**, *24*, 46–54. [CrossRef] [PubMed]
4. Haass, C.; Selkoe, D.J. Soluble protein oligomers in neurodegeneration: Lessons from the Alzheimer's amyloid beta-peptide. *Nat. Rev. Mol. Cell Biol.* **2007**, *8*, 101–112. [CrossRef] [PubMed]
5. Tönnies, E.; Trushina, E. Oxidative stress, synaptic dysfunction, and alzheimer's disease. *J. Alzheimers Dis.* **2017**, *57*, 1105–1121. [CrossRef] [PubMed]
6. Castro, A.; Martinez, A. Targeting beta-amyloid pathogenesis through acetylcholinesterase inhibitors. *Curr. Pharm. Des.* **2006**, *12*, 4377–4387. [CrossRef] [PubMed]
7. Mangialasche, F.; Solomon, A.; Winblad, B.; Mecocci, P.; Kivipelto, M. Alzheimer's disease: Clinical trials and drug development. *Lancet Neurol.* **2010**, *9*, 702–716. [CrossRef]
8. Akyuz, E.; Mega Tiber, P.; Beker, M.; Akbas, F. Expression of cardiac inwardly rectifying potassium channels in pentylenetetrazole kindling model of epilepsy in rats. *Cell. Mol. Biol. (Noisy-le-grand)* **2018**, *64*, 47–54. [CrossRef]
9. Villa, C.; Combi, R. Potassium Channels and Human Epileptic Phenotypes: An Updated Overview. *Front. Cell. Neurosci.* **2016**, *10*, 81. [CrossRef]
10. Binda, A.; Rivolta, I.; Villa, C.; Chisci, E.; Beghi, M.; Cornaggia, C.M.; Giovannoni, R.; Combi, R. A Novel KCNJ2 Mutation Identified in an Autistic Proband Affects the Single Channel Properties of Kir2.1. *Front. Cell. Neurosci.* **2018**, *12*, 76. [CrossRef]
11. Akyuz, E.; Villa, C. A novel role of cardiac inwardly rectifying potassium channels explaining autonomic cardiovascular dysfunctions in a cuprizone-induced mouse model of multiple sclerosis. *Auton. Neurosci.* **2020**, *225*, 102647. [CrossRef] [PubMed]
12. Villa, C.; Suphesiz, H.; Combi, R.; Akyuz, E. Potassium channels in the neuronal homeostasis and neurodegenerative pathways underlying Alzheimer's Disease: An update. *Mech. Ageing Dev.* **2019**, *185*, 111197. [CrossRef] [PubMed]
13. Hibino, H.; Inanobe, A.; Furutani, K.; Murakami, S.; Findlay, I.; Kurachi, Y. Inwardly rectifying potassium channels: Their structure, function, and physiological roles. *Physiol. Rev.* **2010**, *90*, 291–366. [CrossRef] [PubMed]
14. Mayordomo-Cava, J.; Yajeya, J.; Navarro-Lopez, D.J.; Jimenez-Diaz, L. Amyloidbeta(25-35) modulates the expression of GirK and KCNQ channel genes in the Hippocampus. *PLoS ONE* **2015**, *10*, e0134385. [CrossRef] [PubMed]
15. Xu, X.H.; Pan, Y.P.; Wang, X.L. mRNA expression alterations of inward rectifier potassium channels in rat brain with cholinergic impairment. *Neurosci. Lett.* **2002**, *322*, 25–28. [CrossRef]

16. Serpente, M.; Fenoglio, C.; Villa, C.; Cortini, F.; Cantoni, C.; Ridolfi, E.; Clerici, F.; Marcone, A.; Benussi, L.; Ghidoni, R.; et al. Role of OLR1 and its regulating hsa-miR369-3 p in Alzheimer's disease: Genetics and expression analysis. *J. Alzheimers Dis.* **2011**, *26*, 787–793. [CrossRef]
17. Zangerl-Plessl, E.M.; Qile, M.; Bloothooft, M.; Stary-Weinzinger, A.; van der Heyden, M.A.G. Disease Associated Mutations in KIR Proteins Linked to Aberrant Inward Rectifier Channel Trafficking. *Biomolecules.* **2019**, *9*, 650. [CrossRef]
18. Vitvitsky, V.M.; Garg, S.K.; Keep, R.F.; Albin, R.L.; Banerjee, R. Na+ and K+ ion imbalances in Alzheimer's disease. *Biochim. Biophys. Acta.* **2012**, *1822*, 1671–1681. [CrossRef]
19. Anumonwo, J.M.; Lopatin, A.N. Cardiac strong inward rectifier potassium channels. *J. Mol. Cell. Cardiol.* **2010**, *48*, 45–54. [CrossRef]
20. D'Adamo, M.C.; Catacuzzeno, L.; Di Giovanni, G.; Franciolini, F.; Pessia, M. K(+) channelepsy: Progress in the neurobiology of potassium channels and epilepsy. *Front. Cell. Neurosci.* **2013**, *7*, 134. [CrossRef]
21. Haider, S.; Antcliff, J.F.; Proks, P.; Sansom, M.S.; Ashcroft, F.M. Focus on Kir6.2: A key component of the ATP-sensitive potassium channel. *J. Mol. Cell Cardiol.* **2005**, *38*, 927–936. [CrossRef] [PubMed]
22. Griffith, C.M.; Xie, M.X.; Qiu, W.Y.; Sharp, A.A.; Ma, C.; Pan, A.; Yan, X.X.; Patrylo, P.R. Aberrant expression of the pore-forming KATP channel subunit Kir6.2 in hippocampal reactive astrocytes in the 3 xTg-AD mouse model and human Alzheimer's disease. *Neuroscience* **2016**, *336*, 81–101. [CrossRef] [PubMed]
23. Héron-Milhavet, L.; Xue-Jun, Y.; Vannucci, S.; Wood, T.L.; Willing, L.B.; Stannard, B.; Hernandez-Sanchez, C.; Mobbs, C.; Virsolvy, A.; LeRoith, D. Protection against hypoxic-ischemic injury in transgenic mice overexpressing Kir6.2 channel pore in forebrain. *Mol. Cell Neurosci.* **2004**, *25*, 585–593. [CrossRef] [PubMed]
24. Choeiri, C.; Staines, W.A.; Miki, T.; Seino, S.; Renaud, J.M.; Teutenberg, K.; Messier, C. Cerebral glucose transporters expression and spatial learning in the K-ATP Kir6.2(-/-) knockout mice. *Behav. Brain. Res.* **2006**, *172*, 233–239. [CrossRef] [PubMed]
25. Betourne, A.; Bertholet, A.M.; Labroue, E.; Halley, H.; Sun, H.S.; Lorsignol, A.; Feng, Z.P.; French, R.J.; Penicaud, L.; Lassalle, J.M.; et al. Involvement of hippocampal CA3 K(ATP) channels in contextual memory. *Neuropharmacology* **2009**, *56*, 615–625. [CrossRef]
26. May, L.M.; Anggono, V.; Gooch, H.M.; Jang, S.E.; Matusica, D.; Kerbler, G.M.; Meunier, F.A.; Sah, S.; Coulson, E.J. G-protein-Coupled inwardly rectifying potassium (GIRK) channel activation by the p75 neurotrophin receptor is required for amyloid beta toxicity. *Front. Neurosci.* **2017**, *11*, 455. [CrossRef]

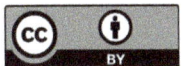

© 2020 by the authors. Licensee MDPI, Basel, Switzerland. This article is an open access article distributed under the terms and conditions of the Creative Commons Attribution (CC BY) license (http://creativecommons.org/licenses/by/4.0/).

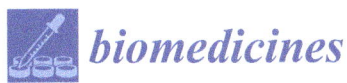

Article

Monopolar Spindle 1 Kinase (MPS1/TTK) mRNA Expression is Associated with Earlier Development of Clinical Symptoms, Tumor Aggressiveness and Survival of Glioma Patients

Almuth F. Kessler [1,†], Jonas Feldheim [1,†], Dominik Schmitt [1], Julia J. Feldheim [1], Camelia M. Monoranu [2], Ralf-Ingo Ernestus [1], Mario Löhr [1] and Carsten Hagemann [1,*]

[1] Tumorbiology Laboratory, Department of Neurosurgery, University of Würzburg, Josef-Schneider-Str. 11, D-97080 Würzburg, Germany; Kessler_A1@ukw.de (A.F.K.); Jonas.Feldheim@googlemail.com (J.F.); Schmitt_D8@ukw.de (D.S.); Feldheim.Julia@gmail.com (J.J.F.); Ernestus_R@ukw.de (R.-I.E.); Loehr_M1@ukw.de (M.L.)

[2] Department of Neuropathology, Intsitute of Pathology, University of Würzburg, Josef-Schneider-Str. 2, D-97080 Würzburg, Germany; camelia-maria.monoranu@mail.uni-wuerzburg.de

* Correspondence: hagemann_c@ukw.de; Tel.: +49-931-201-24644

† AFK and JF share the first authorship.

Received: 29 May 2020; Accepted: 30 June 2020; Published: 3 July 2020

Abstract: Inhibition of the protein kinase MPS1, a mitotic spindle-checkpoint regulator, reinforces the effects of multiple therapies against glioblastoma multiforme (GBM) in experimental settings. We analyzed *MPS1* mRNA-expression in gliomas WHO grade II, III and in clinical subgroups of GBM. Data were obtained by qPCR analysis of tumor and healthy brain specimens and correlated with the patients' clinical data. *MPS1* was overexpressed in all gliomas on an mRNA level (ANOVA, $p < 0.01$) and correlated with tumor aggressiveness. We explain previously published conflicting results on survival: high *MPS1* was associated with poorer long term survival when all gliomas were analyzed combined in one group (Cox regression: t < 24 months, $p = 0.009$, Hazard ratio: 8.0, 95% CI: 1.7–38.4), with poorer survival solely in low-grade gliomas (LogRank: $p = 0.02$, Cox regression: $p = 0.06$, Hazard-Ratio: 8.0, 95% CI: 0.9–66.7), but not in GBM (LogRank: $p > 0.05$). This might be due to their lower tumor volume at the therapy start. GBM patients with high *MPS1* mRNA-expression developed clinical symptoms at an earlier stage. This, however, did not benefit their overall survival, most likely due to the more aggressive tumor growth. Since *MPS1* mRNA-expression in gliomas was enhanced with increasing tumor aggressiveness, patients with the worst outcome might benefit best from a treatment directed against MPS1.

Keywords: glioblastoma multiforme; low-grade glioma; astrocytoma; recurrence; multifocal growth; mRNA expression; MPS1; TTK; therapy

1. Introduction

Glial tumors encompass a group of primary brain tumors that are classified into different subgroups by the World Health Organization (WHO) [1]. The natural history of these tumors varies greatly. Pilocytic astrocytomas WHO grade I (PA) represent a benign form, mainly found in children, with a 10-year survival of over 90% [2–4]. In comparison, low-grade astrocytomas WHO grade II and III grow faster and more infiltrative. Formerly, these tumors were mainly classified due to their histological behavior. With the recent update of the WHO classification, however, molecular markers are now considered as well [1]. For instance, the diagnosis "gliomatosis cerebri" no longer exists, as those widespread tumors with infiltration of three or more lobes show a methylation profile comparable to the other glial tumor entities [5]. *Isocitrate dehydrogenase* (IDH) mutant gliomas of WHO grade II or III (IDHmut glioma) are a slowly growing subcategory, with a comparatively good prognosis.

In contrast, *IDH*-wildtype gliomas of WHO grade II and III (IDHwt glioma), show a growth pattern and patients' clinical course that resembles those of glioblastoma multiforme (GBM), and therefore might even be an early form of a GBM [6–8]. GBM is not only the most common but also the most aggressive form of primary brain tumor [9]. The current standard therapy, consisting of tumor resection, irradiation, concomitant temozolomide (TMZ) chemotherapy, and adjuvant TMZ-treatment, was established in 2005, with a median patient survival of only 14.6 months [10].

After 12 years with mainly negative clinical phase III trials, Tumor Treating Fields (TTFields) raised new hopes for an improvement of the standard therapy [11–13]. Recently, we demonstrated that the effects of TTFields are augmented and accelerated by mitotic checkpoint inhibition of the protein kinase monopolar spindle 1 (MPS1, also known as TTK) in vitro [14], indicating the potential for a combined treatment advantage. MPS1-inhibition reduces cell proliferation of GBM when combined with the antimitotic agent vincristine in vitro and in vivo [15]. It is a dual-specificity protein kinase that regulates the mitotic spindle checkpoint by monitoring proper chromosome alignment and attachment to spindle microtubuli [16–21]. Dysregulation of MPS1 activity has been reported to lead to chromosomal instability and cancerogenesis [19]. It is overexpressed in astrocytic tumors, with overexpression correlating with tumor grade and patients' survival [15]. However, to our knowledge, there are no data published on astrocytic tumors of different growth patterns or on glioma recurrence. Interestingly, aberrant *MPS1* expression and its effects appear to be hugely influenced by their dysregulation of *MPS1* mRNA and its regulator miR-132 [22]. Therefore, it appears promising to explore connections between *MPS1* mRNA expression and patients' clinical course, to lead the way from experimental observations to a translational implementation into clinical research and hopefully, ultimately, patient care. The purpose of this study was (1) to confirm and extend the qPCR-results reported by us previously [15] and (2) to provide information on the expression of *MPS1* in gliomas of different biological behavior and clinical course on an mRNA level. We show that *MPS1* mRNA was indeed dysregulated and overexpressed in gliomas, associated with earlier development of patients' clinical symptoms, correlated to tumor aggressiveness, and associated with the survival of patients with low-grade gliomas.

2. Experimental Section

2.1. Tissue Samples and Clinical Data

All included patients were treated at the Department of Neurosurgery, University Hospital Würzburg, University of Würzburg. All subjects gave their informed consent for inclusion before they participated in the study. The study was conducted in accordance with the declaration of Helsinki, and the protocol was approved on 16-July-2014 by the Institutional Review Board of the University of Würzburg (#103/14). After gaining the tissue during surgery, equal shares were frozen in liquid nitrogen for molecular analyses and embedded in paraffin for immunohistochemistry. The tumors were classified by routine histology in accordance with WHO criteria [1]. Only tumor samples with a typical histological appearance according to the evaluation by an experienced neuropathologist and originating from central, viable tumor areas were included. In addition, GBM samples with an estimated tumor cell content of less than 80% were excluded. The Brain Bank of the Department of Neuropathology, Institute of Pathology, University of Würzburg, Germany was the source for autopsy/biopsy samples of non-pathological brain tissue (normal brain, NB) (approval #78/99 from 09-July-1999 and 04-October-2016). Clinical information of the patients such as tumor localization and growth (e.g., local or multifocal), treatment modalities, recurrence, and outcome were collected retrospectively (Table 1). The tumor volume and extent of surgical resection were measured by evaluating pre- and post-operative Magnetic Resonance Imaging (MRI) images. The IDH mutation status was determined by immunohistochemistry and pyrosequencing, the Ki67 status by immunohistochemistry and the *MGMT* promoter methylation status by high resolution melting real-time polymerase chain reaction. Since some of the specimens were already analyzed for a previous project, the methodology has been described in detail elsewhere [23,24].

2.2. RNA Extraction and qPCR

mRNA was extracted from frozen tissue samples by the TRIzol® Reagent (Thermo Fisher Scientific, Waltham, MA, USA) and converted to DNA, as previously described [23]. qPCR (Quantitative Real-Time Polymerase Chain Reaction) was performed on a StepOnePlus Real-time PCR System (Applied Biosystems, Foster City, CA, USA) to determine the *MPS1* mRNA expression in a duplex setting utilizing the TaqMan Universal PCR Master Mix, TTK_FAM (Hs01009870_m1,) and GAPDH_VIC_PL (Hs99999905_m1) (all from Applied Biosystems, Foster City, CA, USA) according to the manufacturer's instruction. Each sample was tested in technical triplets with 20 ng cDNA each. The PCR's cycling started at 50°C for 2 min, followed by enzyme activation at 95°C for 10 min and 50 cycles of 15 s at 95°C and 1 min at 60°C. If the technical replicates exceeded a standard deviation of 0.5 Cq, the qPCR was repeated. Cq-values were adjusted to a relative standard curve following the manufacturer's instructions.

2.3. Statistics

The analyses were based on the ΔΔCq-values, which were directly obtained from the qPCR [25] and normalized to the expression of the housekeeping gene *Glyceraldehyde 3-phosphate dehydrogenase* (*GAPDH*). As autopsy- and biopsy-derived NB specimens had a similar expression, they were combined into one group. In addition, we analyzed *MPS1* mRNA expression data available from the IVY-GAP database [26] (https://glioblastoma.alleninstitute.org), accessed in March 2020. Statistical calculations were performed with IBM SPSS Statistics 23 (IBM Corporation, Armonk, NY, USA). Boxplots show the relative quantity calculated from the ΔΔCq-values. A comparison of expression and regression analysis was performed with ANOVA (Levene's test, Post-hoc: Scheffe-test or Dunnet-T3), correlation analysis with Spearman's Rho. The patients' outcome was compared by Kaplan–Meier (LogRank), as well as cox regression on time-dependent variables. We refrained from the survival analysis of IDHwt gliomas due to low sample quantity.

Table 1. Clinical parameters of glioblastoma multiforme (GBM) patients ($n = 27$).

Patients' characteristics			
Sex	female: 10/37.0%		male: 17/63.0%
Age (median, quartiles)		56 years (49–65 years)	
ECOG	0: 15/55.6%	1: 10/37.0%	>1: 2/7.4%
Tumor characteristics			
Volume (median, quartiles)		30.9 cm^3 (16.0–54.6 cm^3)	
Localization	left hemisphere: 16/59.3%	right hemisphere: 9/33.3%	both hemispheres: 2/7.4%
Localization (lobe)	frontal: 5/18.5%	occipital: 5/18.5%	temporal: 6/22.2%
	parietal: 4/14.8%	multiple: 6/22.2%	cerebellar: 1/3.7%
IDH mutation status [1]	IDHwt: 21/87.5%		IDHmut: 3/12.5%
MGMT promoter methylation [1]	unmethylated: 7/30.4%		methylated: 16/69.6%
Ki67 staining (median, quartiles)		25% (20–30)	
Therapy			
Time from diagnosis to therapy	0–7 days: 18/66.7%	8–14 days: 5/18.5%	>14 days: 4/14.8%
Surgical intervention [2]	biopsy: 4/15.4%	complete resection: 4/15.4%	incomplete resection: 18/69.2%
Radiation therapy		yes: 25/92.6%	no: 2/7.4%
TMZ chemotherapy		yes: 22/81.5%	no: 5/18.5%

Table 1. Cont.

	Relapse and Outcome		
PFS [3] (median, quartiles)	8 months (6–13 months)		
Relapse	primarily multifocal: 4/14.8%	local: 15/55.6%	multifocal: 8/29.6%
Therapy in relapse [2]	surgical resection followed by radiation and/or TMZ: 12/52.2%	radiation and/or TMZ: 5/21.7%	best supportive care: 6/26.1%
OS (median, quartiles)	19 months (9–13 months)		

Absolute numbers and the respective percentages are shown. [1] Due to a lack of sufficient tissue samples, the IDH mutation and the *MGMT* promoter methylation status could not be re-evaluated for some patients. [2] For some patients partly treated in external institutions, information about therapeutic interventions was limited. [3] Some patients did not match the criteria for tumor progression and, therefore, were excluded from the PFS analysis. ECOG = Eastern Cooperative Oncology Group score [27]; IDH = isocitrate dehydrogenase; IDHmut = IDH-mutated tumors; IDHwt = IDH wildtype tumors; MGMT = O^6-methylguanine-DNA methyltransferase; TMZ = Temozolomide; PFS = progression-free survival; OS = overall survival.

3. Results

3.1. Patient Cohort

We assessed the MPS1 mRNA expression of 7 normal brain (NB) (epilepsy surgery: $n = 3$, autopsy: $n = 4$), 4 PA, 25 IDHmut glioma, 11 IDHwt glioma and 57 GBM specimens with different growth patterns at first diagnosis and relapse. Additionally, we retrospectively collected clinical data of 58 of these patients. Unfortunately, some patients were partly treated in external institutions, limiting access to their clinical information. A low amount of tumor material prevented us from performing all analyses with some samples. Therefore, information on the extent of tumor resection ($n = 1$), *MGMT* promoter methylation ($n = 14$), and Ki67 staining ($n = 3$) is missing for some patients. The available characteristics, molecular and prognostic parameters, outcome results, etc. are summarized in Table 1 (GBM) and Table 2 (IDHmut and IDHwt glioma).

Table 2. Clinical parameters of IDHmut ($n = 20$) and IDHwt glioma ($n = 11$) patients.

Patients' Characteristics	IDHmut Glioma	IDHwt Glioma
Sex	female: 6/30.0% male: 14/70.0%	female: 2/18.2% male: 9/81.8%
Age (median, quartiles)	37 years (33–45 years)	53 years (26–58 years)
OS (median, quartiles)	37.5 months (23.75–42.65 months)	32.0 months (14.0–48.0 months)
Growth pattern	local: 10/50.0% highly diffuse: 10/50.0%	local: 6/54.5% highly diffuse: 5/45.5%

Absolute numbers and the respective percentages are shown. The infiltration of fewer than three lobes was defined as local and the infiltration of three or more lobes as highly diffuse growth. OS = overall survival; IDH = isocitrate dehydrogenase; IDHmut glioma = IDH-mutated tumors with the histological appearance of WHO grade II and III gliomas; IDHwt gliomas = IDH wildtype tumors with the histological appearance of WHO grade II and III gliomas.

3.2. MPS1 mRNA was Overexpressed in Gliomas and Correlated with Tumor Aggressiveness

In comparison to NB, MPS1 mRNA was significantly overexpressed in IDHmut glioma ($p < 0.001$, median: 73-fold) IDHwt glioma ($p < 0.001$, median: 96-fold) as well as in GBM ($p < 0.001$, 91-fold). However, there was no significant difference in the *MPS1* mRNA expression between these three groups ($p > 0.05$) (Figure 1a and Table 3). Benign PA displayed a statistically non-significant tendency towards overexpression (Figure 1a). Nevertheless, by sorting these entities according to their malignancy, a highly significant correlation of MPS1 mRNA expression and tumor aggressiveness was detectable ($p < 0.001$, $R^2 = 0.263$) (Figure 1b). When we analyzed the different GBM-subgroups distinguished by their growth pattern (primary local tumors leading to local relapse, primary local tumors leading to multifocal relapse and primary multifocal tumors) and compared primary tumors and relapses, we did not observe any statistically significant difference in *MPS1* mRNA expression ($p > 0.05$) (Figure 1c and Table 3). Nevertheless, despite different growth and relapse patterns, all tumors displayed significant

MPS1 overexpression compared to NB ($p < 0.001$). Only the local relapses of GBM, although displaying a stronger expression, were not significantly different from NB ($p = 0.06$) (Figure 1c and Table 3). Similarly, both IDHmut glioma with local growth and IDHmut gliomas with highly diffuse growth (infiltration of three or more lobes, formerly classified as "gliomatosis cerebri") had significantly overexpressed *MPS1* mRNA in comparison to NB (both $p < 0.001$), but not between each other (Table 3). The IVY Glioblastoma Atlas Project (IVC-GAP) database allows the examination of regional differences in mRNA expression within the tumor [26]. It revealed enhanced *MPS1* expression in the cellular tumor mass, hyperplastic blood vessels, and microvascular proliferation, but not in the leading edge, infiltrating tumor, the perinecrotic zone, or pseudopalisading cells around necrosis (Figure 1d).

Table 3. Statistical data of the *MPS1* mRNA expression analysis.

NB Compared to:	Difference in ΔΔCq-Values (Median)	95%-CI	*p*-Value
PA	2.5	−1.4–6.4	0.42
IDHmut glioma	4.4	1.7–7.0	**<0.001**
IDHmut glioma with local growth	4.4	1.7–7.2	**0.001**
IDHmut glioma with highly diffuse growth	4.8	2.1–7.5	**<0.001**
IDHwt glioma	5.1	2.1–8.1	**<0.001**
GBM	5.3	2.8–7.8	**<0.001**
GBM with local relapse	5.5	2.7–8.2	**<0.001**
Local relapse of GBM	3.4	−0.1–6.9	0.06
GBM with multifocal relapse	6.3	3.2–9.4	**<0.001**
Multifocal relapse of GBM	6.4	1.6–11.2	**<0.001**
Primary multifocal GBM	5.9	2.8–9.1	**<0.001**

Groups were compared by ANOVA with Levene's test to assess the equality of variances and Scheffe procedure or Dunnet-T3 as posthoc tests. P-values are based on differences of ΔΔCq-values. *p*-values below 0.05 are shown in bold. Local growth was defined as the infiltration of fewer than three lobes and highly diffuse growth as the infiltration of three or more lobes. NB = normal brain; CI = confidence interval; PA = pilocytic astrocytoma; IDH = isocitrate dehydrogenase; IDHmut glioma = IDH-mutated tumors with the histological appearance of WHO grade II and III gliomas; IDHwt gliomas = IDH wildtype tumors with the histological appearance of WHO grade II and III gliomas; GBM = glioblastoma.

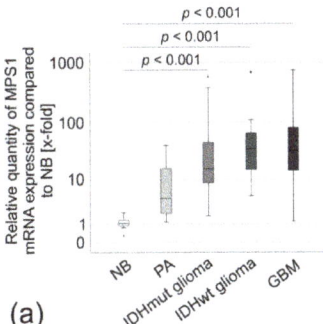
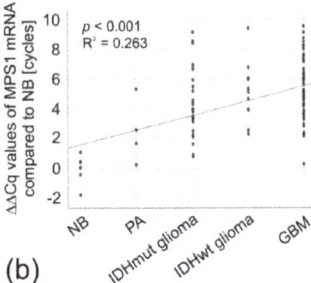

(a) (b)

Figure 1. *Cont.*

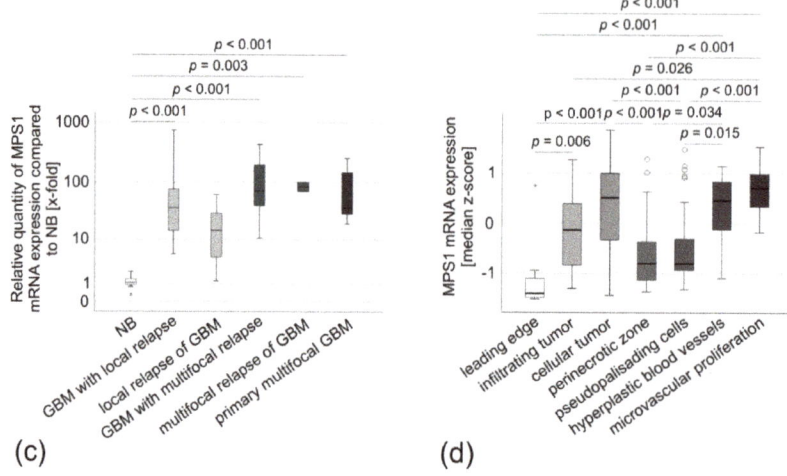

Figure 1. *MPS1* mRNA expression in glioma specimens. (**a**) Box-plot comparing *MPS1* mRNA expression in NB ($n = 7$), PA ($n = 4$, median expression 12-fold), IDHmut glioma ($n = 25$, median expression 73-fold), IDHwt glioma ($n = 11$, median expression 96-fold), and GBM ($n = 57$, median expression 91-fold). The median is displayed by the middle line. The quartiles are represented by the hinges, extreme values, up to 1.5 times the height of the box, are shown by whiskers and outliners represented by points. NB was set as the reference. Groups were compared by ANOVA with Levene's test to assess the equality of variances and Scheffe procedure or Dunnet-T3 as post hoc tests. *p*-values are based on differences of ΔΔCq-values. (**b**) Scatter diagram of tumor aggressiveness and *MPS1* mRNA expression, linear regression, *p*-values were calculated by ANOVA based on ΔΔCq-values. The global effect size was determined by Cohen's *f*. (**c**) Boxplot of *MPS1* mRNA expression in GBM with local relapse (n=14, median expression 112-fold), local relapse of GBM ($n = 5$, median expression 21-fold, $p = 0.06$), GBM with multifocal relapse ($n = 8$, median expression 130-fold), multifocal relapse of GBM ($n = 2$, median expression 84-fold), and primary multifocal GBM ($n = 7$, median expression 94-fold) compared to NB ($n = 7$). The analysis was performed as described in (a). (**d**) IVY-GAP database [26] analysis of *MPS1* mRNA expression in different areas of GBM: leading edge ($n = 16$), infiltrating tumor ($n = 24$), cellular tumor ($n = 110$), perinecrotic zone ($n = 25$), pseudopalisading cells around necrosis ($n = 40$), hyperplastic blood vessels in cellular tumor ($n = 22$), and microvascular proliferation ($n = 28$).

3.3. MPS1 mRNA Expression Correlated with Earlier Development of Clinical Symptoms, Tumor Volume and Long Term Survival of Patients

Having confirmed that *MPS1* mRNA was generally overexpressed in gliomas and particularly in conjunction with glioma aggressiveness, we wondered whether the clinical course of the patients also reflected this. The median *MPS1* expression was 49-fold. Interestingly, when looking at the initial reasons for hospitalization (epileptic seizures, focal neurological symptoms, cognitive decline and/or general symptoms, or incidental finding), GBM patients with *MPS1* expression above this threshold more often had focal neurological symptoms or epileptic seizures (11 of 14, 79%), compared to those with *MPS1* expression below the median (8 of 13, 62%) (Figure 2a). In addition, their tumors were frequently localized solely in the left hemisphere (above median MPS1 expression: 10 of 14, 71%; below median MPS1 expression: 6 of 13, 46%), especially in the temporal or parietal lobe (above median *MPS1* expression: 7 of 14, 50%; below median *MPS1* expression: 3 of 13, 23%) (Figure 2a). In addition, GBM patients with *MPS1* mRNA expression below the median had a significantly higher tumor volume at diagnosis (45 vs. 25 cm^3, $p = 0.043$, unpaired two-tailed *t*-test). This observation was confirmed by regression analysis. *MPS1* mRNA expression correlated negatively with the tumor volume ($p = 0.029$, $R^2 = 0.199$, $f = 0.50$) (Figure 2b). Other clinical parameters did not show any correlation with MPS1 mRNA expression (Table 4).

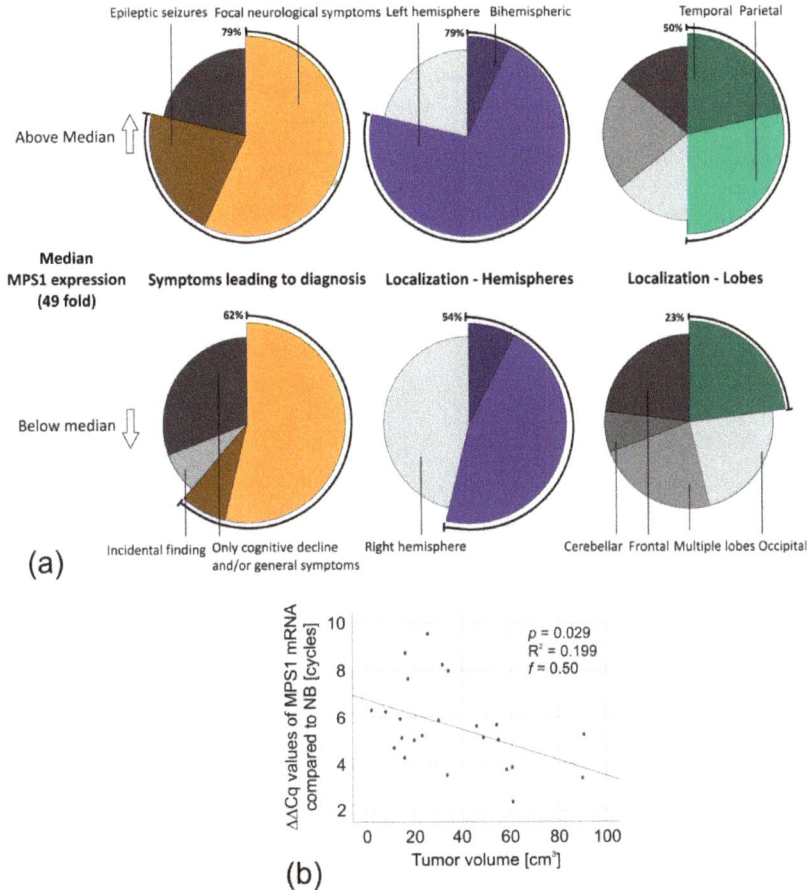

Figure 2. Association of *MPS1* mRNA expression with GBM-patients' symptoms, tumor localization, and tumor volume. (**a**) Pie charts of the reason for initial hospitalization and tumor localization of GBM patients with *MPS1* mRNA expression below and above the median expression (49-fold). Shown is the percentage of patients belonging to each group. (**b**) Scatter diagram of *MPS1* mRNA expression compared to the GBM tumor volume. Linear regression, *p*-values were calculated by ANOVA based on ΔΔCq-values. The global effect size was determined by Cohen's *f*.

Table 4. Correlation of patient and tumor characteristics with *MPS1* mRNA expression.

	IDHmut Glioma		GBM				
	Age (years)	OS (months)	Age (years)	OS (months)	PFS (months)	Tumor Volume (cm³)	Ki67 Staining (%)
Correlation coefficient	0.20	−0.01	0.37	−0.17	−0.27	**0.43**	−0.27
p-value	0.41	0.96	0.06	0.40	0.21	**0.04**	0.19

Non-parametric tests (Spearman's Rho) were utilized to correlate *MPS1* mRNA expression with the selected patient and tumor characteristics. Significant results are highlighted in bold. IDH = isocitrate dehydrogenase; IDHmut glioma = IDH-mutated tumors with the histological appearance of WHO grade II and III gliomas; GBM = glioblastoma; OS = overall survival; PFS = progression-free survival.

To assess patients' survival, we combined all gliomas in one group independently of their WHO grading, as performed in a previous publication by Tannous et al. [15]. After separating them according to the median *MPS1* mRNA expression, there was no significant difference in the overall survival of patients exposed to Kaplan–Meier analysis (Figure 3a). However, closer examination revealed that both curves ran close to parallel for two years, before significantly diverging when it came to long-time survival (Cox regression: t < 24 months, $p = 0.009$, Hazard ratio = 8.0 (95% CI: 1.7–38.4)) (Figure 3a). The GBM subgroup analyses of the progression-free (Figure 3b) and overall survival (Figure 3c) indicated a comparable clinical course of the groups with *MPS1* mRNA expression above or below the median. Interestingly, IDHmut gliomas did not mirror this course. The IDHmut glioma patients with low *MPS1* mRNA expression had a significantly longer survival (LogRank: $p = 0.02$, Cox regression: $p = 0.06$, Hazard-Ratio: 8.0 (95% CI: 0.9–66.7)) than those with high *MPS1* mRNA expression (Figure 3d).

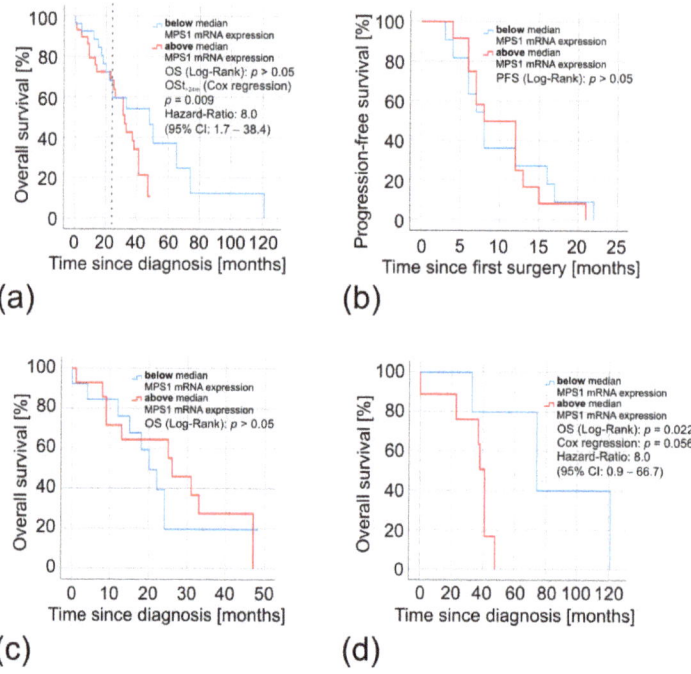

Figure 3. Kaplan–Meier analyses of patients with high and low *MPS1* mRNA expression in their gliomas. Survival of patients with *MPS1* mRNA expression below (**blue**) and above (**red**) the median expression of 49-fold was compared. Hazard ratios and time-dependent effects were calculated by applying the Cox proportional hazards model, p-values by the Log Rank test. (**a**) Overall survival of all glioma patients combined independently of their WHO grade (*MPS1* mRNA expression high $n = 27$, low $n = 29$). The dashed line indicates a survival time of 24 months. (**b**) Progression-free and (**c**) overall survival of GBM patients (*MPS1* mRNA expression high $n = 12$ and $n = 14$, respectively, low $n = 11$ and $n = 13$, respectively). (**d**) Overall survival of patients with IDHmut gliomas (*MPS1* mRNA expression high and low $n = 9$, each).

4. Discussion

MPS1 has been reported to be overexpressed in glioma tissue on an mRNA level, increasing concomitantly with tumor malignancy [15,28,29], and shows potential as a therapeutic target for the treatment of central nervous system tumors [14,30–32]. So far, there are only few publications providing information about MPS1 expression in patients' tissue [15,22,28,29,32]. Therefore, it was vital to confirm and extend those data to validate MPS1 as a future therapeutic target.

Bie et al. and Tannous et al. were the first to analyze *MPS1* mRNA expression in gliomas of different grades, revealing that *MPS1* mRNA was dysregulated and overexpressed in glial tumors grade II-IV [15,28]. Further, the extent of overexpression rose with increasing tumor malignancy [15,29]. Their observations are mirrored by Chen et al., who further suggest a dysregulation of the HLF/miR-132/MPS1 axis to be causal for the malignancy-dependent expression differences [22]. Alimova et al. reported similar results for 90 pediatric brain tumors [32]. *MPS1* mRNA was weakly expressed in cerebellar tissue, as well as cerebral and fetal brain tissue, while the malignant entities atypical teratoid rhabdoid tumors, GBM, and medulloblastomas displayed a high level of *MPS1* mRNA. Interestingly, the authors observed a tendency towards overexpression in benign pediatric PA.

Our analyses confirm the previous observations. The malignant glial tumors strongly expressed *MPS1* mRNA, increasing concomitantly with tumor malignancy/aggressiveness, while the benign adult PA only mildly overexpressed *MPS1*. In the GBM subgroups, we did not detect significant differences between primary tumors and their respective relapses nor between tumors of different growth patterns. The same was true for IDHwt glioma and IDHmut glioma. Therefore, we conclude that the *MPS1* mRNA dysregulation in glial tumors is associated with tumor malignancy but occurs independently of recurrence or growth pattern. Interestingly, the IVY-GAP database [26] revealed that its expression was regionally enhanced in the cellular tumor mass, hyperplastic blood vessels, and microvascular proliferation. These cells are highly proliferative [9,33], while the cells in tumor areas with low *MPS1* expression, the leading edge, infiltrating tumor, the perinecrotic zone, and pseudopalisading cells are mainly migrating [34,35]. This expression pattern is in accordance with the role of MPS1 as a spindle assembly checkpoint regulator during the mitosis of cells [16–21].

Consequently, we wondered whether such association with proliferation and malignancy was also reflected by the patients' clinical characteristics. We divided our panel by the median *MPS1* mRNA expression and could subsequently observe that patients with high expression were numerically more often hospitalized with epileptic seizures and focal neurological symptoms. In addition, their tumors were frequently localized in the left hemisphere, as well as the temporal and parietal lobe. In right-handed patients, who represent the majority in the population, the left hemisphere is dominant. The temporal and parietal lobes are known for critical neurological pathways and, among other areas, are responsible for the tactile sense and speech [36]. Therefore, lesions in these areas can lead to earlier and more prominent symptoms. This misdistribution could be a further indication of *MPS1* mRNA expression being associated with aggressive tumor growth. However, additional confirmation is required to rule out the possibility of a statistical coincidence.

Interestingly, patients with high expression had less than half of the tumor volume at initial diagnosis. As diagnosis predominantly occurs after symptoms of a certain severity (neurological deficits, epileptic seizures, changes of personality, etc.) led to hospitalization, this raises the question of whether *MPS1* overexpression might lead to more dominant and severe clinical deficits at an earlier stage. Since the tumor volume is a prognostic predictor, we investigated the patients' survival.

Previous analyses on MPS1 correlation with patients' survival resulted in contrasting conclusions. Tannous et al. describe a significant difference in survival between a group of high and intermediate MPS1 expression in gliomas of all WHO grades combined [15]. A similar observation was made by Wang et al. for *MPS1* mRNA and protein expression by analyzing the Rembrandt database and immunohistochemically stained tissue slides, respectively [29]. In contrast, Alimova et al. did not detect a difference in outcome in different pediatric high-grade tumor entities (GBM, medulloblastoma, atypical teratoid rhabdoid tumor) [32], an observation confirmed by Bie et al. for GBM from adult patients [28]. We aimed to evaluate these conflicting results.

To reproduce the Kaplan–Meier analysis performed by Tannous et al. [15], we combined all glioma patients and divided them by their median *MPS1* expression. Similarly to these authors, both curves ran almost parallel for approximately two years before they significantly separated, as confirmed by time-dependent cox regression ($p = 0.009$). However, this effect seems to be primarily based on a group of long-term survivors consisting of grade II/III glioma patients. While these low-grade glioma patients benefitted from low *MPS1* mRNA expression, there was no significant difference in the overall or progression-free survival of GBM patients. This observation confirms the results of Bie et al. and Alimova et al. and sheds light on the apparent contrast between these previous publications [15,28,32]. Remarkably, the survival time of the GBM patients was equal, although the group with low MPS1 expression at diagnosis had almost twice the tumor volume of the group with high expression. High pretreatment tumor volume at diagnosis of the primary tumor and relapse is usually associated with poorer survival [37–39]. This mismatch in tumor volume may provide another explanation for the significant effect in outcome when all tumor entities are analyzed together, while subgroup analyses provided negative results. All three previous reports did not consider the tumor volume as a prognostic factor [15,28,32].

To correctly interpret our results, it should be noted that the number of specimens in some subgroups is rather small (e.g., multifocal relapse of GBM), which restrained us from performing multivariable analyses. However, samples of some of the examined tumor sub-entities and data on the role of MPS1 in brain tumors in general, are scarce. Therefore, we consider our results highly valuable, notably, as we observed distinct and statistically significant differences in mRNA expression regardless of the limited number of samples.

Multiple sources have recently suggested MPS1-inhibition to be a viable treatment option for brain tumors, either alone [31,32] or in combination with other therapeutics such as radiation therapy [30], chemotherapy [15], or TTFields [14]. We report MPS1 overexpression in all analyzed tumor entities and subgroups. Therefore, all patients with glial tumors might potentially benefit from such combination therapies, independently of the growth pattern or patient characteristics. At least four different MPS1-inhibitors (BOS-172722, CFI-402257, S81694, and BAY-1217389) are currently tested in Phase I trials on various advanced malignancies [40]. Though the permeability of the blood–brain barrier of these drugs has not been reported in detail, the first preliminary results of their application look promising, and the authors declare good tolerability and manageable adverse effects [41]. Consequently, the inhibition of MPS1 might soon be generally available as a treatment option.

MPS1 expression in gliomas is enhanced with increasing tumor aggressiveness. Therefore, we hypothesize that patients with gliomas WHO grade II/III and high MPS1 expression and especially glioma patients with the worst expected outcome might benefit most from a treatment directed against MPS1. As the dysregulation of MPS1 expression begins at the mRNA level, qPCR-based tests might help to further narrow the pre-selection of suitable patients.

Author Contributions: Conceptualization, C.H., A.F.K., J.F., and M.L.; methodology, J.F., D.S., and C.H.; software, J.F. and J.J.F.; validation, J.F., C.H., M.L., C.M.M., and A.F.K.; formal analysis, J.F., J.J.F., D.S., C.M.M., A.F.K., M.L., and C.H.; investigation, A.F.K., J.F., M.L., and C.H.; resources, C.H., A.F.K., R.-I.E., and M.L.; data curation, C.H. and M.L.; writing—original draft preparation, J.F.; writing—review and editing, C.H., M.L., J.F., A.F.K., and R.-I.E.; visualization, J.F. and C.H.; supervision, C.H., A.F.K., M.L., and R.-I.E.; project administration, C.H., A.F.K., M.L., J.F., and R.-I.E.; funding acquisition, J.F. and R.-I.E.. All authors have read and agreed to the published version of the manuscript.

Funding: This research received no external funding. However, Jonas Feldheim has been supported by the German Academic Foundation (Studienstiftung des Deutschen Volkes), the "Elite Network" of the State of Bavaria and the Graduate School of Life Sciences (GSLS) in Würzburg. This publication was supported by the Open Access Publication Fund of the University of Würzburg.

Acknowledgments: We are very grateful to Elisabeth Karl and Siglinde Kühnel (University of Würzburg, Department of Neurosurgery, Würzburg, Germany) for their excellent technical assistance. We thank Ellaine Salvador (University of Würzburg, Department of Neurosurgery, Würzburg, Germany) for language editing.

Conflicts of Interest: The authors declare no conflict of interest. The funders had no role in the design of the study; in the collection, analyses, or interpretation of data; in the writing of the manuscript; or in the decision to publish the results.

Abbreviations

GBM	Glioblastoma
WHO	World Health Organization
IDH	Isocitrate dehydrogenase
IDHwt glioma	IDH-wild-type gliomas of WHO grade II and III
IDHmut glioma	IDH-mutated gliomas of WHO grade II and III
TMZ	Temozolomide
TTFields	Tumor Treating Fields
MPS1/TTK	Protein kinase Monopolar spindle 1
qPCR	Quantitative real-time polymerase chain reaction
mRNA	Messenger ribonucleic acid
NB	Normal brain
MGMT	O^6-methylguanine-DNA methyltransferase
ECOG	Eastern Cooperative Oncology Group score
PFS	Progression-free survival
OS	Overall survival
ANOVA	Analysis of variance
PCR	Polymerase Chain reaction
GAPDH	Glyceraldehyde 3-phosphate dehydrogenase
MRI	Magnetic Resonance Imaging

References

1. Louis, D.N.; Perry, A.; Reifenberger, G.; von Deimling, A.; Figarella-Branger, D.; Cavenee, W.K.; Ohgaki, H.; Wiestler, O.D.; Kleihues, P.; Ellison, D.W. The 2016 World Health Organization Classification of Tumors of the Central Nervous System: A summary. *Acta Neuropathol.* **2016**, *131*, 803–820. [CrossRef] [PubMed]
2. Sadighi, Z.; Slopis, J. Pilocytic astrocytoma: A disease with evolving molecular heterogeneity. *J. Child Neurol.* **2013**, *28*, 625–632. [CrossRef] [PubMed]
3. Bikowska-Opalach, B.; Szlufik, S.; Grajkowska, W.; Jozwiak, J. Pilocytic astrocytoma: A review of genetic and molecular factors, diagnostic and prognostic markers. *Histol. Histopathol.* **2014**, *29*, 1235–1248. [PubMed]
4. Collins, V.P.; Jones, D.T.; Giannini, C. Pilocytic astrocytoma: Pathology, molecular mechanisms and markers. *Acta Neuropathol.* **2015**, *129*, 775–788. [CrossRef]
5. Herrlinger, U.; Jones, D.T.W.; Glas, M.; Hattingen, E.; Gramatzki, D.; Stuplich, M.; Felsberg, J.; Bahr, O.; Gielen, G.H.; Simon, M.; et al. Gliomatosis cerebri: No evidence for a separate brain tumor entity. *Acta Neuropathol.* **2016**, *131*, 309–319. [CrossRef]
6. Delgado-Lopez, P.D.; Corrales-Garcia, E.M.; Martino, J.; Lastra-Aras, E.; Duenas-Polo, M.T. Diffuse low-grade glioma: A review on the new molecular classification, natural history and current management strategies. *Clin. Transl. Oncol.* **2017**, *19*, 931–944. [CrossRef]
7. Schiff, D. Low-grade Gliomas. *Contin. Minneap. Minn.* **2017**, *23*, 1564–1579. [CrossRef]
8. Hasselblatt, M.; Jaber, M.; Reuss, D.; Grauer, O.; Bibo, A.; Terwey, S.; Schick, U.; Ebel, H.; Niederstadt, T.; Stummer, W.; et al. Diffuse Astrocytoma, IDH-Wildtype: A Dissolving Diagnosis. *J. Neuropathol. Exp. Neurol.* **2018**, *77*, 422–425. [CrossRef]
9. Reifenberger, G.; Collins, V.P. Pathology and molecular genetics of astrocytic gliomas. *J. Mol. Med. (Berl)* **2004**, *82*, 656–670. [CrossRef]
10. Stupp, R.; Mason, W.P.; van den Bent, M.J.; Weller, M.; Fisher, B.; Taphoorn, M.J.; Belanger, K.; Brandes, A.A.; Marosi, C.; Bogdahn, U.; et al. Radiotherapy plus concomitant and adjuvant temozolomide for glioblastoma. *N. Engl. J. Med.* **2005**, *352*, 987–996. [CrossRef]
11. Hottinger, A.F.; Pacheco, P.; Stupp, R. Tumor treating fields: A novel treatment modality and its use in brain tumors. *Neuro Oncol.* **2016**, *18*, 1338–1349. [CrossRef] [PubMed]
12. Mehta, M.; Wen, P.; Nishikawa, R.; Reardon, D.; Peters, K. Critical review of the addition of tumor treating fields (TTFields) to the existing standard of care for newly diagnosed glioblastoma patients. *Crit. Rev. Oncol./Hematol.* **2017**, *111*, 60–65. [CrossRef]

13. Stupp, R.; Taillibert, S.; Kanner, A.A.; Kesari, S.; Steinberg, D.M.; Toms, S.A.; Taylor, L.P.; Lieberman, F.; Silvani, A.; Fink, K.L.; et al. Maintenance Therapy With Tumor-Treating Fields Plus Temozolomide vs Temozolomide Alone for Glioblastoma: A Randomized Clinical Trial. *JAMA* **2015**, *314*, 2535–2543. [CrossRef]
14. Kessler, A.F.; Frombling, G.E.; Gross, F.; Hahn, M.; Dzokou, W.; Ernestus, R.I.; Lohr, M.; Hagemann, C. Effects of tumor treating fields (TTFields) on glioblastoma cells are augmented by mitotic checkpoint inhibition. *Cell Death Discov.* **2018**, *5*, 12. [CrossRef] [PubMed]
15. Tannous, B.A.; Kerami, M.; Van der Stoop, P.M.; Kwiatkowski, N.; Wang, J.; Zhou, W.; Kessler, A.F.; Lewandrowski, G.; Hiddingh, L.; Sol, N.; et al. Effects of the selective MPS1 inhibitor MPS1-IN-3 on glioblastoma sensitivity to antimitotic drugs. *J. Natl. Cancer Inst.* **2013**, *105*, 1322–1331. [CrossRef]
16. Fisk, H.A.; Mattison, C.P.; Winey, M. A field guide to the Mps1 family of protein kinases. *Cell Cycle* **2004**, *3*, 439–442. [CrossRef] [PubMed]
17. Maciejowski, J.; George, K.A.; Terret, M.E.; Zhang, C.; Shokat, K.M.; Jallepalli, P.V. Mps1 directs the assembly of Cdc20 inhibitory complexes during interphase and mitosis to control M phase timing and spindle checkpoint signaling. *J. Cell Biol.* **2010**, *190*, 89–100. [CrossRef] [PubMed]
18. Maure, J.F.; Kitamura, E.; Tanaka, T.U. Mps1 kinase promotes sister-kinetochore bi-orientation by a tension-dependent mechanism. *Curr. Biol.* **2007**, *17*, 2175–2182. [CrossRef]
19. Jelluma, N.; Brenkman, A.B.; McLeod, I.; Yates, J.R., 3rd; Cleveland, D.W.; Medema, R.H.; Kops, G.J. Chromosomal instability by inefficient Mps1 auto-activation due to a weakened mitotic checkpoint and lagging chromosomes. *PLoS ONE* **2008**, *3*, e2415. [CrossRef] [PubMed]
20. Jelluma, N.; Brenkman, A.B.; van den Broek, N.J.; Cruijsen, C.W.; van Osch, M.H.; Lens, S.M.; Medema, R.H.; Kops, G.J. Mps1 phosphorylates Borealin to control Aurora B activity and chromosome alignment. *Cell* **2008**, *132*, 233–246. [CrossRef]
21. Santaguida, S.; Tighe, A.; D'Alise, A.M.; Taylor, S.S.; Musacchio, A. Dissecting the role of MPS1 in chromosome biorientation and the spindle checkpoint through the small molecule inhibitor reversine. *J. Cell Biol.* **2010**, *190*, 73–87. [CrossRef] [PubMed]
22. Chen, S.; Wang, Y.; Ni, C.; Meng, G.; Sheng, X. HLF/miR-132/TTK axis regulates cell proliferation, metastasis and radiosensitivity of glioma cells. *Biomed. Pharmacother. Biomed. Pharmacother.* **2016**, *83*, 898–904. [CrossRef] [PubMed]
23. Feldheim, J.; Kessler, A.F.; Schmitt, D.; Wilczek, L.; Linsenmann, T.; Dahlmann, M.; Monoranu, C.M.; Ernestus, R.I.; Hagemann, C.; Lohr, M. Expression of activating transcription factor 5 (ATF5) is increased in astrocytomas of different WHO grades and correlates with survival of glioblastoma patients. *Onco Targets* **2018**, *11*, 8673–8684. [CrossRef]
24. Feldheim, J.; Kessler, A.F.; Schmitt, D.; Salvador, E.; Monoranu, C.M.; Feldheim, J.J.; Ernestus, R.I.; Löhr, M.; Hagemann, C. Ribosomal Protein S27/Metallopanstimulin-1 (RPS27) in Glioma-A New Disease Biomarker? *Cancers* **2020**, *12*, 1085. [CrossRef]
25. Livak, K.J.; Schmittgen, T.D. Analysis of relative gene expression data using real-time quantitative PCR and the 2(-Delta Delta C(T)) Method. *Methods* **2001**, *25*, 402–408. [CrossRef]
26. Puchalski, R.B.; Shah, N.; Miller, J.; Dalley, R.; Nomura, S.R.; Yoon, J.G.; Smith, K.A.; Lankerovich, M.; Bertagnolli, D.; Bickley, K.; et al. An anatomic transcriptional atlas of human glioblastoma. *Science* **2018**, *360*, 660–663. [CrossRef]
27. Oken, M.M.; Creech, R.H.; Tormey, D.C.; Horton, J.; Davis, T.E.; McFadden, E.T.; Carbone, P.P. Toxicity and response criteria of the Eastern Cooperative Oncology Group. *Am. J. Clin. Oncol.* **1982**, *5*, 649–655. [CrossRef]
28. Bie, L.; Zhao, G.; Cheng, P.; Rondeau, G.; Porwollik, S.; Ju, Y.; Xia, X.Q.; McClelland, M. The accuracy of survival time prediction for patients with glioma is improved by measuring mitotic spindle checkpoint gene expression. *PLoS ONE* **2011**, *6*, e25631. [CrossRef]
29. Wang, J.; Xie, Y.; Bai, X.; Wang, N.; Yu, H.; Deng, Z.; Lian, M.; Yu, S.; Liu, H.; Xie, W.; et al. Targeting dual specificity protein kinase TTK attenuates tumorigenesis of glioblastoma. *Oncotarget* **2018**, *9*, 3081–3088. [CrossRef]
30. Maachani, U.B.; Kramp, T.; Hanson, R.; Zhao, S.; Celiku, O.; Shankavaram, U.; Colombo, R.; Caplen, N.J.; Camphausen, K.; Tandle, A. Targeting MPS1 Enhances Radiosensitization of Human Glioblastoma by Modulating DNA Repair Proteins. *Mol. Cancer Res. Mcr.* **2015**, *13*, 852–862. [CrossRef]
31. Maachani, U.B.; Tandle, A.; Shankavaram, U.; Kramp, T.; Camphausen, K. Modulation of miR-21 signaling by MPS1 in human glioblastoma. *Oncotarget* **2016**, *7*, 52912–52927. [CrossRef]

32. Alimova, I.; Ng, J.; Harris, P.; Birks, D.; Donson, A.; Taylor, M.D.; Foreman, N.K.; Venkataraman, S.; Vibhakar, R. MPS1 kinase as a potential therapeutic target in medulloblastoma. *Oncol. Rep.* **2016**, *36*, 2633–2640. [CrossRef] [PubMed]
33. Zhou, J.; Li, N.; Yang, G.; Zhu, Y. Vascular patterns of brain tumors. *Int. J. Surg. Pathol.* **2011**, *19*, 709–717. [CrossRef] [PubMed]
34. Rong, Y.; Durden, D.L.; Van Meir, E.G.; Brat, D.J. 'Pseudopalisading' necrosis in glioblastoma: A familiar morphologic feature that links vascular pathology, hypoxia, and angiogenesis. *J. Neuropathol. Exp. Neurol.* **2006**, *65*, 529–539. [CrossRef] [PubMed]
35. Kim, C.S.; Jung, S.; Jung, T.Y.; Jang, W.Y.; Sun, H.S.; Ryu, H.H. Characterization of invading glioma cells using molecular analysis of leading-edge tissue. *J. Korean Neurosurg. Soc.* **2011**, *50*, 157–165. [CrossRef] [PubMed]
36. Trepel, M. *Neuroanatomie—Struktur und Funktion*, 5th ed.; Elsevier GmbH: München, Germany, 2012.
37. Ellingson, B.M.; Kim, H.J.; Woodworth, D.C.; Pope, W.B.; Cloughesy, J.N.; Harris, R.J.; Lai, A.; Nghiemphu, P.L.; Cloughesy, T.F. Recurrent glioblastoma treated with bevacizumab: Contrast-enhanced T1-weighted subtraction maps improve tumor delineation and aid prediction of survival in a multicenter clinical trial. *Radiology* **2014**, *271*, 200–210. [CrossRef] [PubMed]
38. Ellingson, B.M.; Kim, E.; Woodworth, D.C.; Marques, H.; Boxerman, J.L.; Safriel, Y.; McKinstry, R.C.; Bokstein, F.; Jain, R.; Chi, T.L.; et al. Diffusion MRI quality control and functional diffusion map results in ACRIN 6677/RTOG 0625: A multicenter, randomized, phase II trial of bevacizumab and chemotherapy in recurrent glioblastoma. *Int. J. Oncol.* **2015**, *46*, 1883–1892. [CrossRef]
39. Ellingson, B.M.; Harris, R.J.; Woodworth, D.C.; Leu, K.; Zaw, O.; Mason, W.P.; Sahebjam, S.; Abrey, L.E.; Aftab, D.T.; Schwab, G.M.; et al. Baseline pretreatment contrast enhancing tumor volume including central necrosis is a prognostic factor in recurrent glioblastoma: Evidence from single and multicenter trials. *Neuro-Oncology* **2017**, *19*, 89–98. [CrossRef]
40. NIH. ClinicalTrials.gov. Available online: https://clinicaltrials.gov/ (accessed on 18 March 2020).
41. Lorusso, P.; Chawla, S.; Bendell, J.; Shields, A.; Shapiro, G.; Rajagopalan, P.; Cyris, C.; Bruns, I.; Mei, J.; Souza, F. 422P First-in-human study of the monopolar spindle 1 (Mps1) kinase inhibitor BAY 1161909 in combination with paclitaxel in subjects with advanced malignancies. *Ann. Oncol.* **2018**, *29*, mdy279. 410. [CrossRef]

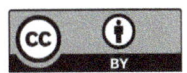

© 2020 by the authors. Licensee MDPI, Basel, Switzerland. This article is an open access article distributed under the terms and conditions of the Creative Commons Attribution (CC BY) license (http://creativecommons.org/licenses/by/4.0/).

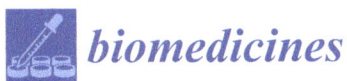

Article

EDTA Chelation Therapy in the Treatment of Neurodegenerative Diseases: An Update

Alessandro Fulgenzi, Daniele Vietti and Maria Elena Ferrero *

Department of Biomedical Sciences for Health, Università degli Studi di Milano, Via Mangiagalli, 31, 20133 Milan, Italy; alessandro.fulgenzi@unimi.it (A.F.); danielevietti@gmail.com (D.V.)
* Correspondence: mariaelena.ferrero@unimi.it; Tel.: +39-025-031-5348

Received: 11 June 2020; Accepted: 1 August 2020; Published: 3 August 2020

Abstract: We have previously described the role played by toxic-metal burdens in the etiology of neurodegenerative diseases (ND). We herein report an updated evaluation of toxic-metal burdens in human subjects affected or not affected by ND or other chronic diseases. Each subject underwent a chelation test with the chelating agent calcium disodium ethylenediaminetetraacetic acid ($CaNA_2EDTA$ or EDTA) to identify the presence of 20 toxic metals in urine samples using inductively coupled plasma mass spectrometry. Our results show the constant presence of toxic metals, such as lead, cadmium, cesium, and aluminum, in all examined subjects but the absence of beryllium and tellurium. Gadolinium was detected in patients undergoing diagnostic magnetic resonance imaging. The presence of toxic metals was always significantly more elevated in ND patients than in healthy controls. Treatment with EDTA chelation therapy removes toxic-metal burdens and improves patient symptoms.

Keywords: EDTA chelation therapy; neurodegenerative diseases; metal detoxification

1. Introduction

Multiple mechanisms are involved in the pathogenesis of neurodegenerative diseases (ND), and knowing how these mechanisms work is of paramount relevance to identify a proper therapeutic strategy. The four most important ND, where both genetic predisposition and environmental factors play important roles, are Parkinson's disease (PD), Alzheimer's disease (AD), multiple sclerosis (MS), and amyotrophic lateral sclerosis (ALS). We have previously described the possible major causes and the related mechanisms involved in direct (toxic metals, air pollution, air and electromagnetic fields, pesticides, neurotoxins, and pathogens) and indirect (proinflammatory cytokines and free oxygen radical productions) neurotoxicity associated to ND [1]. Accumulated evidence of toxic metal cellular damage is now disposable. In particular, recent advances in understanding the role of mitochondrial dysfunction in the pathophysiology of both sporadic and familial PD have already been discussed [2]. More generally, mitochondrial dysfunction is present in ND due to an excessive production of reactive nitric oxide-dependent species, which can trigger post-translational protein modification [3]. Bioenergetic deficits related to mitochondrial dysfunction might be responsible for neuron death and the clinical expression of dementia and are possibly associated to late-onset AD [4]. In addition, the function of some neurotrophic receptors, and their involvement in the pathogenesis, diagnosis, and therapy of PD and AD, has been shown [5].

Moreover, the role of intestinal microbiota in ND has been discussed on more than one occasion [6]. Changes in intestinal microbiota, with consequent microorganism-induced modifications in both intestinal and blood-brain barrier permeability, have been linked to an increased risk of developing AD, PD, and ALS. Furthermore, there is evidence showing a correlation between obesity and the development of AD and PD [7]. Indeed, obese patients frequently display type 2 diabetes mellitus (characterized by neuropathies); insulin resistance is related to dementia, while proinflammatory cytokines in adipose tissue contribute to neuroinflammation [7]. The role played by the inflammatory process in the pathogenesis of neurodegeneration, particularly in the elderly, can be explained by the link between inflammation and mental-function impairment [8]. Alongside these important causes of neuron damage or death, we have focused our studies on the role of toxic metals in the pathogenesis of ND and have described the molecular mechanisms of each toxic metal leading to impaired biological functions in multiple organs, which are cumulatively related to the excessive production of detrimental free oxygen/nitrogen radicals [9].

Many epidemiological studies suggest a role of chronic exposure to toxic metals in the development and propagation of cardiovascular disease [10] and in the generation of vascular complications, especially in diabetic patients [11]. Moreover, it has been shown an association between PD and an exposure to metals such as mercury, lead, manganese, copper, iron, aluminum, bismuth, thallium, and zinc [12] and the potential role of mercury in AD [13]. Exposure to heavy metals such as cadmium and arsenic correlates with glutathione-S-transferase polymorphism in Iranian MS patients, due to the enzyme's ability to remove toxic products [14]. Overall, these findings provide the rationale for the management of ethylenediaminetetraacetic acid (EDTA) chelation therapy [9] as a successful option in the treatment of ND and other diseases associated with metal burdens [1,9]. Notably, chelation therapy has been recently demonstrated a well-tolerated and effective treatment method for post-myocardial infarction patients [15]. The present report is an update and extension on the relationship between toxic-metal burdens and ND, non-ND, and healthy controls [16], with particular focus on the profile of toxic metals in ALS patients. Our study, aimed to investigate the potential and the efficacy of chelation therapy in the cure of subjects affected by toxic metal burden, encouraging its employment in removing toxic-metal poisoning and related symptoms, also through an extensive clinical description of a representative case.

2. Materials and Methods

2.1. Patients

We studied 379 doctors' office patients, age ranging from 13 to 87 years. They gave their consent to undergo chelation therapy, with the chelating agent calcium disodium ethylenediaminetetraacetic acid (EDTA) as unique therapy to treat the disease. Many patients were affected by ND, while others were affected by non-ND (cardiovascular disease, fibromyalgia, rheumatoid arthritis, and peripheral neuropathies); other subjects exposed to occupational or environmental toxic metals, but unaffected by ND or non-ND, acted as healthy controls. The experimental protocol was approved by Milan University's Ethics Advisory Committee (number 64/14). All procedures were performed in accordance with the ethical standard of the responsible committee of human experimentation and with the Helsinki declaration revised in 2000. Informed consent was obtained from each patient included in the study.

2.2. Study Design

All of the patients carried out a "chelation test" (see below) to investigate their possible toxic-metal burdens. Thereafter, they underwent chelation therapy for almost three months. The chelation test was repeated after ten applications to assess the body-burden modifications. The patients were monitored throughout therapy.

2.3. Chelation Test

This was performed as previously described [16]. Briefly, EDTA (2 g) diluted in 500-mL physiological saline (Farmax srl, Brescia, Italy) was slowly (over 2 h) administered intravenously to patients. They were invited to collect urine samples before and for 12 h after the initial intravenous EDTA treatment. Urine samples accurately enveloped in sterile vials were sent to the Laboratory of Toxicology (Doctor's Data Inc., St. Charles, IL, USA) for analysis, as previously reported [16]. Samples were acid-digested with certified metal-free acid, diluted with ultrapure water, and examined via inductively coupled plasma mass spectrometry (ICP-MS), a reliable method to reduce interference. Urine standards, both certified and in-house, were used for quality control and data validation. To avoid a potential error due to fluid intake and sample volume, the results were reported in micrograms (µg) per g of creatinine. Patients showing toxic-metal burdens at the chelation test underwent chelation therapy.

2.4. Chelation Therapy

Chelation therapy was performed by a weekly intravenous infusion of 2-g EDTA in physiological saline. Each patient underwent almost 30 chelation therapy applications. After ten applications, a further chelation test was carried out. Toxic-metal burden values in urine samples are referred to as mineralograms.

2.5. Toxic-Metal Analysis

Twenty toxic metals were analyzed: aluminum (Al), antimony (Sb), arsenicum (As), barium (Ba), beryllium (Be), bismuth (Bi), cadmium (Cd), cesium (Cs), gadolinium (Gd), lead (Pb), mercury (Hg), nickel (Ni), palladium (Pd), platinum (Pt), tellurium (Te), thallium (Tl), thorium (Th), tin (Sn), titanium (Ti), tungsten (W) and uranium (U). Gadolinium is frequently used as a contrast agent in magnetic resonance imaging to diagnose ND.

2.6. Statistical Analysis

Results were expressed as standard error mean of mean (mean ± SEM). They were analyzed using t-tests. Statistical tests were two-sided, and significance was assumed at $p < 0.05$. We used IBM SPSS Statistics. We used also ANOVA to compare the groups (HC vs. ND, non-ND, and ALS).

3. Results

3.1. Patient Characteristics

The patient population was classified as ND, non-ND, and healthy controls (HC) (see Materials and Methods section) (Figure 1). We examined 179 men (mean age = 50.61 years) and 200 women (mean age = 50.82 years). The majority of ND patients were affected by MS.

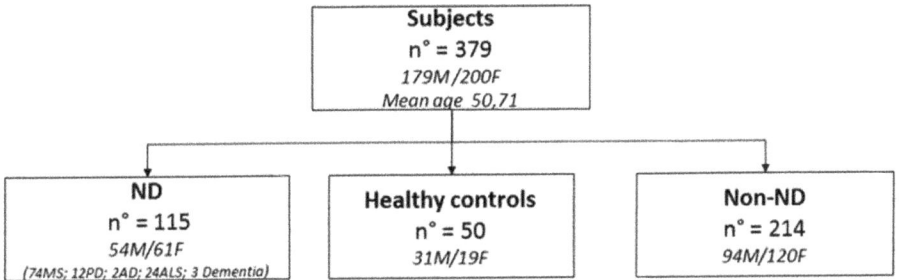

Figure 1. Characteristics of enrolled subjects. ND: neurogenerative diseases, MS: multiple sclerosis, AD: Alzheimer's disease, and ALS: amyotrophic lateral sclerosis.

3.2. Percentage of Patients Affected by Each Toxic-Metal Burden vs. Total Poisoned Population

Figure 2 shows the percentage of ND and HC subjects within the total population: each of the twenty metals known as toxic are analyzed: aluminum (Al), antimony (Sb), arsenicum (As), barium (Ba), beryllium (Be), bismuth (Bi), cadmium (Cd), cesium (Cs), gadolinium (Gd), lead (Pb), mercury (Hg), nickel (Ni), palladium (Pd), platinum (Pt), tellurium (Te), thallium (Tl), thorium (Th), tin (Sn), tungsten (W), and uranium (U). With the exception of thorium, all ND patients presented a more elevated toxic-metal burden compared with HC. Of note, only one HC patient was intoxicated by thorium, possibly due to accidental exposure.

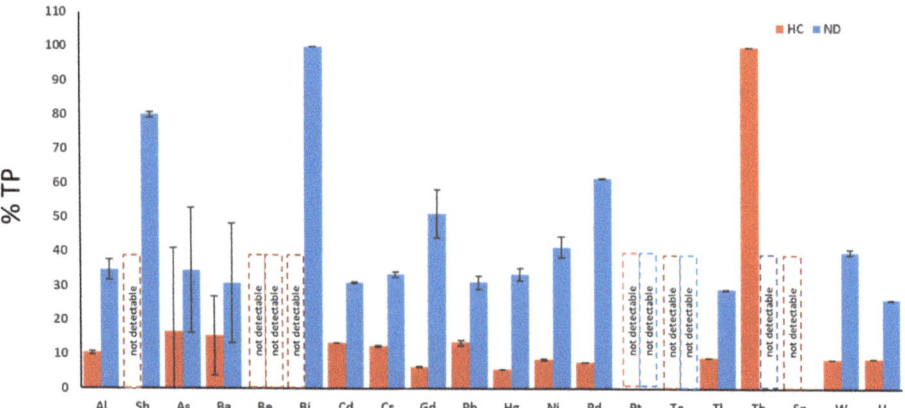

Figure 2. Percentage of total patients (TP) affected by toxic-metal burdens (mean ± SEM). ND = patients affected by neurodegenerative diseases. HC = healthy controls. Aluminum (Al), antimony (Sb), arsenicum (As), barium (Ba), beryllium (Be), bismuth (Bi), cadmium (Cd), cesium (Cs), gadolinium (Gd), lead (Pb), mercury (Hg), nickel (Ni), palladium (Pd), platinum (Pt), tellurium (Te), thallium (Tl), thorium (Th), tin (Sn), tungsten (W), and uranium (U).

3.3. Toxic-Metal Burdens in Patient Urine Samples Following Chelation Test

Patient urine samples collected before the chelation test did not reveal significant toxic-metal contents (data not shown). Toxic-metal burden values assessed in the urine samples taken from patients following the chelation test (e.g., after the first treatment with EDTA) are shown in Table 1. The cut-off represents the limit values of toxic metals, as higher values indicate toxicity. Patients with toxic-metal values above the cut-off are reported in column 3 of Table 1 and indicated as A for each toxic metal in the total population (TP = all patients examined). The percentage of intoxication by each toxic metal with respect to the TP is reported in column 4. Columns 5 and 6 respectively show the mean and standard error of the mean (SEM) of the metal level values above the cut-off. Columns 7 and 8 show the number of ND patients burdened with each toxic metal and the percentage of those patients vs. A. Columns 9 and 10 show the mean values of toxic-metal levels above the cut-off and the SEM in ND patients. Albeit MS is the most frequent ND, we here consider the ALS patients separately from the others ND patients to assess whether they exhibit a different profile of toxic metals in both quality and quantity. Columns 11 and 12 show the number of ALS patients affected by toxic-metal burdens (i.e., levels of toxic metals above the cut-off) and their percentage vs. A. Columns 13 and 14 show the mean values and SEM of toxic-metal levels above the cut-off in ALS patients. Columns 14 and 15 show the number of patients affected by each toxic-metal burden and their percentage vs. A in non-ND patients. Columns 16 and 17 show the mean values of toxic-metal levels above the cut-off and SEM in non-ND patients. Columns 18 and 19 show the number of patients affected by toxic-metal burdens relative to each toxic metal and their percentage vs. A in HC patients. Columns 20 and 21 show the mean values and SEM of toxic-metal levels above the cut-off in HC patients.

Table 1. Toxic-metal burden values assessed in the urine samples taken from patients following the chelation test. The cutoff represents the limit values of toxic metals, as higher values indicate toxicity. Patients with toxic-metal values above the cut-off are reported in the column 3 and indicated as A for each toxic metal in the total population (TP = all patients examined). The percentage of intoxication by each toxic metal with respect to the TP is reported in column 4. Columns 5 and 6 respectively show the mean and standard error of the mean (SEM) of the metal level values above the cut-off. Columns 7 and 8 show the number of ND patients burdened with each toxic metal and the percentage of those patients vs. A. Columns 9 and 10 show the mean values of toxic-metal levels above the cut-off and the SEM in ND patients. Columns 11 and 12 show the number of ALS patients affected by toxic-metal burdens (i.e., levels of toxic metals above the cut-off) and their percentage vs. A. Columns 13 and 14 show the mean values and SEM of toxic-metal levels above the cut-off in ALS patients. Columns 14 and 15 show the number of patients affected by each toxic-metal burden and their percentage vs. A in non-ND patients. Columns 16 and 17 show the mean values of toxic-metal levels above the cut-off and SEM in non-ND patients. Columns 18 and 19 show the number of patients affected by toxic-metal burdens relative to each toxic metal and their percentage vs. A in HC patients. Columns 20 and 21 show the mean values and SEM of toxic-metal levels above the cut-off in HC patients. * $p < 0.05$ HC vs. A and ° $p < 0.05$ HC vs. non-ND. A = number of patients with toxic metal levels > cut-off for each toxic metal. TP = total population, e.g., all patients examined. ND = patients affected by neurodegenerative diseases. Non-ND = patients affected by non-neurodegenerative diseases. HC = healthy controls. ALS = patients affected by amyotrophic lateral sclerosis.

	Cutoff	N° Pz > Cutoff (A)	% TP	Mean (>Cutoff)	SEM	N° Pz > Cutoff ND	% Vs A	Mean (>Cutoff)	SEM	N° Pz > Cutoff ALS	% Vs A	Mean (>Cutoff)	SEM	N° Pz > Cutoff non ND	% Vs A	Mean (>Cutoff)	SEM	N° Pz > Cutoff HC	% Vs A	Mean (>Cutoff)	SEM
Aluminum	25.00	135	36.4	41.93	1.74	47	35	46.70	2.90 *	14	10	56.86	2.21	65	48	47.67	2.11 °	14	10	32.43	0.53 *°
Antimony	0.30	5	1.6	1.25	0.27	4	80	1.53	0.73	1	20	0.07	nd	1	20	1.80	nd	0	nd	nd	nd
Arsenic	108.00	55	15.3	252.07	13.85	19	35	269.47	18.34	1	2	77.95	nd	25	45	317.27	21.35	9	16	288.89	24.73
Barium	7.00	13	3.7	76.43	7.42	4	31	52.83	17.49	2	15	3.05	23.43	6	46	43.78	48.45	2	15	40.50	11.53
Beryllium	1.00	0	nd	nd	nd	nd	nd	nd	nd	0	0	0.00	nd	0	nd	nd	nd	0	nd	nd	nd
Bismuth	10.00	1	0.3	11.00	2.87	1	100	11.00	nd	1	100	0.00	nd	0	nd	1.20	nd	0	nd	nd	nd
Cadmium	0.80	346	92.9	3.49	0.16	107	31	3.96	0.21 *	24	7	3.08	0.16	179	52	4.30	0.14	46	13	2.52	0.08 *
Cesium	9.00	177	47.5	14.63	0.53	59	33	16.00	0.82 *	16	9	8.78	0.64	86	49	16.78	0.53	22	12	12.88	0.25 *
Gadolinium	0.30	172	45.9	31.19	5.41	88	51	41.55	6.96	7	4	8.83	0.81	65	38	8.48	4.34	11	6	2.62	0.18
Lead	2.00	370	99.7	26.76	1.56	115	31	28.00	1.91 *	24	6	22.92	1.75	192	52	38.79	1.53 °	50	14	20.16	0.77 *°
Mercury	3.00	18	5.0	7.58	0.66	6	33	7.17	1.78	3	17	1.55	0.12	11	61	7.53	2.57	1	6	4.60	nd
Nickel	10.00	58	16.1	16.84	0.99	24	41	21.50	3.07 *	7	12	8.80	0.96	29	50	21.93	0.58	5	9	12.00	0.16 *
Palladium	0.30	13	3.4	0.48	0.04	8	62	0.48	0.05	1	8	nd	0.03	5	38	0.65	0.03	1	8	0.40	nd
Platinum	1.00	2	0.5	10.65	9.35	nd	nd	nd	nd	0	0	nd	nd	2	nd	nd	9.35	0	nd	nd	nd
Tellurium	0.80	0	0.0	nd	nd	nd	nd	nd	nd	0	0	nd	nd	0	nd	nd	nd	0	nd	nd	nd
Thallium	0.50	55	14.8	1.20	0.06	16	29	1.33	0.12	8	15	nd	0.03	31	56	1.13	0.12	5	9	0.72	0.02
Thorium	0.03	1	0.3	0.08	0.04	nd	nd	nd	nd	0	0	nd	nd	0	nd	nd	nd	1	100	0.08	nd
Tin	9.00	4	1.1	24.00	1.47	nd	nd	nd	nd	0	0	nd	nd	3	75	48.00	2.29	0	nd	nd	nd
Tungsten	0.40	35	9.5	1.18	0.18	14	40	2.06	0.82	7	20	nd	1.14	19	54	2.88	0.04	3	9	0.60	0.03
Uranium	0.03	23	6.3	0.39	0.24	6	26	0.25	0.076	1	4	nd	nd	15	65	0.31	0.299	2	9	0.09	0.004

Aluminum. Patients affected by Al burdens totaled 135, representing the 36.4% of the TP. The cut-off value for Al is 25 µg/g creatinine, measured in the urine samples, and the mean value of Al > cut-off was 41.95 ± 1.74. Neurodegenerative disease patients affected by Al burdens totaled 47 (35% of A), with a mean value of Al > cut-off = 46.70 ± 2.90. Of some ND patients affected by ALS presenting Al burdens: they were 14 (10% of A), with a mean value of Al > cut-off = 56.86% ± 2.21. Non-ND patients affected by Al burdens totaled 65 (48% of A), with a mean value of Al > cut-off = 47.67 ± 2.11. Patients classified as HC affected by Al burdens totaled 14 (10% of A), with a mean value of Al > cut-off = 32.43% ± 0.53.

Antimony. Five patients were affected by Sb burdens, representing 1.6% of the TP. The cut-off value for Sb was 0.30 µg/g creatinine in the urine samples, and the mean value of Sb > cut-off was 1.25 ± 0.27. Neurodegenerative patients affected by Sb burdens totaled four (80% of A), with a mean value of Sb > cut-off = 1.53 ± 0.73. One patient affected by ALS presented a Sb burden (20% of A), with a value of Sb > cut-off = 0.07. Only one non-ND patient was affected by a Sb burden (20% vs. A), with the value of Sb > cut-off = 1.80. No HC patient was affected by a Sb burden.

Arsenic. Patients affected by As burdens totaled 55 (15.3% of TP). The cut-off value for As was 108.00 µg/g creatinine in the urine samples, with a mean value of As > cut-off = 252.07 ± 13.85. Nineteen ND patients were affected by As burdens (35% of A), with a mean value of As > cut-off = 269.47 ± 18.34. One ALS patient only was affected by an As burden, with a value > cut-off = 77.95%. Twenty-five non-ND patients were affected by As burdens (45% vs. A), with a mean value of As > cut-off = 317.17 ± 21.35. Patients classified as HC affected by As burdens were nine (15% vs. A), with a mean value of As > cut-off = 288.89 ± 24.73.

Barium. Thirteen patients were affected by Ba burdens (3.7 of TP). The cut-off value for Ba was 7.00 µg/g creatinine, and the mean value of Ba > cut-off was = 76.43 ± 7.42. Four ND patients were affected by Ba burdens (31% of A), with a mean value of Ba > cut-off of 52.83 ± 17.49. Two ALS patients were affected by Ba burdens (25% of A), with a not statistically significant mean value of Ba > cut-off. Six non-ND patients and two HC patients only were affected by Ba burdens.

Beryllium. No patients displayed Be intoxication.

Bismuth. One patient only was affected by a Bi burden and was an ALS patient.

Cadmium. Patients affected by Cd burdens totaled 346 (92.9% of TP). The cut-off value for Cd was 0.80 µg/g creatinine, and the mean value of Cd > cut-off was = 3.49 ± 0.16. Neurodegenerative patients affected by Cd burdens totaled 107 (31% of A), with a mean value of Cd > cut-off = 3.96 ± 0.21. Patients affected by ALS and bearing Cd burdens were 24 (7% of A), with a mean value of Cd > cut-off = 3.08 ± 0.16. Non-ND patients affected by Cd burdens totaled 179 (52% of A), with a mean value of Cd > cut-off = 4.30 ± 0.14). Finally, HC totaled 46 (15% of A), with a mean value of Cd > cut-off = 2.52 ± 0.08).

Cesium. Patients affected by Cs burdens totaled 177 (47.5% of TP). The cut-off value for Cs was 9.00 µg/g creatinine, and the mean value of Cs > cut-off was = 14.63 ± 0.53. Neurodegenerative disease patients affected by Cs burdens were 59 (33% of A), with a mean value of Cs > cut-off = 16.00 ± 0.82. Patients affected by ALS with Cs burdens were 16 (9% of A), and the mean value of Cs > cut-off was = 8.78 ± 0.64. Non-ND patients affected by Cs burdens totaled 86 (49% of A), with a mean value of Cs > cut-off 16.78 ± 0.53. Healthy controls with Cs burdens totaled 22 (12% of A), with a mean value of Cs > cut-off = 12.88 ± 0.25.

Gadolinium. Patients affected by Gd intoxication totaled 172 (45.9% of TP). The cut-off value for Gd was 0.30 µg/g creatinine, and the mean value of Gd > cut-off was 31.19 ± 5.41. Neurodegenerative disease patients affected by Gd burdens were 88 (51% of A), with a mean value of Gd > cut-off = 41.55 ± 6.96. Seven patients affected by Gd intoxications were ALS patients (4% of A), with a mean value of Gd > cut-off = 58.83 ± 0.81. Non-ND patients affected by Gd intoxications were 65 (38% of A), with a mean value of Gd > cut-off = 8.48 ± 4.34. Healthy control patients affected by Gd intoxications were 11 (6% of A), with a mean value of Gd > cut-off = 2.62 ± 0.18.

Lead. Patients affected by Pb intoxications totaled 370 (99.7% of TP). The cut-off value for Pb was 2.0 µg/g creatinine, and the mean value of Pb > cut-off was 26.76 ± 1.56. Neurodegenerative disease patients affected by Pb burdens totaled 115 (31% of A), with a mean value of Pb > cut-off = 28.00 ± 1.91. Patients with ALS affected by Pb burdens were 24 (6% of A), with a mean value of Pb > cut-off = 22.92 ± 1.75. Non-ND patients affected by Pb burdens were 192 (52% of A), with a mean value of Pb > cut-off = 38.79 ± 1.53. Healthy controls affected by Pb burdens totaled 50 (14% of A), with a Pb value > cut-off = 20.16 ± 0.77.

Mercury. Patients affected by Hg intoxications totaled 18 (5% of TP). The cut-off value for Hg was 3.00 µg/g creatinine, and the mean value of Hg > cut-off was 7.58 ± 0.66. Neurodegenerative disease patients affected by Hg burdens totaled six (33% of A), with a mean value of Hg > cut-off = 7.17 ± 1.78. Of the ND patients, three ALS patients (17% of A) were intoxicated by Hg, with a mean value of Hg > cut-off = 1.55 ± 0.12. Non-ND patients bearing Hg burdens were 11 (61% of A), with a mean value of Hg > cut-off = 7.53 ± 2.57. Only one HC patient was affected by a Hg burden.

Nickel. Patients affected by Ni intoxications totaled 58 (16.1% of TP). The cut-off value for Ni was 10.00 µg/g creatinine, and the mean value of Ni > cut-off was 16.84 ± 0.99. Patient with ND affected by Ni burdens were 24 (41% of A), with a mean value of Ni > cut-off = 21.50 ± 3.07. Seven patients with ALS were affected by Ni burdens (12% of A), with a mean value of Ni > cut-off = 8.80 ± 0.96. Non-ND patients affected by Ni burdens were 29 (50% of A), with a mean value of Ni > cut-off = 21.93 ± 0.58. Healthy controls bearing Ni burdens were five (9% of A), with a mean value of Ni > cut-off = 12.00 ± 0.16.

Palladium. Patients affected by Pd intoxications were 13 (3.4% of TP). The cut-off value for Pd was 0.30 µg/g creatinine, and the mean value of Pd > cut-off was 0.48 ± 0.04. Eight ND patients were affected by Pd burdens (62% of A), with a mean value of Pd > cut-off = 0.48 ± 0.05. Only one ALS patient was affected by a Pd burden. Five non-ND patients displayed Pd burdens (38% of A), with a mean value of Pd > cut-off = 0.65 ± 0.03. Only one HC patient displayed a Pd burden.

Platinum. Only two patients were affected by Pt intoxications and were non-ND patients.

Tellurium. No patient was affected by a Te intoxication.

Thallium. Patients affected by Tl intoxications totaled 55 (14.8% of TP). The cut-off value for Tl was 0.50 µg/g creatinine, with a mean value of Tl > cut-off = 1.20 ± 0.06. Patients affected ND and by Tl burdens were 16 (29% of A), with a mean value of Tl > cut-off = 1.13 ± 0.12. Eight ALS patients (15% of A) were affected by Tl burdens. Thirty-one non-ND patients were affected by Tl burdens (56% of A), with a mean value of Tl > cut-off = 1.15 ± 0.12. Five HC patients were affected by Tl burdens (9% of A), with a mean value of Tl > cut-off = 0.72 ± 0.02.

Thorium. Only one patient was affected by a Th intoxication and was a HC patient.

Tin. Patients affected by Sn burdens were four (11% of TP). The cut-off value for Sn was 9.00 µg/g creatinine, and the mean value of Sn > cut-off was 24.00 ± 1.47. No ND patients nor HC patients were affected by Sn intoxications. Three non-ND patients were affected by Sn intoxications (75% of A), with a mean value of Sn > cut-off = 48.00 ± 2.29.

Tungsten. Patients affected by W intoxications were 35 (9.5% of TP). The cut-off value for W was 0.40 µg/g creatinine, and the mean value of W > cut-off was 1.18 ± 0.18. Neurodegenerative patients affected by W burdens totaled 14 (40% of A), with a mean value of W > cut-off = 2.06 ± 0.82. Seven ALS patients were affected by W intoxications. Nineteen non-ND patients were affected by W intoxications (54% of A), with a mean value of W > cut-off = 2.88 ± 0.04. Finally, three HC patients were affected by W intoxications (9% of A), with a mean value of W > cut-off = 0.60 ± 0.03.

Uranium. Patients affected by U intoxications were 23 (6.3% of A). The cut-off for U was 0.03 µg/g creatinine, with a mean value of U > cut-off = 0.39 ± 0.24. Neurodegenerative disease patients affected by U burdens were six (26% of A), with a mean value of U > cut-off = 0.25 ± 0.076. Only one ALS patient was affected by a U burden. Non-ND patients affected by U burdens were 15 (65% of A), with a mean value of U > cut-off = 0.31 ± 0.299. Two HC patients were affected by U burdens (9% of A), with a mean value of U > cut-off = 0.09 ± 0.004.

The results obtained deserve consideration. Firstly, no one was affected by beryllium or tellurium intoxications. Patients were mainly intoxicated by lead, cadmium, cesium, gadolinium, aluminum, and, to a lesser extent, nickel, arsenic, thallium, and tungsten. Patients affected by ND were intoxicated by lead, cadmium, gadolinium, cesium, and aluminum. In particular, those affected by ALS were intoxicated by lead, cadmium, cesium and aluminum. Gadolinium intoxications were related to the elevated number of MRI examinations undergone by ND patients, especially by MS patients and also by some non-ND patients. Patients affected by non-ND also showed elevated levels of lead, cadmium, cesium, gadolinium, and aluminum. Healthy controls displayed elevated levels of lead, cadmium, and cesium. All examined ALS patients were intoxicated by lead and cadmium and, to a lesser extent, by gadolinium and aluminum. Maximum levels of lead and cadmium intoxications were reached by non-ND patients. The levels of aluminum, cadmium, cesium, lead, and nickel were significantly more elevated in ND patients than in HC. The levels of aluminum and lead were significantly higher in non-ND patients than in HC. Obviously, the levels of gadolinium were significantly more elevated in ND and non-ND patients than in HC due to many MRI performed. No ND patient was affected by a Sn intoxication.

Interestingly, we found that non-ND patients displaying elevated levels of some toxic metals were affected by the following diseases: cardiovascular diseases, fibromyalgia, rheumatoid arthritis, and peripheral neuropathies.

We then compared the levels of toxic metals measured in urine samples following a chelation test in ND, non-ND, and ALS vs. HC. With an ANOVA test, we could appreciate that Al was significantly higher in ND, non-ND, and ALS, with respect to HC. Moreover, Pb was higher in ALS patients with respect to HC.

3.4. Reduction of Poisoning Following Chelation Therapy

Poisoned patients who underwent chelation therapies exhibited a significant reduction of toxic-metal levels (data not shown), as previously reported [16], accompanied by a consistent alleviation of related symptoms (headache, paresthesia, tingling, difficulty to walking, memory and visus loss, hypertension, and asthenia) [9]. In particular, ALS patients displayed improved weaknesses, as well as upper and lower motor dysfunctions. The results here described are superimposable to the previous ones [16]. ND patients displayed a reduction of toxic-metal levels following about 20–30 chelation therapies and constantly ameliorated with repeated chelations. As an exemplification, we report the case of a patient affected by MS. Figure 3 shows the toxic-metal levels following the chelation test. High levels of gadolinium, owing to MRI, cadmium, and lead, are evident. The patient underwent 60 chelation therapy applications over a 20-month period. Figure 4 shows a dramatic reduction in gadolinium levels (from 82 microg/g creatinine to 17 microg/g creatinine), as well as reduced lead and cadmium levels. Of note, reductions over time of gadolinium levels permits the elimination of those toxic metals present in minimal quantities unaffected by previous chelation therapy, such as mercury and cesium.

TOXIC METALS		RESULT µg/g creat	REFERENCE INTERVAL	WITHIN REFERENCE	OUTSIDE REFERENCE
Aluminum	(Al)	16	< 25		
Antimony	(Sb)	< dl	< 0.2		
Arsenic	(As)	52	< 75		
Barium	(Ba)	1.2	< 7		
Beryllium	(Be)	< dl	< 1		
Bismuth	(Bi)	< dl	< 2		
Cadmium	(Cd)	3.2	< 0.8		
Cesium	(Cs)	9.1	< 9		
Gadolinium	(Gd)	82	< 0.5		
Lead	(Pb)	25	< 2		
Mercury	(Hg)	2.4	< 3		
Nickel	(Ni)	7.6	< 8		
Palladium	(Pd)	< dl	< 0.1		
Platinum	(Pt)	< dl	< 0.1		
Tellurium	(Te)	< dl	< 0.5		
Thallium	(Tl)	0.2	< 0.5		
Thorium	(Th)	< dl	< 0.03		
Tin	(Sn)	0.5	< 4		
Tungsten	(W)	0.5	< 0.4		
Uranium	(U)	< dl	< 0.03		

Figure 3. Toxic-metal levels measured by inductively coupled plasma mass spectrometry in patient urine collected during the 12 h following the ethylenediaminetetraacetic acid (EDTA) challenge (chelation test) reported in µg/g creatinine. The black lines indicate the levels of each toxic metal. Whitin the green column the values are considered normal, while in the yellow and in the red columns high and very high values are reported, respectively. The 42-year-old male patient was affected by multiple sclerosis and was a smoker.

TOXIC METALS		RESULT µg/g creat	REFERENCE INTERVAL	WITHIN REFERENCE	OUTSIDE REFERENCE
Aluminum	(Al)	17	< 25		
Antimony	(Sb)	< dl	< 0.2		
Arsenic	(As)	63	< 75		
Barium	(Ba)	1.3	< 7		
Beryllium	(Be)	< dl	< 1		
Bismuth	(Bi)	< dl	< 2		
Cadmium	(Cd)	1.7	< 0.8		
Cesium	(Cs)	12	< 9		
Gadolinium	(Gd)	17	< 0.5		
Lead	(Pb)	9.8	< 2		
Mercury	(Hg)	3.8	< 3		
Nickel	(Ni)	3.7	< 8		
Palladium	(Pd)	< dl	< 0.1		
Platinum	(Pt)	< dl	< 0.1		
Tellurium	(Te)	< dl	< 0.5		
Thallium	(Tl)	0.2	< 0.5		
Thorium	(Th)	< dl	< 0.03		
Tin	(Sn)	0.4	< 4		
Tungsten	(W)	< dl	< 0.4		
Uranium	(U)	< dl	< 0.03		

Figure 4. Toxic-metal levels measured by inductively coupled plasma mass spectrometry in the patient urine collected over 12 h reported in µg/g creatinine. The black lines indicate the levels of each toxic metal. Whitin the green column the values are considered normal, while in the yellow and in the red columns high and very high values are reported, respectively. The patient was affected by multiple sclerosis and underwent 60 chelation therapy applications over a 20-month period.

4. Discussion

The involvement of toxic substances in the pathogenesis and progression of ND is widely debated. The neuroinflammation hypothesis regarding the link between air pollution and ND supports the concept that inhaled pollutants activate the microglial production of cytokines and reactive oxygen species in the brain that can progressively damage the neurons [17]. The contributing role of miRNA alterations in the pathogenesis of neurodegenerative processes in response to environmental stimuli, such as metals and pesticides, has already been described [18]. Although genetic mutations are known to be responsible for the onset of ND, new evidence suggests that ALS, AD, and PD are caused by complex gene-environment interactions involving metal neurotoxicity [19]. Even excessive exposure to essential metals, such as iron and manganese, might lead to pathological conditions, such as neurodegeneration through impaired homeostasis, in essential metal metabolisms [20]. High levels of copper, manganese, and iron, responsible for Wilson's disease, manganism, and hemochromatosis, respectively, exert an important role also in the pathogenesis of ND participating in the formation of α-synuclein aggregates in intracellular inclusions in the central nervous system (CNS); in particular, the accumulation of iron is responsible for PD and AD [21]. On the other hand, transition metals act as catalysts in oxidative reactions, causing oxidative tissue damage. In particular, redox-active metals, such as iron, copper, and chromium, undergo redox-cycling, whereas redox-inactive toxic metals, like lead, cadmium, and mercury, deplete major cell antioxidants, such as thiol-containing antioxidants and enzymes [22–24]. More recently, mercury and lead, in a concentration-dependent way, have been shown to induce an increase in amyloid beta protein (Aβ42) misfolding and aggregation with toxic properties, suggesting their implication in AD [25]. The potential relationship between mercury exposure and AD has also been further described [16]. In a neuronal cell human model, exposure to cadmium has highlighted gene deregulation, carcinogenicity, perturbations of essential metals, interference with calcium regulation, and other effects involved in neurodegeneration [26]. Moreover, metal-induced neurotoxicity has been linked to autophagic dysfunction, as the deficient elimination of abnormal or toxic protein aggregates can promote cellular stress, failure, and death [27]. Some heavy metals (e.g., lead, cadmium, and aluminum) used at subtoxic concentrations can lead to oligodendrocyte dysfunction, especially when oligodendrocytes are cocultured with neurons. The most important dysfunctions relate to imbalanced intracellular calcium ion regulation, altered lipid formation, and imbalanced myelin formation [28]. Aluminum toxicity in humans due to chronic inevitable exposure has already been described [29,30]. Furthermore, mercury neurotoxicity seems to be potentiated by the presence of apolipoprotein E4 [31].

We previously demonstrated that, unlike in HC, high levels of toxic metals are present in ND patients and in non-ND patients [16]. We extend this notion, showing that ND patients are affected by higher levels of each considered toxic metal compared with HC (Figure 2), except for thorium, which was found only in one HC. Moreover, here, we demonstrate that the profile of toxic metals is similar in ND and non-ND groups, which both display high levels of lead, cadmium, gadolinium, cesium, aluminum, and nickel, and that EDTA chelation therapy is effective in removing metal burdens. Of note, all patients (24/24) in the group of ALS were intoxicated by lead and cadmium; moreover, 14/24 were intoxicated by Al and 16/24 by Cs. Of note, Pb was significantly higher in ALS patients with respect to HC. Maximal levels of lead and cadmium intoxications were reached in non-ND patients, which we have examined in a greater number than before [16]. This observation is not surprising, because our cohort of non-ND patients was affected by either cardiovascular disease or by fibromyalgia, both diseases whose pathogenic mechanisms might be related to toxic-metal burdens [10,32,33] and whose detrimental effects we have shown to impact on and damage not only neurons but, also, other cell types—in particular, endothelial cells [34] Patient intoxication is a chronic event and requires several chelation therapy applications to reduce the toxic-metal burdens and improve symptoms (Figures 3 and 4). The elevated levels of Gd in ND and, also, in non-ND patients are important to be considered as responsible for neurotoxicity. Our therapeutic approach relies in the administration of two grams once a week. After ten chelations, the therapy is able to reduce all toxic metals and to improve the patient symptoms, listed in the Results section; subsequent chelations progressively improve their reductions, often reaching physiologic levels. In particular, we measured in patients treated with EDTA chelation therapy the blood levels of Na, K, Mg, Cl, Ca, P, and Fe, which were not affected (data not shown). The therapy is well-tolerated and not associated with side effects.

The beneficial effect exerted by EDTA therapy can be supported by our experimental evidences, suggesting that EDTA may revert cellular endothelial damage induced in vitro by the cytokine TNF-alpha [35]. Moreover, in patients treated with EDTA chelation therapy, the levels of ROS in blood samples, as well as of oxLDL, were reduced and associated with an increase of the total antioxidant capacity, overall suggesting the role of EDTA as an antioxidant compound [36,37]. Finally, in patients affected by ND, the low levels of free glutathione (GSH) in erythrocytes were increased by EDTA chelation therapy, reaching those of control patients [38].

Author Contributions: Conceptualization, M.E.F.; data curation, A.F. and D.V.; formal analysis, A.F.; Supervision, M.E.F.; and writing—review and editing, M.E.F. All authors have read and agreed to the published version of the manuscript.

Funding: This research received no external funding.

Conflicts of Interest: The authors declare no conflicts of interest.

Abbreviations

ND	Neurodegenerative diseases
Non-ND	Non neurodegenerative diseases
HC	Healthy controls
EDTA	calcium disodium ethylenediaminetetraacetic acid
AD	Alzheimer's disease
ALS	Amyotrophic lateral sclerosis
MS	Multiple sclerosis
PD	Parkinson's disease
ICP	MS inductively coupled plasma mass spectrometry
Al	aluminum
Sb	antimony
As	arsenicum
Ba	barium
Be	beryllium
Bi	bismuth
Cd	cadmium
Cs	cesium
Gd	gadolinium
Pb	lead
Hg	mercury
Ni	nickel
Pd	palladium
Pt	platinum
Te	tellurium
Tl	thallium
Th	thorium
Sn	tin
W	tungsten
U	uranium

References

1. Fulgenzi, A.; Ferrero, M.E. EDTA Chelation Therapy for the Treatment of Neurotoxicity. *Int. J. Mol. Sci.* **2019**, *20*, 1019.
2. Park, J.-S.; Davis, R.L.; Sue, C.M. Mitochondrial Dysfunction in Parkinson's Disease: New Mechanistic Insights and Therapeutic Perspectives. *Curr. Neurol. Neurosci. Rep.* **2018**, *18*, 21. [CrossRef] [PubMed]
3. Nakamura, T.; Lipton, S.A. Nitric Oxide-Dependent Protein Post-Translational Modifications Impair Mitochondrial Function and Metabolism to Contribute to Neurodegenerative Diseases. *Antioxid. Redox Signal.* **2020**, *32*, 817–833. [CrossRef] [PubMed]
4. Mecocci, P.; Baroni, M.; Senin, U.; Boccardi, V. Brain Aging and Late-Onset Alzheimer's Disease: A Matter of Increased Amyloid or Reduced Energy? *J. Alzheimer's Dis.* **2018**, *64*, S397–S404. [CrossRef] [PubMed]
5. Meldolesi, J. Neurotrophin receptors in the pathogenesis, diagnosis and therapy of neurodegenerative diseases. *Pharmacol. Res.* **2017**, *121*, 129–137. [CrossRef]
6. Spielman, L.J.; Gibson, D.L.; Klegeris, A. Unhealthy gut, unhealthy brain: The role of the intestinal microbiota in neurodegenerative diseases. *Neurochem. Int.* **2018**, *120*, 149–163. [CrossRef]
7. Mazon, J.N.; de Mello, A.H.; Ferreira, G.K.; Rezin, G.T. The impact of obesity on neurodegenerative diseases. *Life Sci.* **2017**, *182*, 22–28. [CrossRef]
8. Chen, W.W.; Zhang, X.; Huang, W.J. Role of neuroinflammation in neurodegenerative diseases (Review). *Mol. Med. Rep.* **2016**, *13*, 3391–3396. [CrossRef]
9. Ferrero, M.E. Rationale for the Successful Management of EDTA Chelation Therapy in Human Burden by Toxic Metals. *Biomed Res. Int.* **2016**. [CrossRef]
10. Lamas, G.A.; Navas-Acien, A.; Mark, D.B.; Lee, K.L. Heavy Metals, Cardiovascular Disease, and the Unexpected Benefits of Chelation Therapy. *J. Am. Coll. Cardiol.* **2016**, *67*, 2411–2418. [CrossRef]
11. Peguero, J.G.; Arenas, I.; Lamas, G.A. Chelation therapy and cardiovascular disease: Connecting scientific silos to benefit cardiac patients. *Trends Cardiovasc. Med.* **2014**, *24*, 232–240. [CrossRef] [PubMed]
12. Bjorklund, G.; Stejskal, V.; Urbina, M.A.; Dadar, M.; Chirumbolo, S.; Mutter, J. Metals and Parkinson's Disease: Mechanisms and Biochemical Processes. *Curr. Med. Chem.* **2018**, *25*, 2198–2214. [CrossRef] [PubMed]
13. Bjørklund, G.; Tinkov, A.A.; Dadar, M.; Rahman, M.M.; Chirumbolo, S.; Skalny, A.V.; Skalnaya, M.G.; Haley, B.E.; Ajsuvakova, O.P.; Aaseth, J. Insights into the Potential Role of Mercury in Alzheimer's Disease. *J. Mol. Neurosci.* **2019**, *67*, 511–533. [CrossRef] [PubMed]
14. Aliomrani, M.; Sahraian, M.A.; Shirkhanloo, H.; Sharifzadeh, M.; Khoshayand, M.R.; Ghahremani, M.H. Correlation between heavy metal exposure and GSTM1 polymorphism in Iranian multiple sclerosis patients. *Neurol. Sci.* **2017**, *38*, 1271–1278. [CrossRef] [PubMed]
15. Avila, M.D.; Escolar, E.; Lamas, G.A. Chelation therapy after the Trial to Assess Chelation Therapy: Results of a unique trial. *Curr. Opin. Cardiol.* **2014**, *29*, 481. [CrossRef] [PubMed]
16. Fulgenzi, A.; Vietti, D.; Maria Elena, F. Chronic toxic-metal poisoning and neurodegenerative diseases. *Int. J. Curr. Res.* **2017**, *9*, 57899–57999.
17. Jayaraj, R.L.; Rodriguez, E.A.; Wang, Y.; Block, M.L. Outdoor Ambient Air Pollution and Neurodegenerative Diseases: The Neuroinflammation Hypothesis. *Curr. Environ. Health Rep.* **2017**, *4*, 166–179. [CrossRef]
18. Ferrante, M.; Conti, G.O. Environment and Neurodegenerative Diseases: An Update on miRNA Role. *MicroRNA* **2017**, *6*, 157–165. [CrossRef]
19. Cicero, C.E.; Mostile, G.; Vasta, R.; Rapisarda, V.; Signorelli, S.S.; Ferrante, M.; Zappia, M.; Nicoletti, A. Metals and neurodegenerative diseases. A systematic review. *Environ. Res.* **2017**, *159*, 82–94. [CrossRef]
20. Farina, M.; Avila, D.S.; Da Rocha, J.B.T.; Aschner, M. Metals, oxidative stress and neurodegeneration: A focus on iron, manganese and mercury. *Neurochem. Int.* **2013**, *62*, 575–594. [CrossRef]
21. Mezzaroba, L.; Alfieri, D.F.; Colado Simão, A.N.; Vissoci Reiche, E.M. The role of zinc, copper, manganese and iron in neurodegenerative diseases. *Neurotoxicology* **2019**, *74*, 230–241. [CrossRef] [PubMed]
22. Nuran Ercal, B.S.P.; Hande Gurer-Orhan, B.S.P.; Nukhet Aykin-Burns, B.S.P. Toxic Metals and Oxidative Stress Part I: Mechanisms Involved in Metal induced Oxidative Damage. *Curr. Top. Med. Chem.* **2005**. [CrossRef] [PubMed]
23. Jamilian, M.; Mirhosseini, N.; Eslahi, M.; Bahmani, F.; Shokrpour, M.; Chamani, M.; Asemi, Z. The effects of magnesium-zinc-calcium-vitamin D co-supplementation on biomarkers of inflammation, oxidative stress and pregnancy outcomes in gestational diabetes. *BMC Pregnancy Childbirth* **2019**, *19*, 107. [CrossRef] [PubMed]

24. Ouyang, Y.; Peng, Y.; Li, J.; Holmgren, A.; Lu, J. Modulation of thiol-dependent redox system by metal ions via thioredoxin and glutaredoxin systems. *Metallomics* **2018**, *10*, 218–228. [CrossRef]
25. Meleleo, D.; Notarachille, G.; Mangini, V.; Arnesano, F. Concentration-dependent effects of mercury and lead on Aβ42: Possible implications for Alzheimer's disease. *Eur. Biophys. J.* **2019**, *48*, 173–187. [CrossRef] [PubMed]
26. Forcella, M.; Lau, P.; Oldani, M.; Melchioretto, P.; Bogni, A.; Gribaldo, L.; Fusi, P.; Urani, C. Neuronal specific and non-specific responses to cadmium possibly involved in neurodegeneration: A toxicogenomics study in a human neuronal cell model. *Neurotoxicology* **2020**, *76*, 162–173. [CrossRef] [PubMed]
27. Zhang, Z.; Miah, M.; Culbreth, M.; Aschner, M. Autophagy in neurodegenerative diseases and metal neurotoxicity. *Neurochem. Res.* **2016**, *41*, 409–422. [CrossRef]
28. Maiuolo, J.; Macrì, R.; Bava, I.; Gliozzi, M.; Musolino, V.; Nucera, S.; Carresi, C.; Scicchitano, M.; Bosco, F.; Scarano, F.; et al. Myelin disturbances produced by sub-toxic concentration of heavy metals: The role of oligodendrocyte dysfunction. *Int. J. Mol. Sci.* **2019**, *20*, 4554. [CrossRef]
29. Fulgenzi, A.; De Giuseppe, R.; Bamonti, F.; Vietti, D.; Ferrero, M.E. Efficacy of chelation therapy to remove aluminium intoxication. *J. Inorg. Biochem.* **2015**, *152*, 214–218. [CrossRef]
30. Exley, C. The toxicity of aluminium in humans. *Morphologie* **2016**, *100*, 51–55. [CrossRef]
31. Crespo-Lopez, M.E. Role for apolipoprotein E in neurodegeneration and mercury intoxication. *Front. Biosci.* **2018**, *10*, 819. [CrossRef] [PubMed]
32. Chowdhury, R.; Ramond, A.; O'Keeffe, L.M.; Shahzad, S.; Kunutsor, S.K.; Muka, T.; Gregson, J.; Willeit, P.; Warnakula, S.; Khan, H.; et al. Environmental toxic metal contaminants and risk of cardiovascular disease: Systematic review and meta-analysis. *BMJ* **2018**, *362*, k3310. [CrossRef] [PubMed]
33. Nigra, A.E.; Ruiz-Hernandez, A.; Redon, J.; Navas-Acien, A.; Tellez-Plaza, M. Environmental Metals and Cardiovascular Disease in Adults: A Systematic Review Beyond Lead and Cadmium. *Curr. Environ. Health Rep.* **2016**, *3*, 416–433. [CrossRef] [PubMed]
34. Fulgenzi, A.; Zito, F.; Marchelli, D.; Colombo, F.; Ferrero, M.E. New Insights into EDTA In Vitro Effects on Endothelial Cells and on In Vivo Labeled EDTA Biodistribution. *J. Heavy Met. Toxic. Dis.* **2016**, *1*, 7.
35. Sabolić, I. Common mechanisms in nephropathy induced by toxic metals. *Nephron-Physiol.* **2006**, *10*, p107–p114. [CrossRef] [PubMed]
36. Foglieni, C.; Fulgenzi, A.; Ticozzi, P.; Pellegatta, F.; Sciorati, C.; Belloni, D.; Ferrero, E.; Ferrero, M.E. Protective effect of EDTA preadministration on renal ischemia. *BMC Nephrol.* **2006**, *7*, 1–12. [CrossRef]
37. Fulgenzi, A.; Giuseppe, R.D.; Bamonti, F.; Ferrero, M.E. Improvement of oxidative and metabolic parameters by cellfood administration in patients affected by neurodegenerative diseases on chelation treatment. *Biomed Res. Int.* **2014**, *2014*, 281510. [CrossRef]
38. Dellanoce, C.; Fulgenzi, A.; Ferrero, M.E. Glutathione Redox Status in Neurodegenerative Diseases. *Austin J. Clin. Neurol.* **2019**, *6*, 6.

© 2020 by the authors. Licensee MDPI, Basel, Switzerland. This article is an open access article distributed under the terms and conditions of the Creative Commons Attribution (CC BY) license (http://creativecommons.org/licenses/by/4.0/).

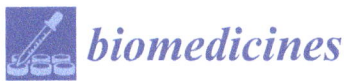

Article

Lupeol, a Plant-Derived Triterpenoid, Protects Mice Brains against Aβ-Induced Oxidative Stress and Neurodegeneration

Riaz Ahmad, Amjad Khan, Hyeon Jin Lee, Inayat Ur Rehman, Ibrahim Khan, Sayed Ibrar Alam and Myeong Ok Kim *

Division of Life Sciences and Applied Life Science (BK 21plus), College of Natural Science, Gyeongsang National University, Jinju 52828, Korea; riazk0499@gnu.ac.kr (R.A.); amjadkhan@gnu.ac.kr (A.K.); dlguswls363@naver.com (H.J.L.); inayaturrehman201516@gnu.ac.kr (I.U.R.); ibrahimbiotech11@gmail.com (I.K.); ibrar@gnu.ac.kr (S.I.A.)
* Correspondence: mokim@gnu.ac.kr; Tel.: +82-55-772-1345; Fax: +82-55-772-2656

Received: 25 August 2020; Accepted: 25 September 2020; Published: 26 September 2020

Abstract: Alzheimer's disease (AD) is a progressive neurodegenerative disorder that represents 60–70% of all dementia cases. AD is characterized by the formation and accumulation of amyloid-beta (Aβ) plaques, neurofibrillary tangles, and neuronal cell loss. Further accumulation of Aβ in the brain induces oxidative stress, neuroinflammation, and synaptic and memory dysfunction. In this study, we investigated the antioxidant and neuroprotective effects of the natural triterpenoid lupeol in the $Aβ_{1-42}$ mouse model of AD. An Intracerebroventricular injection (i.c.v.) of Aβ (3 μL/5 min/mouse) into the brain of a mouse increased the reactive oxygen species (ROS) levels, neuroinflammation, and memory and cognitive dysfunction. The oral administration of lupeol at a dose of 50 mg/kg for two weeks significantly decreased the oxidative stress, neuroinflammation, and memory impairments. Lupeol decreased the oxidative stress via the activation of nuclear factor erythroid 2-related factor-2 (Nrf-2) and heme oxygenase-1 (HO-1) in the brain of adult mice. Moreover, lupeol treatment prevented neuroinflammation by suppressing activated glial cells and inflammatory mediators. Additionally, lupeol treatment significantly decreased the accumulation of Aβ and beta-secretase-1 (BACE-1) expression and enhanced the memory and cognitive function in the Aβ-mouse model of AD. To the best of our knowledge, this is the first study to investigate the anti-oxidative and neuroprotective effects of lupeol against $Aβ_{1-42}$-induced neurotoxicity. Our findings suggest that lupeol could serve as a novel, promising, and accessible neuroprotective agent against progressive neurodegenerative diseases such as AD.

Keywords: Alzheimer's disease; reactive oxygen species (ROS); neuroinflammation; neurodegeneration; cognitive dysfunction

1. Introduction

Neurodegenerative diseases are incurable conditions that result in the progressive loss of neuronal cells. There are several neurodegenerative disorders including Alzheimer's disease (AD), which is the most common and represents approximately 60–70% of all dementia cases [1,2]. AD is a chronic and progressive neurodegenerative disorder that affects synaptic and cognitive functions. The pathophysiology of AD is the formation and accumulation of extracellular amyloid-beta (Aβ), plaques, intracellular neurofibrillary tangles, and a loss of connection among the nerve cells in the brain [3–5] Aβ-peptide is generated from a transmembrane protein called the amyloid precursor protein (APP) by the action of a beta secretase-1 enzyme (BACE-1) [6,7]. The increased activity of these enzymes is responsible for the sequential cleavage of APP, resulting in the formation and aggregation of the Aβ-peptide [7,8].

The accumulation of Aβ in the brain enhances oxidative stress and neuroinflammation and affects the memory function of the brain [9]. The elevated level of reactive oxygen species (ROS) disrupts the normal functioning of various biomolecules (lipid and DNA) in the brain [10,11]. The higher oxidative stress is responsible for the progression of the pathophysiology of AD by several mechanisms such as the activation of the innate immune system and the release of inflammatory mediators. Boosting the antioxidant defense mechanisms may counteract the progression of AD and its consequences.

Aβ and oxidative stress in the brain are responsible for the activation of glial cells, which are involved in the production of inflammatory cytokines and mediators, resulting in neuroinflammation [12]. The activated glial cells are an important component of chronic neuroinflammation, neuronal loss, and the progression of AD [13,14]. Increased levels of oxidative stress and neuroinflammation disturb the proper structure and function of neurons as well as the synaptic, memory, and cognitive function of the brain [15,16].

Natural products played important role in human disease therapy. Terpenoids, also known as terpenes are the largest group belonging from natural compounds synthesized in plants [17,18]. Among them, triterpenoids are a highly diverse group of natural products broadly distributed in plants [19]. The majority of the known triterpenoids arise from the dammarenyl cation [20] having broad range of biological activities including anti-inflammatory, anti-tumour, anti-HIV antiviral, insecticidal activities and for the treatment of metabolic diseases [21].

Lupeol is a pentacyclic triterpenoid and biologically active compound, naturally found in fruits, vegetables, and several medicinal plants [22]. In vegetables, it is mainly found in white cabbage, pepper, cucumber, and tomato, and in fruits, it is mainly found in mango, fig, strawberry, and red grapes [23]. Lupeol has a wide range of biological effects including anti-cancer, anti-microbial, anti-diabetic, cardio, and hepatoprotective effects [24]. Lupeol has also been shown to exhibit anti-oxidant and anti-inflammatory effects [25,26]. The purpose of the current study was to evaluate the effects of lupeol against $Aβ_{1-42}$-induced oxidative stress-mediated neuroinflammation, neurodegeneration, and cognitive dysfunctions in mice. The amyloid-beta-induced AD mouse model is a known and accepted model of Alzheimer's disease, produced by an intracerebroventricular injection of the amyloid-beta-peptide into the brain of mice [27]. The amyloid fibrils are formed from the Aβ peptide, which occurs in different forms of varying sizes. The $Aβ_{1-42}$ represents the most expressed form in several types of AD cases. The $Aβ_{1-42}$ accumulates to form mini dimers, oligomers, and other insoluble fibrils. To show all amyloid-beta forms, we injected the $Aβ_{1-42}$ peptides into the brains of mice. For biochemical studies, we conducted western blot and immunofluorescence analysis for the $Aβ_{1-42}$-mediated oxidative stress and neuroinflammation. For the behavioral analysis, we performed the Morris water maze (MWM) test and Y-maze tests.

2. Materials and Methods

2.1. Chemical

Aβ and lupeol (CAS Number*: 545-47-1) were purchased from Sigma Co. (St. Louis, MO, USA).

2.2. Animals

Wild-type male C57BL/12N mice (12 mice for western blot and immunofluorescence each) (n = 36) that were eight weeks old and 25–30 g in weight were purchased from Samtako Bio Usan South Korea. All mice were processed according to the protocol approved by the Animal Ethics Committee of the Division of Applied Life Sciences, Gyeongsang National University, South Korea (Approval ID: 125, 3 Jun 2020). Mice were adapted for one week in the university animal house to a 12 h light/dark cycle at 23–25 °C with 60 ± 10% humidity and were provided with standard food and water. We used male mice in this study, according to the literature, male mice are more resistant to stress, hard environment, and hormonal changes.

2.3. Drug Treatment

The mice were randomly divided into three groups, and the mice received the treatment as described in Figure 1. The $A\beta_{1-42}$ peptide of human origin was reconstituted in sterile saline solution as a stock solution at a concentration of 1 mg/mL, followed by incubation at 37 °C for four days. Stereotaxically $A\beta_{1-42}$ peptide aggregates or a vehicle (0.9%NaCl, 3 µL/5 min/mouse) were injected into the ventricles (i.c.v.), by using a Hamilton micro-syringe, 2.4 mm dorsoventral (DV), 0.2 mm anteroposterior (AP), and 1 mm mediolateral (ML) to the bregma. After 24 h of i.c.v. $A\beta_{1-42}$ and the vehicle, mice were divided into the following groups: (1) The control group, which received saline for two weeks as a vehicle; (2) the $A\beta_{1-42}$ group; and (3) and the $A\beta_{1-42}$ + lupeol (50 mg/kg/day/mice/p.o.) group. Dosages of lupeol were selected following previously published studies [28]. The lupeol alone group was not considered in the current study, as previously no unwanted effects of lupeol have been reported in the brain [29]. Lupeol was dissolved in dimethyl sulfoxide (DMSO) to prepare a stock solution. Each day, fresh lupeol solution was prepared in normal saline, according to the required volume of injection, and was employed to treat the mice.

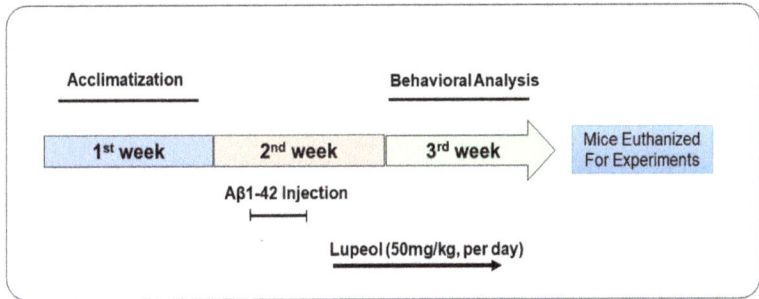

Figure 1. Schematic diagram of experimental design showing duration of lupeol treatment to Aβ mouse model of Alzheimer's disease and their behavioral analysis.

2.4. Behavior Studies

To analyze the effect of lupeol on memory function, we performed the Morris water maze (MWM) test and the Y-maze test. The MWM equipment consisted of a round tank (100 cm in diameter, 40 cm high, and 15.5 cm deep) filled with water, which was made opaque with white ink. A transparent platform with a diameter of 10 cm and a height of 20 cm was hidden 1 cm below the surface of the water in one quadrant of the apparatus during the experiment. The MWM test was carried out for four days, with each mouse being trained by using a hidden platform in one quadrant with three quadrants starting to rotate. After the training session, a probe test was conducted by removing the hidden platform and the mice were allowed to swim freely for 60 s in the water tank. In the probe trial, the number of crossings over the hidden platform and the time spent in the area where the hidden platform was present were calculated. All of the data were recorded using video-tracking software (SMART, Panlab Harvard Apparatus Bioscience Company, MA, USA).

For the evaluation of spatial working memory, we performed the Y-maze test, which was built of black painted plastic. Each arm of the maze was 50 cm long, 20 cm high, and 10 cm wide at both the bottom and top. The mouse was placed at the center of the apparatus and allowed to explore the apparatus for 8 min. The number of arm entries was observed visually. A spontaneous alteration was defined as the successive entry of the mice in three arms in an overlapping set of triplets. The percentage (%) of spontaneous alternation behavior was calculated as [successive triplet sets (entries in three different arms consecutively)/total number of arm entries − 2] × 100. A higher percentage of spontaneous alternation behavior was considered for showing the improved spatial working memory and vice versa.

2.5. Protein Extraction and Homogenization of the Brain of Mice

After the behavioral study, all mice were anesthetized with ketamine/xylazine and the brain tissues were immediately removed and the cortex and hippocampus were separated. The tissues were homogenized in a PRO-PREP™ extraction solution (iNtRON Biotechnology, Dallas Texas MA USA) and centrifuged at a speed of 13,000 rpm for 25 min at 4 °C. The supernatant was collected and stored at −80 °C.

2.6. Western Blot Analysis

Western blotting was performed as described previously, with some modification [30,31]. The protein concentrations were quantified by using a Bio-Rad Protein Assay Kit (Bio-Rad Laboratories, CA, USA). Equal amounts of protein samples (15–30 mg) were electrophoresed on a 12–15% SDS PAGE gel and transferred to a polyvinylidene difluoride (PVDF) membrane. A protein marker (GangNam-STAIN, iNtRON Biotechnology, CA USA) was loaded in parallel for the determination of the molecular weights of the proteins. To reduce the nonspecific bindings, the membranes were blocked in skim milk (5% *w/v* skim milk in 1X Tris-Buffered Saline, 0.1% Tween®20 Detergent (1xTBST), and the membranes were then incubated with the required primary antibodies at 4 °C (1:1000 dilutions, as optimized) for 16 h. After the primary antibody treatment, the membranes were washed with 1× TBST and blocked with horseradish peroxidase-conjugated secondary antibodies, as appropriate. After washing, the bands were detected using an Enhanced chemiluminescent (ECL) detection reagent (EzWestLumiOne, ATTO, Tokyo, Japan). The optical densities of the bands were evaluated with ImageJ (v. 1.50, NIH, Bethesda, MD, USA).

2.7. Immunofluorescence

Immunofluorescence staining was performed as described previously [32,33]. After washing with 1% 1x Phosphate-Buffered Saline (PBS), the slides were treated with proteinase K for 5 min and incubated with a blocking solution (2% normal serum, 0.3% Triton X-100). After blocking, the slides were incubated with primary antibodies (1:100) for 24 h. After incubation with primary antibodies, slides were treated with fluorescein isothiocyanate (FITC) labeled secondary antibodies for 2 h. After the completion of the secondary antibody treatment, the slides were treated with 4,6-diamidino-2-phenylindole (DAPI), for visualizing the nucleus. The slides were then rinsed and mounted with coverslips by using a DAKO fluorescent mounting medium. The images were captured using FluoView 1000 (FV 1000 MPE). Through ImageJ, the relative integrated densities were evaluated among the different experimental groups, which sums all of the pixels within a region and gives a total value and the obtained values were compared among the different experimental groups.

2.8. Antibodies

The antibodies used in this study are given in Table 1.

Table 1. Information on the primary antibodies.

Name	Source	Application	Manufacturer	Catalog Number	Concentration
Aβ	Mouse	WB/IF	Santa Cruz Biotechnology, United States	SC: 28365	1:1000/1:100
Bace-1	Mouse	WB	=	SC: 33711	1:1000
Nrf-2	Mouse	WB/IF	=	SC: 365949	1:1000/1:100
HO-1	Mouse	WB	=	SC: 136961	1:1000
GFAP	Mouse	WB/IF	=	SC: 33673	1:1000/1:100
Iba-1	Rabbit	WB	abcam	Ab: 178846	1:1000
P-NF-kB	Mouse	WB	Santa Cruz Biotechnology, United States	SC: 136548	1:1000
TNF-α	Mouse	WB	=	SC: 52746	1:1000
NOS-2	Rabbit	WB	=	SC: 651	1:1000
IL-1β	Mouse	IF	=	SC: 32294	1:100

2.9. Reactive Oxygen Species (ROS) ssay

The assay was performed to analyze the levels of Reactive Oxygen Species (ROS) in the brains of the experimental groups (n = 6 mice/group). The ROS assay was based on the oxidation of DCFH-DA) to 2'7'-dichlorofluorescein (DCF) [27]. The conversion of 2'-7'dichlorofluorescin diacetate (DCFH-DA to DCF was assessed by a spectrofluorometer at an excitation wavelength of 484 nm and an emission wavelength of 530 nm. To measure the conversion of DCFH-DA to DCF in the absence of homogenate (background fluorescence), parallel blanks were used. The ROS levels were quantified from a DCF standard curve and expressed as relative pmol DCF/mg protein.

2.10. Statistical Analysis

For the analysis of the intensities of the bands, the X-ray films were scanned, and through the ImageJ software (v. 1.50, NIH, Bethesda, MD, USA), the densities were measured. Similarly, for the immunofluorescence analysis, the integrated density was analyzed through ImageJ. The data were been presented as the mean ± standard error of the mean (SEM). For statistical analysis, one-way analysis of variance (ANOVA) followed by the Student's "t" test was used for comparisons of the different groups. The graphs were generated via GraphPad Prism6 (GraphPad Software, San Diego, CA, USA). P values of less than 0.05 were considered to indicate a significant difference between the groups; * indicates a significant difference from the vehicle-treated control group, while # indicates a significant difference from the $A\beta_{1-42}$ treated groups.

3. Results

3.1. Administration of Lupeol Reduced the Aβ and BACE-1 Expression

To analyze the effects of lupeol against the elevated amyloidogenic process, we analyzed the expression of Amyloid beta (Aβ) and beta amyloid cleaving enzyme-1) BACE-1 in the experimental groups. According to our findings, a single intracerebroventricular injection of $A\beta_{1-42}$ increased the expression of Aβ and BACE-1 in the cortex and hippocampus of the mice brains, compared to the saline-treated control group, as shown by the western blot results. Treatment with lupeol significantly reduced the expression of Aβ and BACE-1 compared to $A\beta_{1-42}$ injected mice (Figure 2a). We also analyzed the expression of Aβ through immunofluorescence, and the findings showed an increased immunoreactivity of Aβ in the cortex and hippocampus of $A\beta_{1-42}$-treated mice compared to the control mice. The expression of Aβ was markedly reduced with the administration of lupeol compared to the $A\beta_{1-42}$-injected mice (Figure 2b).

3.2. Oral Administration of Lupeol Decreased Oxidative Stress via the Nrf2/HO1 Signaling Pathway

Oxidative stress is a key factor of AD, and several studies have indicated that Aβ deposition in AD is associated with the generation of reactive oxygen species and oxidative stress [34,35]. Nuclear factor erythroid 2-related factor 2 (Nrf2) is a cytoprotective factor with a protective role against oxidative stress. Nrf2 also regulates the expression of heme oxygenase (HO1), which removes the toxic heme from the cell and plays a protective role against oxidative stress [36,37]. To analyze the effects of lupeol on Nrf2 and HO1, we performed western blot analysis, which showed a reduced expression of Nrf2/HO1 in $A\beta_{1-42}$-induced AD mice brains (cortex and hippocampus) compared to the saline-treated control mice. Treatment with lupeol significantly increased the expression of Nrf2/HO1 (Figure 3a). Similarly, the immunofluorescence analysis also suggested a reduced expression of Nrf2 in $A\beta_{1-42}$-injected mice, which was significantly upregulated with the administration of lupeol, as shown in Figure 3b. To further strengthen our findings, we performed the ROS assay, which showed that the injection of $A\beta_{1-42}$ significantly increased the level of ROS compared to the saline-treated control group. Additionally, this effect was significantly reduced with the administration of lupeol to the treated group (Figure 3c).

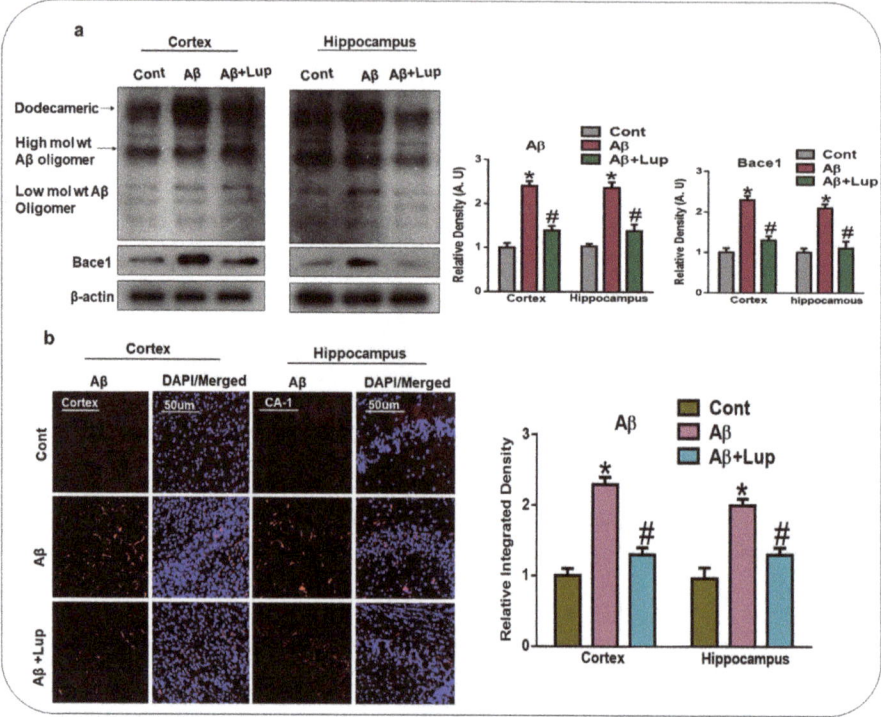

Figure 2. Administration of lupeol reduced the Aβ and BACE-1 expression. (**a**) Western blot analysis and representative histogram of Aβ, and BACE-1 in the cortex and hippocampus of experimental mice. (n = 6 mice/group) the bands were quantified using ImageJ software, and the differences were represented by histograms. β-actin was used as a loading control. (**b**) Confocal microscopy of Aβ (n = 6/mice/group), red, with their representative histogram and stained with DAPI, blue in cortex and hippocampus (CA1 region), in the experimental mice, and are presented relative to the control. Magnification 10×. Scale bar = 50 μm. The expressed data are relative to the control. * significantly different from saline-injected; # significantly different from Aβ-injected. Significance = * $p < 0.05$, # $p < 0.05$. Aβ: Amyloid beta, BACE-1: beta-site amyloid precursor protein cleaving enzyme-1, Lup: Lupeol, DAPI: 4′, 6-Diamidino-2-Phenylindole, Dihydrochloride.

3.3. Lupeol Treatment Attenuated Aβ-Induced Glial Cells in the Brains of Mice

Aβ deposition and oxidative stress in the brain are responsible for the activation of astrocytes and microglial cells [38]. Activated astrocytes and microglia are the main players in neuroinflammation and neurodegeneration [39]. Ionized calcium-binding adaptor molecule-1 (Iba-1) and the glial fibrillary acidic protein (GFAP) are specific markers of activated microglia and astrocytes, respectively. Therefore, we analyzed the expression of Iba-1 and GFAP in the cortex and hippocampus of the experimental mice. Our results showed an elevated expression of Iba-1 and GFAP in the Aβ$_{1-42}$-injected mice brains (cortex and hippocampus) compared to the saline-treated control mice. Interestingly, lupeol treatment significantly decreased the expression of activated Iba-1 and GFAP in the cortex and hippocampus of experimental mice (Figure 4a). We also evaluated the expression of GFAP through immunofluorescence, which showed that Aβ$_{1-42}$ administration increased the expression of GFAP in the cortex and hippocampus compared to the saline-treated control mice. Treatment with lupeol significantly decreased the immunoreactivity of GFAP compared to the Aβ$_{1-42}$-injected mice (Figure 4b).

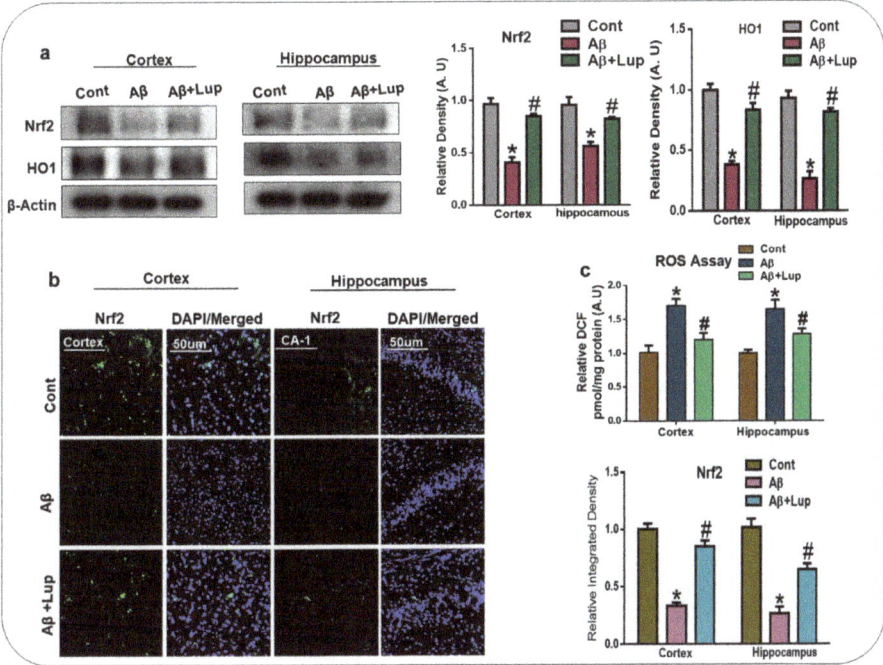

Figure 3. Oral administration of lupeol decreased oxidative stress via Nrf2/HO1 signaling pathway. (**a**) Western blot analysis of Nrf2/HO1, in the cortex and hippocampus of experimental mice (n = 6 mice/group). Western blot bands were quantified by ImageJ software, and the differences were represented by a histogram. β-actin was used as a loading control. (**b**) Immunofluorescence analysis of Nrf2 (green) along with their respective histogram stained with DAPI (blue) in cortex and hippocampus (CA1), in the adult mice (n = 6 mice/group). The data are presented relative to control. Magnification 10×. Scale bar = 50 µm. (**c**) is a representative histogram of the ROS level in the homogenates of the cortex and hippocampus of the adult mice. Aβ$_{1-42}$ increased the levels of ROS, while treatment with lupeol decreased the level of ROS in the adult mice brain. The expressed data are relative to the control. * significantly different from saline-injected; # significantly different from Aβ-injected. Significance = * $p < 0.05$, #, $p < 0.05$. ROS: Reactive Oxygen Species, Nrf-2: nuclear factor erythroid 2–related factor 2, HO-1: Heme Oxygenase-1, DAPI: 4′, 6-Diamidino-2-Phenylindole, Dihydrochloride.

3.4. Oral Administration of Lupeol Reduced the Release of Inflammatory Cytokines in Aβ$_{1-42}$-Injected Mice

It has been reported that activated glial cells and Aβ deposition in the brain are responsible for the release of several inflammatory markers and mediators [40,41]. Therefore, in this study, we evaluated the expressions of p-NF-κB, TNF-α, and NOS-2 in the cortex and hippocampus of adult mice of the experimental groups, which showed an upregulation of p-NF-κB, TNF-α, and NOS-2 in the Aβ$_{1-42}$-induced mice compared to the vehicle-treated control mice. Interestingly, the expressions of these activated cytokines were significantly downregulated with the treatment of lupeol (Figure 5a). We also examined the expression of IL-1β through confocal microscopy. Our result indicated an increased immunoreactivity of IL-1β in the cortex and hippocampus of the Aβ-mouse model of AD compared to the control mice. Interestingly, the expression of IL-1β was markedly reduced with the administration of lupeol (Figure 5b). These results showed that lupeol plays an important role against inflammation by suppressing these inflammatory mediators and cytokines in the Aβ$_{1-42}$-mouse model of AD.

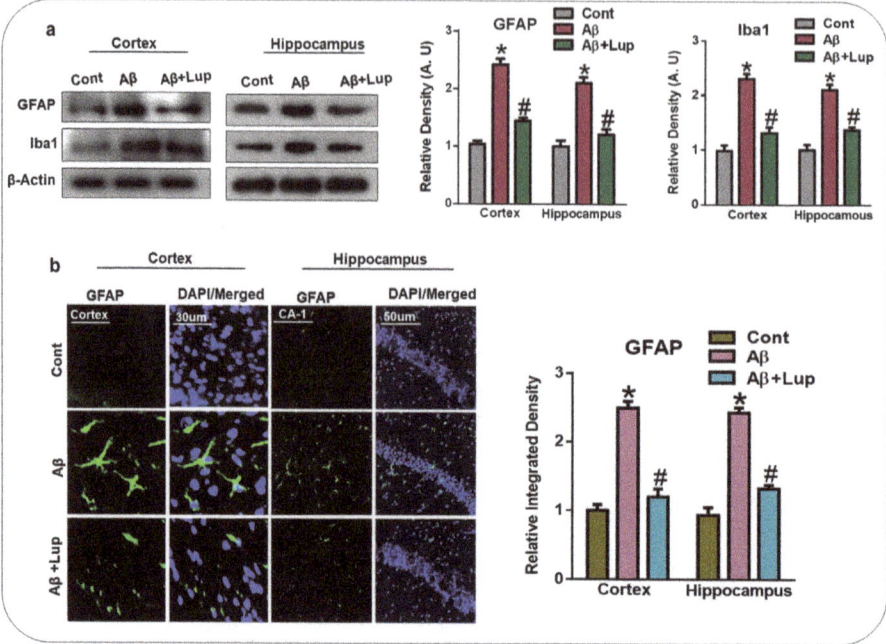

Figure 4. Lupeol treatment attenuated Aβ-induced glial cell in mice brain. (**a**) Western blot analysis shows the increased expression of Iba1 and GFAP in the Aβ-injected mice whereas lupeol treatment, reduced the expression of these markers (n = 6 mice/group). The bands were quantified using ImageJ software, and the differences are represented by a histogram. β-actin was used as a loading control. The density values are expressed in arbitrary units (A.U) as the means ± SEM for the respective indicated cortex and hippocampus proteins (n = 6 mice/group). (**b**) Immunofluorescence analysis GFAP (green) along with their respective histogram stained with DAPI (blue) in cortex and hippocampus (CA1 region) in the adult mice (n = 6 mice/group). The data are presented relative to control. Magnification 10×. Scale bar = 50 μm. The expressed data are relative to the control. * significantly different from saline-injected; # significantly different from Aβ-injected. Significance = * $p < 0.05$, #, $p < 0.05$.

3.5. Lupeol Treatment Enhanced Memory Impairments in Aβ$_{1-42}$-Induced AD Mice

To examine the effects of lupeol on learning and memory dysfunctions in Aβ$_{1-42}$-injected mice, we performed the Morris water maze and Y-maze tests. In MWM, after the initial training, the animals were allowed to find the hidden platform and the latency time was recorded in the MWM task. In the training session, the Aβ$_{1-42}$-induced mice showed memory impairments, as it took them longer to find the hidden platform compared to the saline-treated control mice (Figure 6a). After the training session, a probe test was performed, in which the hidden platform was removed, which showed that the Aβ$_{1-42}$-injected mice spent less time in the target quadrant, while lupeol-treated mice improved in terms of the time in the target quadrant as well as the number of crossings in the area where the previously hidden platform was present (Figure 6b,c). The Y-maze result showed that Aβ$_{1-42}$-injected mice exhibited short-term spatial memory impairments, while treatment with lupeol enhanced the percentage of spontaneous alteration behavior, which resulted in an increased function of the spatial working memory (Figure 6d). All of these results showed that lupeol treatment improved learning and memory in the Aβ-mouse model of AD.

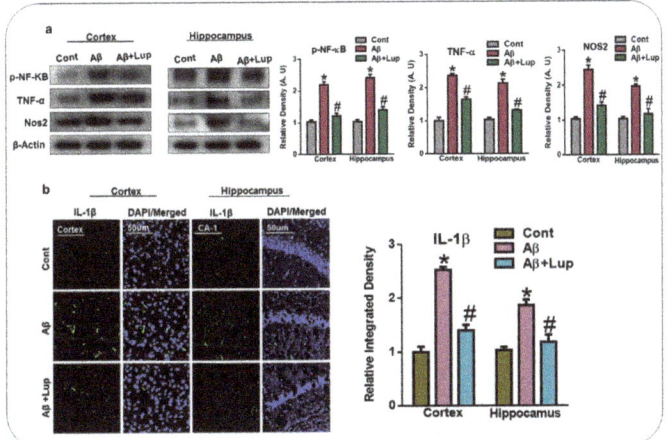

Figure 5. Oral administration of lupeol reduced the release of inflammatory cytokines. (**a**) Western blot analysis of inflammatory cytokines (p-NF-KB, TNF-α, and NOS2), in the cortex and hippocampus of experimental mice (n = 6 mice/group). Western blot bands were quantified by ImageJ software, and the differences were represented by a histogram. β-actin was used as a loading control. (**b**) Immunofluorescence analysis of IL-1β (green) along with their respective histogram stained with DAPI (blue) in cortex and hippocampus (CA-1 region) in the adult mice (n = 6 mice/group). The data are presented relative to the control. Magnification 10×. Scale bar = 50 µm. The expressed data are relative to the control. * Significantly different from saline-injected; # significantly different from Aβ-injected. Significance = * $p < 0.05$, # $p < 0.05$. NF-kB: Nuclear Factor kappa-light-chain- B, TNF-α: Tumor necrosis factor alpha, NOS-2: Nitric oxide synthase 2, IL-1β: Interleukin 1 beta.

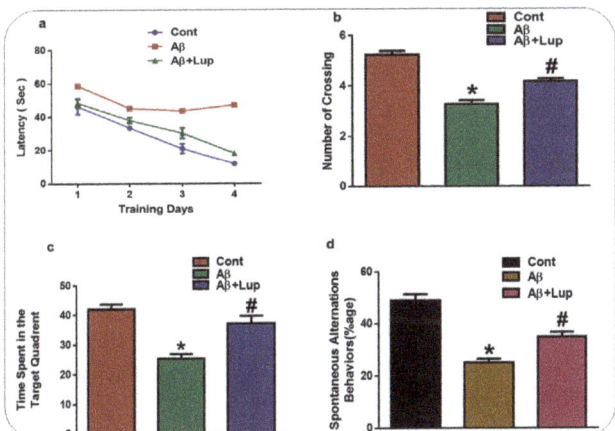

Figure 6. Lupeol treatment enhanced memory impairments in the Aβ-mouse model of AD. To examine the memory function of the experimental mice, the MWM and Y-maze were performed (n = 15 mice/group). (**a**) Average escape latency time for experimental mice to reach the hidden platform. (From day 1 to 4 days). (**b**) The average number of crossing in the MWM in the hidden platform during the probe test. (**c**) Time in the quadrant was previously the hidden platform was placed during the training session. (**d**) Spontaneous alteration behavior % of the mice during the Y-maze test. The data are shown as a mean ± S.E.M. * Significantly different from normal saline-treated mice and # significantly different from Aβ-injected mice, respectively; * $p < 0.05$, # $p < 0.05$. Cont: Control, Aβ: Amyloid beta, Lup: Lupeol.

4. Discussion

In the present study, we investigated the neuroprotective mechanism of lupeol in the Aβ-mouse model of AD, which suggested that lupeol suppressed the elevated oxidative stress, neuroinflammation, and memory and cognitive dysfunctions. The pathogenesis of AD occurred due to the accumulation of toxic Aβ-peptide in the central nervous system, causing synaptic dysfunction, neuronal cell death, and memory and cognitive impairments [42,43]. The amyloid precursor protein (APP) can be cleaved by the beta-amyloid cleaving enzyme (BACE-1), which accelerates the production of Aβ-peptide in the brain. BACE-1 is a potential target for the prevention and treatment of AD [44,45]. In our findings, the level of Aβ and BACE-1 in the $Aβ_{1-42}$-mouse model of AD was significantly reduced with the administration of lupeol, as shown by the western blot and immunofluorescence analysis (Figure 2a,b). Inhibition of the amyloidogenic process may be achieved by different mechanisms, one of which is rescuing the brains against elevated oxidative stress [46]. Oxidative stress is a key factor of AD, and several studies have indicated that Aβ deposition in AD is associated with the generation of reactive oxygen species and oxidative stress [47]. Nuclear factor erythroid 2-related factor2 (Nrf2) is a member of the cap 'n' colon family, which is a master regulator of oxidative stress. It plays a protective role against oxidative stress, and also regulates several other signaling pathways and important anti-oxidant genes [48,49]. Heme oxygenase (HO1) is the target gene of Nrf2, which removes toxic heme, carbon oxide, and iron, and plays a protective role against oxidative injury [48]. The effects of lupeol against the elevated oxidative stress indicates that lupeol may reduce the amyloidogenic process by reducing the oxidative stress, as indicated previously [50]. To unveil this, we examined the oxidative stress-related parameters in the experimental groups, which suggested that lupeol markedly reduced the elevated oxidative stress compared to the $Aβ_{1-42}$-injected mice (Figure 3a–c). To analyze the effects of lupeol against the amyloid-beta-induced activated astrocytes and microglia, we checked the expression of Iba-1 and GFAP in the experimental groups, which showed the reduced expression of these markers with the administration of lupeol (Figure 4a,b). The activated microglial cells further aggravated the phosphorylation and nuclear translocation of p-NF-κB, which further facilitated the release of inflammatory cytokines and mediators [51]. The p-NF-κB is a large family of innate immunity and a major regulator in the initiation of inflammation [52]. Tumor necrosis factor-alpha (TNF-α) is a potent pro-inflammatory cytokine that ameliorates neuroinflammation in neurodegenerative diseases [53]. Nitric oxide 2 (NOS-2) plays an important role in neuroinflammation by generating nitric oxide (NO), and the excessive NO production is one of the major causative reagents of neuroinflammation and neurodegeneration [54]. Therefore, we checked, through western bolt analysis, the expression of p-NF-κB, TNF-α, and NOS-2 in the experimental groups. The result showed the elevated expression of these inflammatory cytokines in the cortex and hippocampus of $Aβ_{1-42}$-injected mice, while treatment with lupeol decreased the expression of these inflammatory mediators (Figure 5a). Furthermore, confocal microscopy showed the increased immunoreactivity of IL-1β in the Aβ-mouse model of AD; however, treatment with lupeol reduced the expression of IL-1β in the experimental animals (Figure 5b). The overall findings suggested that lupeol suppressed the activated microglial cells and inflammatory mediators, and thereby conferred neuroprotection to the brains of mice against $Aβ_{1-42}$-induced neuroinflammation. Aβ accumulation, oxidative stress, and inflammation in the brain accelerate the cognitive and spatial working memory [55]. Therefore, we performed the MWM and Y-maze tests, which suggested that with the inhibition of oxidative stress and neuroinflammation, there was a significant improvement in the cognitive functions of the mice (Figure 6a–c). Similarly, in the Y-maze test, the $Aβ_{1-42}$-injected mice exhibited a lower percentage of spontaneous alternation behaviors, while lupeol enhanced the spontaneous alteration behavior and reduced the spatial working memory (Figure 6d). The overall findings are in accordance with our previous study conducted on lupeol, where we demonstrated that lupeol suppresses neuroinflammation [28].

5. Conclusions

In conclusion, we suggest that lupeol has strong anti-oxidant, anti-neuroinflammatory, and anti-amyloidogenic effects. Moreover, this study also indicated that lupeol reverses the memory deficits in the Aβ-mouse model of AD. Based on current and previous studies, lupeol may protect the brains of mice against Aβ-induced oxidative stress-mediated neuroinflammation and cognitive dysfunctions. Our findings may be fruitful for the advancement of new therapeutic approaches for the management of AD-like conditions.

Author Contributions: R.A. designed, and conducted the experiments, wrote the manuscript, and performed the statistical analysis; A.K., H.J.L., I.U.R., I.K., and S.I.A. conducted experiments, reviewed, and edited the manuscript; M.O.K. supplied all of the chemicals reagents, supervised, and approved the final version of the manuscript. All authors have read and agreed to publish the manuscript.

Funding: This research was supported by the Neurological Disorder Research Program of the National Research Foundation (NRF) funded by the Korean Government (MSIT) (2020M3E5D9080660).

Conflicts of Interest: The funders had no role in the design of the study; in the collection, analyses, or interpretation of data; in the writing of the manuscript, or in the decision to publish the results.

References

1. Ikram, M.; Park, T.J.; Ali, T.; Kim, M.O. Antioxidant and Neuroprotective Effects of Caffeine against Alzheimer's and Parkinson's Disease: Insight into the Role of Nrf-2 and A2AR Signaling. *Antioxidants (Basel)* **2020**, *9*, 902. [CrossRef]
2. Niu, X.; Chen, J.; Gao, J. Nanocarriers as a powerful vehicle to overcome blood-brain barrier in treating neurodegenerative diseases: Focus on recent advances. *Asian J. Pharm. Sci.* **2019**, *14*, 480–496. [CrossRef]
3. Singh, S.K.; Srivastav, S.; Yadav, A.K.; Srikrishna, S.; Perry, G. Overview of Alzheimer's Disease and Some Therapeutic Approaches Targeting Abeta by Using Several Synthetic and Herbal Compounds. *Oxidative Med. Cell. Longev.* **2016**, *2016*, 7361613. [CrossRef] [PubMed]
4. Serrano-Pozo, A.; Frosch, M.P.; Masliah, E.; Hyman, B.T. Neuropathological alterations in Alzheimer disease. *Cold Spring Harb. Perspect. Med.* **2011**, *1*, a006189. [CrossRef]
5. Cho, J.E.; Kim, J.R. Recent approaches targeting beta-amyloid for therapeutic intervention of Alzheimer's disease. *Recent Pat. CNS Drug Discov.* **2011**, *6*, 222–233. [CrossRef] [PubMed]
6. Costa, L.G.; Garrick, J.M.; Roque, P.J.; Pellacani, C. Mechanisms of Neuroprotection by Quercetin: Counteracting Oxidative Stress and More. *Oxid. Med. Cell Longev.* **2016**, *2016*, 2986796. [CrossRef]
7. Hosen, S.M.Z.; Rubayed, M.; Dash, R.; Junaid, M.; Mitra, S.; Alam, M.S.; Dey, R. Prospecting and Structural Insight into the Binding of Novel Plant-Derived Molecules of Leea indica as Inhibitors of BACE1. *Curr. Pharm. Des.* **2018**, *24*, 3972–3979. [CrossRef] [PubMed]
8. Vassar, R.; Bennett, B.D.; Babu-Khan, S.; Kahn, S.; Mendiaz, E.A.; Denis, P.; Teplow, D.B.; Ross, S.; Amarante, P.; Loeloff, R.; et al. Beta-secretase cleavage of Alzheimer's amyloid precursor protein by the transmembrane aspartic protease BACE. *Science* **1999**, *286*, 735–741. [CrossRef] [PubMed]
9. Rosales-Corral, S.; Acuna-Castroviejo, D.; Tan, D.X.; Lopez-Armas, G.; Cruz-Ramos, J.; Munoz, R.; Melnikov, V.G.; Manchester, L.C.; Reiter, R.J. Accumulation of exogenous amyloid-beta peptide in hippocampal mitochondria causes their dysfunction: A protective role for melatonin. *Oxid. Med. Cell Longev.* **2012**, *2012*, 843649. [CrossRef] [PubMed]
10. Enogieru, A.B.; Haylett, W.; Hiss, D.C.; Bardien, S.; Ekpo, O.E. Rutin as a Potent Antioxidant: Implications for Neurodegenerative Disorders. *Oxid. Med. Cell Longev.* **2018**, *2018*, 6241017. [CrossRef]
11. Fischer, R.; Maier, O. Interrelation of oxidative stress and inflammation in neurodegenerative disease: Role of TNF. *Oxid. Med. Cell Longev.* **2015**, *2015*, 610813. [CrossRef] [PubMed]
12. Ahmad, A.; Ali, T.; Park, H.Y.; Badshah, H.; Rehman, S.U.; Kim, M.O. Neuroprotective Effect of Fisetin Against Amyloid-Beta-Induced Cognitive/Synaptic Dysfunction, Neuroinflammation, and Neurodegeneration in Adult Mice. *Mol. Neurobiol.* **2017**, *54*, 2269–2285. [CrossRef] [PubMed]
13. Refolo, V.; Stefanova, N. Neuroinflammation and Glial Phenotypic Changes in Alpha-Synucleinopathies. *Front. Cell. Neurosci.* **2019**, *13*, 263. [CrossRef] [PubMed]

14. Panaro, M.A.; Benameur, T.; Porro, C. Extracellular Vesicles miRNA Cargo for Microglia Polarization in Traumatic Brain Injury. *Biomolecules* **2020**, *10*, 901. [CrossRef] [PubMed]
15. Kim, Y.E.; Hwang, C.J.; Lee, H.P.; Kim, C.S.; Son, D.J.; Ham, Y.W.; Hellstrom, M.; Han, S.B.; Kim, H.S.; Park, E.K.; et al. Inhibitory effect of punicalagin on lipopolysaccharide-induced neuroinflammation, oxidative stress and memory impairment via inhibition of nuclear factor-kappaB. *Neuropharmacology* **2017**, *117*, 21–32. [CrossRef]
16. Baierle, M.; Nascimento, S.N.; Moro, A.M.; Brucker, N.; Freitas, F.; Gauer, B.; Durgante, J.; Bordignon, S.; Zibetti, M.; Trentini, C.M.; et al. Relationship between inflammation and oxidative stress and cognitive decline in the institutionalized elderly. *Oxidative Med. Cell. Longev.* **2015**, *2015*, 804198. [CrossRef]
17. Perveen, S. *Introductory Chapter: Terpenes and Terpenoids*; IntechOpen Limited: London, UK, 2018.
18. Wang, G.; Tang, W.; Bidigare, R.R. *Terpenoids as Therapeutic Drugs and Pharmaceutical Agents*; Humana Press: Totowa, NJ, USA, 2005.
19. Vincken, J. P.; Heng, L.; de Groot, A.; Gruppen, H. Saponins, classification and occurrence in the plant kingdom. *Phytochemistry* **2007**, *68*, 275–297.
20. Stephenson, M. J.; Field, R. A.; Osbourn, A. The protosteryl and dammarenyl cation dichotomy in polycyclic triterpene biosynthesis revisited: Has this 'rule' finally been broken? *Nat. Prod. Rep.* **2019**, *36*, 1044–1052.
21. Hill, R. A.; Connolly, J. D. Triterpenoids. *Nat. Prod. Rep.* **2012**, *29*, 780–818.
22. Beserra, F.P.; Vieira, A.J.; Gushiken, L.F.S.; de Souza, E.O.; Hussni, M.F.; Hussni, C.A.; Nobrega, R.H.; Martinez, E.R.M.; Jackson, C.J.; de Azevedo Maia, G.L.; et al. Lupeol, a Dietary Triterpene, Enhances Wound Healing in Streptozotocin-Induced Hyperglycemic Rats with Modulatory Effects on Inflammation, Oxidative Stress, and Angiogenesis. *Oxid. Med. Cell Longev.* **2019**, *2019*, 3182627. [CrossRef] [PubMed]
23. Hajialyani, M.; Hosein Farzaei, M.; Echeverria, J.; Nabavi, S.M.; Uriarte, E.; Sobarzo-Sanchez, E. Hesperidin as a Neuroprotective Agent: A Review of Animal and Clinical Evidence. *Molecules* **2019**, *24*, 648. [CrossRef]
24. Lee, C.; Lee, J.W.; Seo, J.Y.; Hwang, S.W.; Im, J.P.; Kim, J.S. Lupeol inhibits LPS-induced NF-kappa B signaling in intestinal epithelial cells and macrophages, and attenuates acute and chronic murine colitis. *Life Sci.* **2016**, *146*, 100–108. [CrossRef] [PubMed]
25. Saleem, M. Lupeol, a novel anti-inflammatory and anti-cancer dietary triterpene. *Cancer Lett.* **2009**, *285*, 109–115. [CrossRef]
26. Fernandez, M.A.; de las Heras, B.; Garcia, M.D.; Saenz, M.T.; Villar, A. New insights into the mechanism of action of the anti-inflammatory triterpene lupeol. *J. Pharm. Pharmacol.* **2001**, *53*, 1533–1539. [CrossRef] [PubMed]
27. Ikram, M.; Muhammad, T.; Rehman, S.U.; Khan, A.; Jo, M.G.; Ali, T.; Kim, M.O. Hesperetin Confers Neuroprotection by Regulating Nrf2/TLR4/NF-κB Signaling in an Aβ Mouse Model. *Mol. Neurobiol.* **2019**, *56*, 6293–6309. [CrossRef]
28. Badshah, H.; Ali, T.; Shafiq-ur, R.; Faiz-ul, A.; Ullah, F.; Kim, T.H.; Kim, M.O. Protective Effect of Lupeol Against Lipopolysaccharide-Induced Neuroinflammation via the p38/c-Jun N-Terminal Kinase Pathway in the Adult Mouse Brain. *J. Neuroimmune Pharmacol.* **2016**, *11*, 48–60. [CrossRef]
29. Zhang, Z.; Xu, C.; Hao, J.; Zhang, M.; Wang, Z.; Yin, T.; Lin, K.; Liu, W.; Jiang, Q.; Li, Z.; et al. Beneficial consequences of Lupeol on middle cerebral artery-induced cerebral ischemia in the rat involves Nrf2 and P38 MAPK modulation. *Metab. Brain Dis.* **2020**, *35*, 841–848. [CrossRef]
30. Ahmad, A.; Ali, T.; Kim, M.W.; Khan, A.; Jo, M.H.; Rehman, S.U.; Khan, M.S.; Abid, N.B.; Khan, M.; Ullah, R.; et al. Adiponectin homolog novel osmotin protects obesity/diabetes-induced NAFLD by upregulating AdipoRs/PPARalpha signaling in ob/ob and db/db transgenic mouse models. *Metabolism* **2019**, *90*, 31–43. [CrossRef]
31. Idrees, M.; Xu, L.; Song, S.H.; Joo, M.D.; Lee, K.L.; Muhammad, T.; El Sheikh, M.; Sidrat, T.; Kong, I.K. PTPN11 (SHP2) Is Indispensable for Growth Factors and Cytokine Signal Transduction During Bovine Oocyte Maturation and Blastocyst Development. *Cells* **2019**, *8*, 1272. [CrossRef] [PubMed]
32. Rehman, S.U.; Ahmad, A.; Yoon, G.H.; Khan, M.; Abid, M.N.; Kim, M.O. Inhibition of c-Jun N-Terminal Kinase Protects Against Brain Damage and Improves Learning and Memory After Traumatic Brain Injury in Adult Mice. *Cereb. Cortex* **2018**, *28*, 2854–2872. [CrossRef] [PubMed]
33. Ikram, M.; Saeed, K.; Khan, A.; Muhammad, T.; Khan, M.S.; Jo, M.G.; Rehman, S.U.; Kim, M.O. Natural Dietary Supplementation of Curcumin Protects Mice Brains against Ethanol-Induced Oxidative Stress-Mediated

Neurodegeneration and Memory Impairment via Nrf2/TLR4/RAGE Signaling. *Nutrients* **2019**, *11*, 1082. [CrossRef] [PubMed]
34. Smith, M.A.; Hirai, K.; Hsiao, K.; Pappolla, M.A.; Harris, P.L.; Siedlak, S.L.; Tabaton, M.; Perry, G. Amyloid-beta deposition in Alzheimer transgenic mice is associated with oxidative stress. *J. Neurochem.* **1998**, *70*, 2212–2215. [CrossRef] [PubMed]
35. Matsuoka, Y.; Picciano, M.; La Francois, J.; Duff, K. Fibrillar beta-amyloid evokes oxidative damage in a transgenic mouse model of Alzheimer's disease. *Neuroscience* **2001**, *104*, 609–613. [CrossRef]
36. Araujo, J.A.; Zhang, M.; Yin, F. Heme oxygenase-1, oxidation, inflammation, and atherosclerosis. *Front. Pharmacol.* **2012**, *3*, 119. [CrossRef]
37. Cores, A.; Piquero, M.; Villacampa, M.; Leon, R.; Menendez, J.C. NRF2 Regulation Processes as a Source of Potential Drug Targets against Neurodegenerative Diseases. *Biomolecules* **2020**, *10*, 904. [CrossRef]
38. Palpagama, T.H.; Waldvogel, H.J.; Faull, R.L.M.; Kwakowsky, A. The Role of Microglia and Astrocytes in Huntington's Disease. *Front. Mol. Neurosci.* **2019**, *12*, 258. [CrossRef]
39. Block, M.L.; Zecca, L.; Hong, J.S. Microglia-mediated neurotoxicity: Uncovering the molecular mechanisms. *Nat. Rev. Neurosci.* **2007**, *8*, 57–69. [CrossRef]
40. Turner, M.D.; Nedjai, B.; Hurst, T.; Pennington, D.J. Cytokines and chemokines: At the crossroads of cell signalling and inflammatory disease. *Biochimica et biophysica acta* **2014**, *1843*, 2563–2582. [CrossRef]
41. Kinney, J.W.; Bemiller, S.M.; Murtishaw, A.S.; Leisgang, A.M.; Salazar, A.M.; Lamb, B.T. Inflammation as a central mechanism in Alzheimer's disease. *Alzheimer's Dement.* **2018**, *4*, 575–590. [CrossRef]
42. Kim, H.Y.; Lee, D.K.; Chung, B.R.; Kim, H.V.; Kim, Y. Intracerebroventricular Injection of Amyloid-beta Peptides in Normal Mice to Acutely Induce Alzheimer-like Cognitive Deficits. *J. Vis. Exp.* **2016**. [CrossRef]
43. Souza, L.C.; Jesse, C.R.; Antunes, M.S.; Ruff, J.R.; de Oliveira Espinosa, D.; Gomes, N.S.; Donato, F.; Giacomeli, R.; Boeira, S.P. Indoleamine-2,3-dioxygenase mediates neurobehavioral alterations induced by an intracerebroventricular injection of amyloid-beta1-42 peptide in mice. *Brain Behav. Immun.* **2016**, *56*, 363–377. [CrossRef] [PubMed]
44. Ali, T.; Yoon, G.H.; Shah, S.A.; Lee, H.Y.; Kim, M.O. Osmotin attenuates amyloid beta-induced memory impairment, tau phosphorylation and neurodegeneration in the mouse hippocampus. *Sci. Rep.* **2015**, *5*, 11708. [CrossRef] [PubMed]
45. Wagle, A.; Seong, S.H.; Castro, M.J.; Faraoni, M.B.; Murray, A.P.; Jung, H.A.; Choi, J.S. Influence of functional moiety in lupane-type triterpenoids in BACE1 inhibition. *Comput. Biol. Chem.* **2019**, *83*, 107101. [CrossRef]
46. Badshah, H.; Ikram, M.; Ali, W.; Ahmad, S.; Hahm, J.R.; Kim, M.O. Caffeine May Abrogate LPS-Induced Oxidative Stress and Neuroinflammation by Regulating Nrf2/TLR4 in Adult Mouse Brains. *Biomolecules* **2019**, *9*, 719. [CrossRef]
47. Tonnies, E.; Trushina, E. Oxidative Stress, Synaptic Dysfunction, and Alzheimer's Disease. *J. Alzheimers Dis.* **2017**, *57*, 1105–1121. [CrossRef]
48. Loboda, A.; Damulewicz, M.; Pyza, E.; Jozkowicz, A.; Dulak, J. Role of Nrf2/HO-1 system in development, oxidative stress response and diseases: An evolutionarily conserved mechanism. *Cell. Mol. Life Sci.* **2016**, *73*, 3221–3247. [CrossRef]
49. Le, W.D.; Xie, W.J.; Appel, S.H. Protective role of heme oxygenase-1 in oxidative stress-induced neuronal injury. *J. Neurosci. Res.* **1999**, *56*, 652–658. [CrossRef]
50. Cheignon, C.; Tomas, M.; Bonnefont-Rousselot, D.; Faller, P.; Hureau, C.; Collin, F. Oxidative stress and the amyloid beta peptide in Alzheimer's disease. *Redox. Biol.* **2018**, *14*, 450–464. [CrossRef]
51. Mussbacher, M.; Salzmann, M.; Brostjan, C.; Hoesel, B.; Schoergenhofer, C.; Datler, H.; Hohensinner, P.; Basilio, J.; Petzelbauer, P.; Assinger, A.; et al. Cell Type-Specific Roles of NF-kappaB Linking Inflammation and Thrombosis. *Front. Immunol.* **2019**, *10*, 85. [CrossRef]
52. Taniguchi, K.; Karin, M. NF-kappaB, inflammation, immunity and cancer: Coming of age. *Nat. Rev. Immunol.* **2018**, *18*, 309–324. [CrossRef] [PubMed]
53. Frankola, K.A.; Greig, N.H.; Luo, W.; Tweedie, D. Targeting TNF-alpha to elucidate and ameliorate neuroinflammation in neurodegenerative diseases. *CNS Neurol. Disord. Drug Targets* **2011**, *10*, 391–403. [CrossRef] [PubMed]
54. Yuste, J.E.; Tarragon, E.; Campuzano, C.M.; Ros-Bernal, F. Implications of glial nitric oxide in neurodegenerative diseases. *Front. Cell Neurosci.* **2015**, *9*, 322. [CrossRef] [PubMed]

55. Cai, Z.; Hussain, M.D.; Yan, L.J. Microglia, neuroinflammation, and beta-amyloid protein in Alzheimer's disease. *Int. J. Neurosci.* **2014**, *124*, 307–321. [CrossRef] [PubMed]

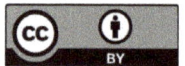 © 2020 by the authors. Licensee MDPI, Basel, Switzerland. This article is an open access article distributed under the terms and conditions of the Creative Commons Attribution (CC BY) license (http://creativecommons.org/licenses/by/4.0/).

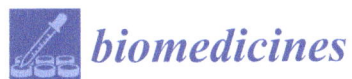

Review

Body Fluid Biomarkers for Alzheimer's Disease—An Up-To-Date Overview

Adrian Florian Bălașa [1], Cristina Chircov [2] and Alexandru Mihai Grumezescu [2,*]

1. Târgu Mures, Emergency Clinical Hospital, "George Emil Palade" University of Medicine, Pharmacy, Science and Technology of Târgu Mures, RO-540142 Târgu Mures, Romania; adrian.balasa@yahoo.fr
2. Faculty of Applied Chemistry and Materials Science, University Politehnica of Bucharest, RO-060042 Bucharest, Romania; cristina.chircov@yahoo.com
* Correspondence: grumezescu@yahoo.com; Tel.: +40-21-402-39-97

Received: 26 August 2020; Accepted: 13 October 2020; Published: 15 October 2020

Abstract: Neurodegeneration is a highly complex process which is associated with a variety of molecular mechanisms related to ageing. Among neurodegenerative disorders, Alzheimer's disease (AD) is the most common, affecting more than 45 million individuals. The underlying mechanisms involve amyloid plaques and neurofibrillary tangles (NFTs) deposition, which will subsequently lead to oxidative stress, chronic neuroinflammation, neuron dysfunction, and neurodegeneration. The current diagnosis methods are still limited in regard to the possibility of the accurate and early detection of the diseases. Therefore, research has shifted towards the identification of novel biomarkers and matrices as biomarker sources, beyond amyloid-β and tau protein levels within the cerebrospinal fluid (CSF), that could improve AD diagnosis. In this context, the aim of this paper is to provide an overview of both conventional and novel biomarkers for AD found within body fluids, including CSF, blood, saliva, urine, tears, and olfactory fluids.

Keywords: neurodegeneration; Alzheimer's disease; neurofibrillary tangles; diagnosis methods; biomarkers

1. Introduction

Neurodegeneration is a complex process that encompasses several different molecular pathways and a multifaceted interplay between a variety of regulatory factors [1,2]. It is characterized by a progressive and irreversible neuronal loss from the specific brain and spinal cord regions, mainly the nuclei of the base within the subcortical areas and the cerebral cortex, consequently leading to damage and dysfunction manifested through cognitive and motor dysfunctions [2–4]. Generally, the causal factors include the following: oxidative stress and free radical formation; protein misfolding, oligomerization and aggregation; mitochondrial dysfunction, axonal transport deficits and abnormal neuron–glial interactions; calcium deregulation, phosphorylation impairment; neuroinflammation; DNA damage and aberrant RNA processing [2,5,6].

Neurodegeneration is the underlying factor for many debilitating and incurable age-dependent disorders [3,7,8]. The prevalence of neurodegenerative disorders is continuously increasing as a consequence of the dramatic rise in life expectancy due to scientific achievements and progress, thus posing a significant threat to human health [5,7,9,10]. Moreover, neurodegeneration is associated with various neurodegenerative, neurotraumatic, and neuropsychiatric disorders, with considerably diverse pathophysiology, including memory and cognitive impairments, muscle weakness and/or paralysis, abnormal control of the voluntary movement, seizures, confusion, and pain [2,4,7,11–13]. Specifically, such diseases vary from progressive degenerative disorders, including Alzheimer's disease (AD), Parkinson's disease, Huntington's disease, amyotrophic lateral sclerosis and multiple sclerosis [4,5,10,14,15], to acute traumatic injuries, such as traumatic brain injury, stroke or spinal cord injury [15,16].

Among them, AD is the most common neurodegenerative disorder, affecting more than 45 million individuals worldwide and is expected to reach 60 million by 2030 due to the increase in the elderly population [17,18]. AD is characterized by the progressive death of cholinergic neurons within the hippocampal and cortical regions, the consequent atrophy, abnormal neurotransmission and loss of synapses, and neurodegeneration [4,18–21]. At molecular levels, the underlying mechanisms of AD involve the extracellular deposition of amyloid-β (Aβ) peptides, known as amyloid plaques, and the intracellular formation of hyperphosphorylated tau (Tubulin Associated Unit) protein aggregates, known as neurofibrillary tangles (NFTs), which subsequently induce oxidative stress, chronic neuroinflammation, neuron dysfunction, and neurodegeneration [4,10,17,19,22,23].

In addition to cognitive tests, the current diagnostic methods rely on imaging techniques [24–27] and cerebrospinal fluid (CSF) assays. On one hand, the purpose of the neuroimaging methods is assessing the hippocampal atrophy through magnetic resonance imaging and the cortical Aβ deposition through positron emission tomography. On the other hand, CSF analyses aim to provide quantitative measurements of Aβ and tau protein levels as AD biomarkers [18]. However, the available methods are expensive, relatively invasive [18,28], and have low sensitivity and specificity, which result in the risks of either overdiagnosis or undiagnosed, misattributed, or dismissed and ignored symptoms [29,30]. Additionally, as there is a serious lack of AD diagnosis assays at all illness stages, patients are generally diagnosed late, which places a great burden on the health systems [17,18]. Therefore, the development of novel methods of AD early detection and accurate diagnosis is essential [17,29].

Detection strategies based on novel biomarkers beyond Aβ and tau protein could represent a promising solution for the early diagnosis of AD [18]. However, as no single biomarker can be used to accurately diagnose AD, a combination of biomarkers could significantly increase diagnostic accuracy [30,31]. Moreover, such biomarkers should ideally be easy to sample and should be measurable through simple and cost-efficient methods and at all stages of the disease, allowing for standardization processes [30,32]. In this context, the aim of this manuscript is to provide an up-to-date overview of both conventional and novel AD biomarkers, which could play fundamental roles in its accurate and timely diagnosis.

2. Cerebrospinal Fluid Biomarkers

Biomarkers can be described as molecules that can be detected and quantified within body fluids, such as blood, CSF, urine or saliva, and changes in their levels or activity are generally associated with different pathologies. Offering the possibility of early disease diagnosis, most biomarkers involve the measurement of structural, metabolic or enzymatic proteins and should be non-invasive, easy to use, and cost-efficient [33,34].

Residing in the subarachnoid space and ventricular system of the brain and spinal cord, the CSF is a fundamental neuropathology indicator as it carries the brain's interstitial fluid across the ventricular ependymal lining, and thus it reflects any biochemical change within the brain [35,36]. Moreover, as the blood–CSF barrier restricts the transport of molecules and proteins, the CSF is isolated from the peripheral system. Thus, it is a useful matrix for the detection of neurodegenerative disorder markers, providing the tools for disease screening, prognosis and monitoring [37–39]. Among them, AD biomarkers have received a great deal of clinical interest, allowing for the depiction of AD pathology [35,39,40]. Furthermore, such biomarkers could also be applied for the diagnosis of mild cognitive impairment (MCI), the transitional phase from normal cognition to dementia, that generally manifests as a silent pre-clinical phase in 6–15% of AD patients [40–42].

The CSF biomarkers most indicative of AD are associated with the main pathological changes in the brain, namely the deposition of extracellular Aβ plaques, the formation of NFTs, and the loss of neurons [37]. Thus, the biomarkers that have received clinical attention for AD diagnosis are Aβ, total-tau (T-tau) and phosphorylated-tau (P-tau), as they are recognized by the International Working

Group (IWG) 2 Criteria for AD and the National Institute on Aging-Alzheimer's Association (NIA-AA) Criteria for AD and MCI associated with AD [35,39].

Generally, the transmembrane protein amyloid precursor protein (APP) predominantly expressed in the brain is enzymatically processed via two routes. Thus, it can be cleaved either by the α-secretase followed by γ-secretase, resulting in the release of soluble APPα through the non-amyloidogenic pathway or by β-secretase followed by γ-secretase, leading to the formation of the highly insoluble $A\beta_{1-42}$ (composed of 42 amino acids) peptide through the amyloidogenic pathway [34,37] (Figure 1). Among the various Aβ isoforms found in the CSF, the levels of $A\beta_{40}$ and $A\beta_{42}$ are the most reliable in terms of assessment for AD diagnosis. Specifically, as $A\beta_{42}$ aggregates into fibrils and plaques within the brain, its concentration in the CSF is considerably reduced, thus serving as an AD indicator [43,44]. However, while $A\beta_{40}$ is the most abundant isoform, there are no significant changes in its levels in AD patients. In this case, its levels are analyzed by the $A\beta_{42}/A\beta_{40}$ ratio, which is more reliable than only assessing $A\beta_{42}$ concentrations due to individual fluctuation compensations [35,42,45]. Specifically, the $A\beta_{42}$ values are normalized, as $A\beta_{40}$ is used as a proxy for the total Aβ values [46]. Moreover, other truncated forms of the $A\beta_{42}$ amyloidogenic peptide, including $A\beta_{37}$, $A\beta_{38}$ and $A\beta_{39}$, could provide additional diagnostic information. Among them, the accuracy of the $A\beta_{42}/A\beta_{38}$ ratio is comparable to that of $A\beta_{42}/A\beta_{40}$ in terms of predicting AD [35,46]. Evidence for these findings relies on autopsy studies, antemortem lumbar CSF analyses, and functional imaging studies based on positron emission tomography using Aβ ligands, e.g., 11c-labelled Pittsburgh Compound [42]. Nonetheless, the use of these biomarkers in routine clinical practice is still in its infancy [40], as there are still some limitations that must be overcome, such as the interindividual differences in the production of Aβ or the overlapping between CSF and $A\beta_{1-42}$ between neurodegenerative disorders, as in Creutzfeldt–Jakob disease, dementia with Lewy bodies, frontotemporal lobar degeneration, and prodromal and manifest (subcortical) vascular dementia [47,48]. As such, most studies analyze Aβ levels in comparison with T-tau and P-tau values in order to increase accuracy [35]. Furthermore, several studies have investigated the levels of APP cleavage metabolites, including soluble APPα, soluble APPβ and total soluble APP, as biomarkers for AD. However, the results are generally inconsistent due to several reasons, including disease heterogeneity, co-morbidities, assay specificity and sensitivity, antibody cross-reactivity, sampling differences, and CSF processing and storage [49,50]. In this context, one study suggested higher levels of soluble APPα in MCI-AD patients compared with non-AD and control groups, and higher levels of APPβ in both AD and MCI-AD patients [50]. Moreover, soluble APPα and soluble APPβ levels have been associated with biomarkers of BACE1 activity.

Tau is a highly important microtubule-regulating protein abundantly expressed in the cytosol of axons. Its activity mainly focuses on microtubule-related functions, namely tubulin assembly promotion, dynamic instability regulation, a spatial organization in a parallel network, and axonal transport of kinesins and dyneins, which contribute to microtubule stabilization [37,51,52]. The kinase and phosphatase imbalances in AD lead to the hyperphosphorylation of tau and its consequent detachment from microtubules and accumulation into NFTs (Figure 2). Subsequently, tau and P-tau proteins are released into the extracellular space of the CSF, resulting in increased levels characteristic for neurodegeneration [37]. On one hand, tau proteins are assessed by using monoclonal antibodies, which detect all isoforms independently of their phosphorylation state. In AD patients, T-tau concentrations increase by 200–300%, which is further associated with the severity of neuronal/axonal damage and neurodegeneration. However, increased levels of T-tau have also been observed in other neurological disorders, including stroke, brain trauma, or Creutzfeldt–Jakob disease [53–55], which makes it less specific for AD. On the other hand, moderately increased levels of P-tau proteins are more accurately associated with AD, as they indicate both the brain phosphorylation state and the NFTs' formation and load [35,42].

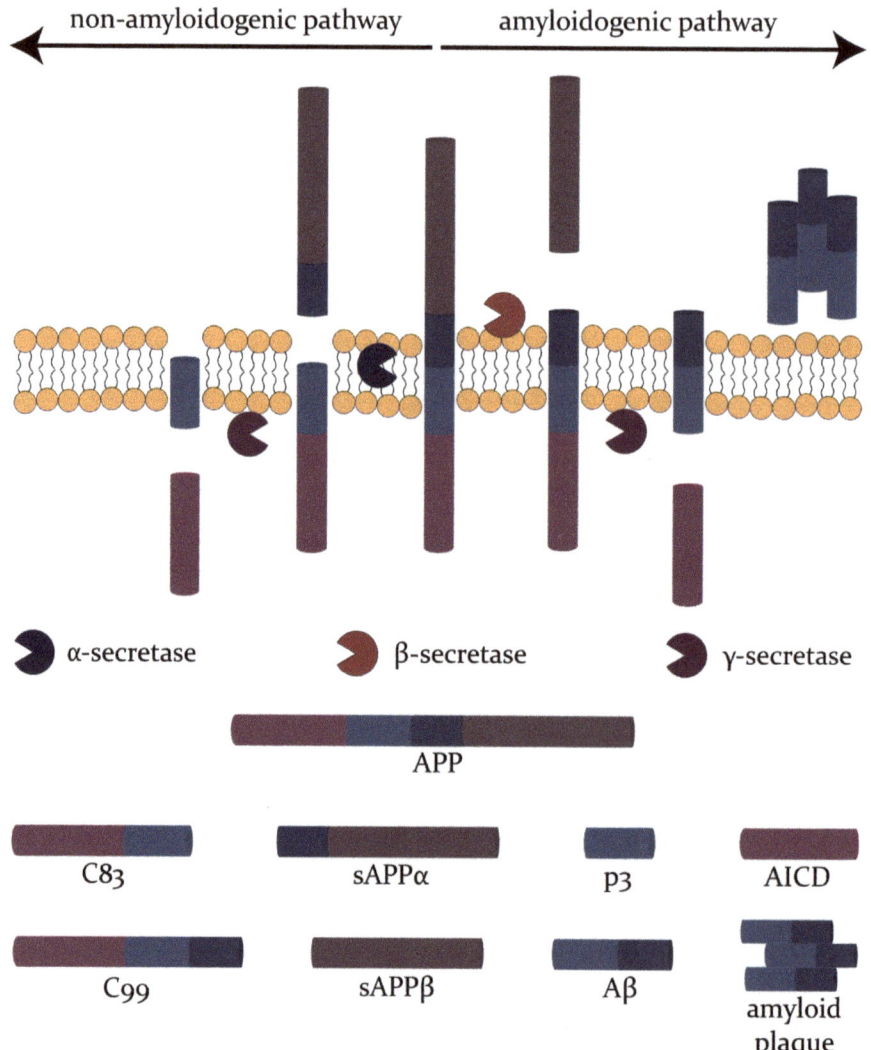

Figure 1. The non-amyloidogenic and amyloidogenic pathways involved in the enzymatic processing of APP.

While the deposition of Aβ plaques occurs years or even decades before the onset of the symptoms, and could be used for early diagnosis, tau biomarkers change later as the disease progresses, and are strongly correlated with local degeneration and cognitive decline [37,56]. The most effective strategy for developing a biomarker-based diagnostic tool is to combine both disease-specific and non-specific biomarkers. In this context, the decrease in $Aβ_{42}$, and concomitant increase in $Aβ_{42}/Aβ_{40}$ and $Aβ_{42}/Aβ_{38}$ ratios and T-tau and P-tau levels is commonly referred to as the Alzheimer profile or signature, as it offers the possibility of detecting AD in its early stages [35,42,57,58]. Additionally, their combined use for AD diagnosis is characterized by sensitivity and specificity of approximately 85–95% [59]. Similarly, by increasing the palette of biomarkers, the discrimination between AD and other differential diagnoses, such as MCI, dementia or depression, could be possible.

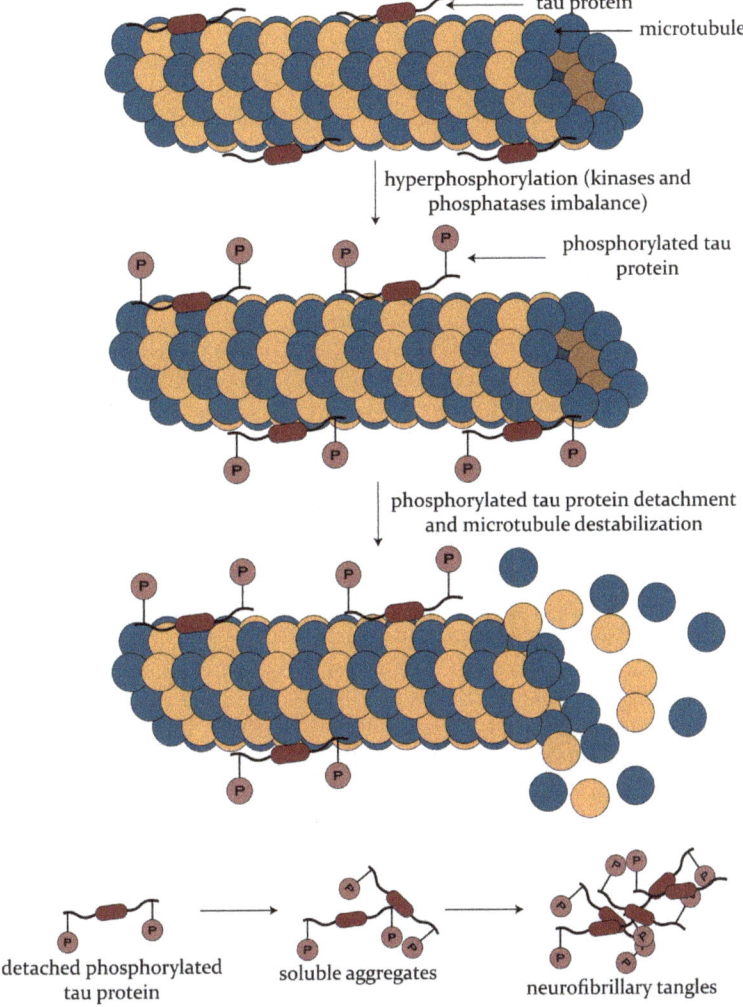

Figure 2. The formation of neurofibrillary tangles through the process of tau protein hyperphosphorylation.

In this context, recent years have witnessed the rise of a new generation of biomarkers related to AD pathological mechanisms, such as neurofilament light (NFL) for neuronal injury, neurogranin, BACE1, SNAP-25 and synaptotagmin for synaptic dysfunction and/or loss, and sTREM2 and YKL-40 for neuroinflammation, due to the activation of microglia and astrocytes [38,60,61].

The neurofilament heteropolymers are the primary cytoskeleton proteins predominantly found in axons. Among the four subunits, namely the three isoforms NFL, neurofilament medium and neurofilament heavy, and alpha-internexin, NFL is the most abundant [59,62]. Forming the core of the neurofilament, NFL is a triplet protein essential to the structure of the myelin that surrounds the axons within the central nervous system [62,63]. As their presence within the CSF is specific for axonal injury, elevated NFL concentrations have been widely reported in neurodegenerative disorders, especially in AD patients [59,62–64]. While the mechanisms of NFL aggregation are still unelucidated, they are thought to be similar to the hyperphosphorylation process of tau proteins [65].

Neurogranin is a small neuron-specific and post-synaptic protein abundantly expressed in the brain, especially in the hippocampal and cerebrocortical dendritic spine [66–68]. Neurogranin has been found to play key roles in synaptic plasticity and long-term potentiation as a major regulator of the calcium-binding protein calmodulin and of calcium-signal transduction and memory formation [66–69]. Autopsy studies revealed a possible correlation between neurogranin and AD, as analyses showed reduced levels of neurogranin in brains and increased levels in the CSF of AD patients [68]. In this regard, there is accumulated evidence confirming the potential of neurogranin as an AD biomarker, both as a full-length molecule and as fragments from the C-terminal half [66,70]. Moreover, it has been shown to be able to detect early-stage pathological changes, even in the MCI stage, and predict and monitor AD-related cognitive decline, thus serving as a promising pre-symptomatic biomarker [67,68]. BACE1 (β-site APP cleaving enzyme-1) is an aspartyl protease discovered in 1999, which, by contrast to other peptidases of the pepsin family, such as cathepsin D and E, is a type I transmembrane protein [69,71]. Commonly expressed in neurons, oligodendrocytes and astrocytes, BACE1 is more abundantly found within certain neuronal cell types [69]. The generation of Aβ monomeric forms is dependent upon the activity of BACE1, this being directly related to synaptic functions, plasticity and homeostasis [69,72]. Studies have shown the significantly increased concentrations and activity rates of BACE1 in AD brains and CSF, which is thought to cause a vicious cycle by producing Aβ peptides near synapses [69,72–75]. Other synaptic dysfunction-associated biomarkers for AD include synaptotagmin, a calcium sensor protein, SNAP-25, a component of the soluble N-ethylmaleimide sensitive factor attachment protein receptor complex, GAP-43, a pre-synaptic membrane protein, and synaptophysin, which has exhibited increased levels in the CSF of AD patients [69,76].

On one hand, TREM2, the triggering receptor expressed on myeloid cells 2, is a type I transmembrane receptor protein of the innate immune system, selectively expressed on the plasma membrane of microglia and dendrocytes within the central nervous system [77–81]. TREM2 plays fundamental roles in microglial functions, including in the phagocytosis of apoptotic neurons, damaged myelin and amyloid plaques, biosynthetic metabolism, proliferation, migration, survival, cytokine release, lipid sensing, and inflammatory signaling inhibition, and it has been proven to be essential in synapse pruning during early development [79–81]. Furthermore, its ectodomain is cleaved in the cell surface and shed at the plasma membrane, thus releasing a soluble fragment (sTREM2) which can be measured in the CSF as an indicator of microglial activity [78–80]. As it is involved in the regulation of microglia dynamics, and the subsequent amyloid plaque formation and synaptic plasticity, increased levels of sTREM2 within the CSF have been related to a protective response against AD pathology, thus serving as a potential biomarker [80–83]. On the other hand, YKL-40, the inflammation-related glycoprotein known as chitinase-3-like protein 1, breast regression protein 39, human cartilage glycoprotein 39 or chondrex, belongs to the family of chitinase-like proteins, but lacks the enzymatic activity of chitinases [84,85]. Normally expressed in the fibrillar astrocytes within the white matter, YKL-40 plays key roles in inflammation, proliferation, angiogenesis and tissue remodeling [84–86], and CSF YKL-40 is a biomarker for astroglial activity [80]. Furthermore, elevated levels of YKL-40 in the brain and CSF are generally associated with neurodegeneration, appearing as a pre-clinical sign of AD pathology [80,86,87].

Another important group of AD biomarkers is the microRNAs (miRNAs), which are small non-coding RNAs with an average length of 22 nucleotides, involved in gene expression at the post-transcriptional level, regulation through binding to mRNA targets, and the subsequent translational repression or degradation of the target by the RNA-induced silencing complex [88–90]. Although recent studies have been intensively focusing on miRNA deregulation associated with AD, the lack of standardization in the quantification methods and protocols used is considerably challenging for establishing the discrimination power of miRNAs as biomarkers for AD [91]. Thus, the available results are generally not comparable since they target different miRNA molecules, which further increases the complexity of the subject [91–96].

The previously described CSF biomarkers for AD and the associated mechanisms of pathology are summarized in Table 1.

Table 1. The major changes of the identified CSF biomarkers for AD and the associated mechanisms of pathology.

Mechanism of AD Pathology	CSF Biomarker	Change in AD Pathology	Sensitivity	Specificity	References
Aβ plaque deposition	$Aβ_{42}$	↓	0.69–0.81	0.44–0.89	[43,97–100]
	$Aβ_{40}$	-	0.72	0.39	[98,101]
	$Aβ_{38}$	-	0.63	0.56	[98,101]
	$Aβ_{42}/Aβ_{40}$	↑	0.81–0.93	0.60–1	[45,97–99]
	$Aβ_{42}/Aβ_{38}$	↑	0.92	0.89	[101]
tau pathology	T-tau	↑↑	0.74–0.77	0.70–0.75	[97,100]
	P-tau	↑	0.66–0.73	0.63–0.82	[97,100]
neuronal injury	NFL	↑	0.81	0.79	[100]
synaptic dysfunction and/or loss	neurogranin	↑	0.73	0.84	[102]
	BACE1	↑	0.87	0.63	[103]
	synaptotagmin	↑	n.r.	n.r.	[69,76]
	SNAP-25	↑	n.r.	n.r.	[69,76]
	GAP-43	↑	n.r.	n.r.	[69,76]
	synaptophysin	↑	n.r.	n.r.	[69,76]
neuroinflammation	sTREM2	↑	n.r.	n.r.	[82,83]
	YKL-40	↑	0.77–0.85	0.81–0.84	[80,86,87,104]

n.r.—not reported; ↓—decrease; ↑—increase; ↑↑—high increase.

3. Blood Biomarkers

Although CSF biomarkers provide significantly more accurate diagnostics of AD and/or MCI, their clinical application is generally limited due to their invasive nature, which is traumatic to patients, and their high costs. Therefore, the scientific focus has shifted towards more accessible biomarkers that could increase their application for clinical practice. In this context, the use of peripheral blood biomarkers for AD diagnosis possesses a series of advantages, namely minimal invasiveness, facile sampling, cost- and time-efficiency, and widespread adoption [67,105].

Nonetheless, although blood communicates with the brain through the blood–brain barrier, the lymph vessels and the glymphatic system, the interchange is indirect. Therefore, the applicability of blood biomarkers in clinical practice is still not possible due to a series of challenges, in terms of both biological and technical issues [60,105–107]. First, the central nervous system is an isolated environment and the concentration of the potential biomarkers might be relatively low, as they must cross the blood–brain barrier as intact molecules [106]. Additionally, the volume ratio between the blood and the CSF will cause a significant analyte dilution [60]. However, there is strong evidence of barrier dysfunction in AD patients, which leads to increased protein and other molecule exchanges [105,106]. Second, as blood is a highly complex fluid comprising various molecules and cells, non-specific biomarkers, such as inflammatory or acute phase proteins, could be expressed by sources other than the central nervous system, which further introduces and increases variability within analyses [60,106]. Additionally, the variety of proteins and heterophilic antibodies present in the blood might potentially cause interference in the analysis [60]. Third, blood biomarkers might undergo liver or plasma proteolytic degradation, matrix effects due to plasma protein or blood cell adhesion, or kidney excretion, which will further substantially lower their concentration [60,106]. Fourth, the sensitivity and specificity of blood biomarkers are still considerably low, as there is a high risk of the overlapping of neurodegenerative disorders and other co-morbidities of AD patients that could also change plasma protein profiles [67,106]. Therefore, blood biomarker assays for AD diagnosis still lack standardization between instruments and laboratories, and the complexity of the blood is associated with a series of variables that are challenging in terms of result replication [60,105].

Among the conventional biomarkers for AD, $A\beta_{42}$, $A\beta_{40}$ and $A\beta_{42}/A\beta_{40}$ have been recognized as potential screening molecules [108]. However, early studies led to inconsistency between results and a lack of correlation between CSF and blood $A\beta$ [46,106,109–111]. Such results were probably due to low $A\beta$ concentrations in blood and the influences of matrix effects, as plasma proteins have a tendency of binding to $A\beta$, and the analytical sensitivity of the assay did not allow for diluting these effects [46,109], as measurements were performed using enzyme-linked immunosorbent assay (ELISA) methods [106,110,112]. However, more recent studies are considerably more promising, as they use ultrasensitive immunoassay techniques, such as single-molecule array or SIMOA, immunoprecipitation coupled with mass spectrometry, and stable isotope labeling kinetics followed by immunoprecipitation coupled with mass spectrometry [46,105,106,109–111]. As such, the results showed the expected decrease in blood $A\beta_{42}$, $A\beta_{40}$ and $A\beta_{42}/A\beta_{40}$ levels in AD and MCI patients [106,109–111,113]. However, the presence of various factors that introduce variability to the results limits the applicability of $A\beta$ as a blood biomarker for AD [105].

Similarly, the introduction of ultrasensitive immunoassay techniques, including SIMOA, mesoscale discovery or MSD, label-free real-time surface plasmon resonance technology, and immunomagnetic reduction, has led to more promising results in terms of T-tau and P-tau blood levels. In this regard, results have shown that increased levels of blood T-tau and P-tau are generally associated with AD [46,106,109]. However, more accurate results have been obtained by using enzymes involved in tau protein hyperphosphorylation processes, such as glycogen synthase kinase 3β (GSK-3β) and dual-specificity tyrosine-phosphorylation regulated kinase A (DYRK1A) [105]. On one hand, GSK-3β is a GSK-3 isoform, part of the serine/threonine kinase family, known for its important roles in neuron polarity and synapse plasticity. Consequently, there is strong evidence of its implications in the pathological mechanisms of neurodegeneration disease development and the progression of tauopathies associated with AD [114–117]. In this context, blood levels of GSK-3β are considerably elevated in AD and MCI patients, which proves its potential as a blood-based AD biomarker [105,118]. On the other hand, DYRK1A, a member of the proline-directed serine/threonine kinases, is widely known for its implications for cell proliferation, as well as various signaling pathways fundamental for brain development and function, namely neuron survival, synaptic plasticity, and actin cytoskeleton and microtubule regulation [119–121]. As AD patients present considerably reduced blood levels, DYRK1A could be used as a potential biomarker [105,122].

The emergence of the ultrasensitive techniques has also allowed for the accurate quantification of blood NFL, which has been shown to closely correlate with CSF results, thus reflecting brain pathology [46,106,110]. Both plasma and serum levels of NFL are elevated in AD and MCI patients years before symptom onset [46,105,109–111,123,124]. Additionally, as NFL levels could also serve as biomarkers for disease severity, namely brain atrophy, cognitive impairment or glucose hypometabolism, it can also be used as a biomarker for disease staging [46]. Although it is among the most consistent blood biomarkers [111,123,125], increased concentrations of NFL are not specific for AD, as they have been observed in other neurodegenerative disorders [105,109].

Moreover, several studies have demonstrated that sustained chronic inflammation is directly related to AD development, as postmortem tissues of AD models exhibited inflammatory responses [126]. Among the mediators involved in the systemic immune response regulation, including transcriptional factors, cytokines, chemokines, complements, coagulation factors, enzymes, various peptides and lipids [127], interleukins (IL-1, IL-4, IL-6 and IL-10), cytokine I-309, interferon-γ, and tumor necrosis factor α (TNF-α) are particularly important biomarkers for the early diagnosis of AD [105].

Furthermore, clusterin, also termed as apolipoprotein J, is a highly sialylated multifunctional glycoprotein that is highly expressed in the brain, liver, testicles and ovaries [128–130]. Studies show that clusterin is involved in a series of pathophysiological states, including cell death, oxidative stress, proteotoxic stress and neurodegenerative processes [130]. As its main function is to act as a chaperone for various extracellular proteins, it has been demonstrated that clusterin is capable of binding Aβ peptides, thus decreasing Aβ toxicity and the associated apoptosis and oxidative stress [105,130,131]. In this context, as it is found in higher concentrations in the blood of AD patients, clusterin could be a promising AD biomarker [105].

The previously described blood biomarkers for AD and the associated mechanisms of pathology are summarized in Table 2.

Table 2. The major changes of the identified blood biomarkers for AD and the associated mechanisms of pathology.

Mechanism of AD Pathology	Blood Biomarker	Change in AD Pathology	Sensitivity	Specificity	References
Aβ plaque deposition	Aβ$_{42}$	↓	0.82	0.77	[35,132,133]
	Aβ$_{40}$	↓	n.r.	n.r.	[133]
	Aβ$_{42}$/Aβ$_{40}$	↓	0.75	0.77	[35,132,133]
tau pathology	T-tau	↑	0.62	0.54	[134]
	P-tau	↑	n.r.	n.r.	[135]
	GSK-3β	↑	n.r.	n.r.	[105,118]
	DYRK1A	↓	n.r.	n.r.	[105,122]
neuronal injury	NFL	↑	0.86	0.76	[136]
inflammation	IL-1, IL-4, IL-6, and IL-10	↑	n.r.	n.r.	[105]
	cytokine I-309	↑	n.r.	n.r.	[105]
	interferon-γ	↑	n.r.	n.r.	[105]
	TNF-α	↑	n.r.	n.r.	[105]
apoptosis	clusterin	↑	0.76	0.63	[105,137]

n.r.—not reported; ↓—decrease; ↑—increase.

4. Saliva Biomarkers

Saliva is a complex biological fluid secreted in the mouth by three main pairs of salivary glands, namely the parotid, the submandibular, and the sublingual, which generate 0.75–1.5 L daily. The compositions of their secretions depend on the sympathetic and parasympathetic stimulation, circadian rhythm, health status, eating habits and drug intake [138,139]. Considering the direct relation between the salivary gland and the nervous system, as the facial nerve innervates the sublingual and submandibular glands through the submandibular ganglion and the glossopharyngeal nerve innervates the parotid gland through the otic ganglion, saliva could represent an important source of biomarkers for nervous system disorders [139,140]. In contrast to blood, saliva is a matrix that can be collected easily and non-invasively, at all ages and many times per day, and assessed through different assays [139,141–144], which is promising for its future clinical application in the timely detection, diagnosis, prognosis and monitoring of neurological disorders [142,145]. In this regard, a novel term has been introduced, salivaomics, which encompasses all biomarkers discovered within the genome, microbiome, epigenome, transcriptome, proteome and metabolome for the development of translational and clinical tools for diagnosis [145,146].

Therefore, due to the capacity of molecules to pass from the blood to the saliva through passive diffusion, active transport or microfiltration, saliva is a promising AD-related biomarker pool that could be used for its early and accurate diagnosis [147,148]. The most important AD biomarkers found within the saliva are Aβ peptides, T-tau and P-tau, acetylcholine, lactoferrin, and trehalose, each related to different AD pathophysiological mechanism.

Owing to the saliva–blood interactions and the buccal cell degradation, Aβ peptides should also be present in the saliva, as APP is a widely expressed protein in the peripheral tissues. Although the number of studies on the matter is still considerably limited, recent results have shown that salivary $Aβ_{42}$ is increased in AD patients, while $Aβ_{40}$ does not change [148–150]. However, there are no studies regarding the $Aβ_{42}/Aβ_{40}$ ratio in the saliva, which should also be validated considering its significant relevance in the CSF [151].

Similarly, studies on salivary T-tau and P-tau are still limited, with preliminary results demonstrating elevated levels of T-tau and P-tau, and also an elevated P-tau/T-tau ratio [152,153]. However, the results are not conclusive, as tau proteins are also expressed and secreted by acinar epithelial cells, the subunits of salivary glands, and released from the cranial nerves [151,154].

Furthermore, as salivary glands are under cholinergic innervation, acetylcholinesterase, a type-B carboxylesterase enzyme mainly found in the synaptic cleft at the post-synaptic neuromuscular junctions, further diffuses into the saliva [151,155,156]. Its primary function is the termination of neuron transmission and signaling, but recent studies have demonstrated its role in the development of AD by promoting Aβ fibril formation [156–158]. In this context, the available studies reported reduced levels of salivary acetylcholinesterase associated with aging and even lower levels for AD patients [139,148,151]. However, while they proved its potential as a salivary AD biomarker, the conclusiveness of the results is still limited due to a lack of standardization [151].

Antimicrobial peptides have been previously proposed as biomarkers for brain infections involved in the AD developmental processes [151]. An example of such biomarkers is lactoferrin, a globular non-hemic iron-binding glycoprotein that belongs to the family of serum transferrin proteins, and it is mostly synthesized by glandular epithelial cells and neutrophils [159–162]. Owing to its iron-binding activity, lactoferrin is a multifunctional protein that exhibits antibacterial, antiviral, antifungal, antioxidant, immunomodulatory, anti-cancer, anti-inflammatory and anti-allergenic properties [160,162–164]. Moreover, while there is evidence of lactoferrin presence within the human brain, its levels are substantially increased in AD patients and those with related neurodegenerative disorders, which could be attributed to its Aβ-binding ability [165–167]. Therefore, lactoferrin has been associated with AD pathogenesis, as it has been detected in the amyloid plaques, NFTs and microglia of AD brains [164,165]. Studies on AD patients are still limited, but there is strong evidence that the salivary levels of lactoferrin significantly decrease when compared to healthy controls and elderly subjects [139,148,164,168]. Moreover, lactoferrin has also demonstrated its potential for early disease detection, as the accuracy of AD diagnosis using it was greater than with CSF T-tau and Aβ42 [139,151].

The previously described saliva biomarkers for AD and the associated mechanisms of pathology are summarized in Table 3.

Table 3. The major changes of the identified saliva biomarkers for AD and the associated mechanisms of pathology.

Mechanism of AD Pathology	Saliva Biomarker	Change in AD Pathology	Sensitivity	Specificity	References
Aβ plaque deposition	$Aβ_{42}$	↑	0.16	0.93	[148–150,169]
	$Aβ_{40}$	-	n.r.	n.r.	[148,149]
	acetylcholinesterase	↓	n.r.	n.r.	[139,148,151,170]
tau pathology	T-tau	↑	n.r.	n.r.	[152,153,171]
	P-tau	↑	n.r.	n.r.	[152,153]
	P-tau/T-tau	↑	0.73–0.83	0.30–0.50	[152,153]
inflammation	lactoferrin	↓	1	0.98	[168]

n.r.—not reported; ↓—decrease; ↑—increase.

5. Emerging Body Fluid Biomarkers

Recent years have witnessed significant advancements in the profiling technologies, which have improved the detection sensitivity and allowed for the quantification of minute samples. In this manner, previously difficult-to-assess body fluids, such as urine, tears or olfactory fluids, have become a rich source of biocompounds that could reflect the pathological state of an individual [171].

Urine has become a highly desirable source of disease biomarkers, as it can easily and non-invasively be collected in relatively large volumes. Additionally, it contains cellular components, biochemical compounds, and proteins originating from plasma glomerular filtration, renal tubule excretion or urogenital tract secretion, thus reflecting the metabolic and pathophysiological condition of an individual. In this context, recent works have focused on the plethora of biomarkers present within the urinary proteins, glycoproteins and exosomes that could allow for the early diagnosis, prognosis, prevention or treatment of various diseases [172,173]. Furthermore, urine can also reflect AD pathology signs, generally associated with modifications in protein and lipid metabolism caused by oxidative stress [174,175]. Moreover, since the concentration of the creatinine waste product is physiologically stable, it can be used for normalizing urine biomarker concentrations [174]. In this context, the most promising urinary biomarkers include isoprostane [176], glycine and total free amino acids [177], and 8-hydroxy-2'-deoxyguanosine [178], which have achieved over 90% accuracy [174,175].

While tears are available in considerably reduced volumes for sampling, they are a neglected key reservoir of biomarkers, with great potential in medical diagnostics [179,180]. Tears are complex protein, lipid, mucin, water and salt mixtures, and the development of novel proteomic, lipidomic and glycomic techniques has allowed for a complete understanding of these components and their changes associated with ocular or non-ocular disorders [171,181,182]. For example, proteomic techniques have revealed the presence of AD-related peptides within aqueous humor samples [183], while tear fluid has proven to be clinically relevant through the discovery of a combination of four tear proteins, namely lipocalin-1, dermicidin, lysozyme C and lactritin, with a sensitivity of 81% and a specificity of 77% for AD [184,185]. Another study suggested the discriminatory power of tear T-tau and $A\beta_{42}$, as their levels increased in AD patients [186]. Additionally, total microRNA abundance was also found at increased levels in AD patients, with microRNA-200b-5p as the most promising AD biomarker [183,187].

Moreover, several studies have reported the isolation of NFTs and identified increased levels of T-tau and P-tau in AD patients' nasal secretions [35], thus proving the potential of olfactory fluids as non-invasive AD biomarkers.

6. Conclusions and Future Perspectives

AD is the most common neurodegenerative disorder that predominantly affects the elderly population. Thus, it is expected that the number of AD patients worldwide will reach 60 million by 2030, which will have a significant impact on the global health system. The current diagnosis methods involve cognitive tests, neuroimaging techniques and CSF assays. However, there is still no clinical strategy available for the accurate and early detection of AD. Recent trends have focused on identifying novel biomarkers beyond Aβ and tau proteins, as well as new matrices as biomarker sources, such as the blood, saliva, urine, tear or olfactory fluids. While there have been considerable advancements in the field, the lack of standardized sampling and assays poses significant challenges for the use of such biomarkers in the clinical practice. In this context, recent trends have been focusing on the identification of protein or lipid panels, which could better reflect the complete mechanisms of AD.

Furthermore, research should also focus on the development of advanced platforms and biosensor devices that could provide real-time information regarding the health status of AD patients [188]. In this context, biosensor-on-chip devices could represent a promising strategy for accurately assessing a great pallet of AD biomarkers.

Author Contributions: A.F.B., C.C., A.M.G. have participated in review writing and revision. All authors have read and agreed to the published version of the manuscript.

Funding: This manuscript received no external funding.

Conflicts of Interest: The authors declare no conflict of interest.

References

1. Mythri, R.B.; Srinivas Bharath, M.M. Chapter 9-Omics and Epigenetics of Polyphenol-Mediated Neuroprotection: The Curcumin Perspective. In *Curcumin for Neurological and Psychiatric Disorders*; Farooqui, T., Farooqui, A.A., Eds.; Academic Press: Cambridge, MA, USA, 2019; pp. 169–189. [CrossRef]
2. Farooqui, A.A. Chapter 1-Classification and Molecular Aspects of Neurotraumatic Diseases: Similarities and Differences With Neurodegenerative and Neuropsychiatric Diseases. In *Ischemic and Traumatic Brain and Spinal Cord Injuries*; Farooqui, A.A., Ed.; Academic Press: Cambridge, MA, USA, 2018; pp. 1–40. [CrossRef]
3. Peña-Bautista, C.; Casas-Fernández, E.; Vento, M.; Baquero, M.; Cháfer-Pericás, C. Stress and neurodegeneration. *Clin. Chim. Acta* **2020**, *503*, 163–168. [CrossRef] [PubMed]
4. Lima, J.A.; Hamerski, L. Chapter 8-Alkaloids as Potential Multi-Target Drugs to Treat Alzheimer's Disease. In *Studies in Natural Products Chemistry*; Atta ur, R., Ed.; Elsevier: Amsterdam, The Netherlands, 2019; Volume 61, pp. 301–334.
5. Sheikh, S.; Safia; Haque, E.; Mir, S.S. Neurodegenerative Diseases: Multifactorial Conformational Diseases and Their Therapeutic Interventions. *J. Neurodegener. Dis.* **2013**, *2013*, 563481. [CrossRef] [PubMed]
6. Zyuz'kov, G.N.; Suslov, N.I.; Miroshnichenko, L.A.; Simanina, E.V.; Polykova, T.Y.; Stavrova, L.A.; Zhdanov, V.V.; Minakova, M.Y.; Udut, E.V.; Udut, V.V. Halogenated (CL-ion) songorine is a new original agonist of fibroblast growth factor receptors of neuronal-committed progenitors possessing neuroregenerative effect after cerebral ischemia and hypoxia in experimental animals. *Biointerface Res. Appl. Chem.* **2019**, *9*, 4317–4326. [CrossRef]
7. Gitler, A.D.; Dhillon, P.; Shorter, J. Neurodegenerative disease: Models, mechanisms, and a new hope. *Dis. Model. Mech.* **2017**, *10*, 499–502. [CrossRef] [PubMed]
8. Farkhondeh, T.; Forouzanfar, F.; Roshanravan, B.; Samarghandian, S. Curcumin effect on non-amyloidogenic pathway for preventing alzheimer's disease. *Biointerface Res. Appl. Chem.* **2019**, *9*, 4085–4089. [CrossRef]
9. Steffen, J. "A Battle You Would Never Choose to Fight": The Management of Neurodegenerative Diseases as a Societal Challenge. *Neurodegener. Dis.* **2019**, *19*, 1–3. [CrossRef] [PubMed]
10. Sardoiwala, M.N.; Kaundal, B.; Roy Choudhury, S. Chapter 37-Development of Engineered Nanoparticles Expediting Diagnostic and Therapeutic Applications Across Blood–Brain Barrier. In *Handbook of Nanomaterials for Industrial Applications*; Mustansar Hussain, C., Ed.; Elsevier: Amsterdam, The Netherlands, 2018; pp. 696–709. [CrossRef]
11. Balasa, A.; Balasa, R.; Egyed-Zsigmond, I.; Chinezu, R.J.T.N. Bilateral thalamic glioma: Case report and review of the literature. *Turk. Neurosurg.* **2016**, *26*, 321–324. [CrossRef]
12. Gherasim, D.N.; Gherman, B.; Balasa, A.J.R.J.O.N. Clinical Evolution of Primary Intramedullary Tumors in Adults. *Rom. J. Neurol.* **2012**, *11*, 165–171.
13. Balasa, A.; Tamas, F.; Hurghis, C.; Maier, S.; Motataianu, A.; Chinezu, R. First-Onset Hypokalemic Periodic Paralysis Following Surgery for Myxopapillary Ependymoma. *World Neurosurg.* **2020**, *141*, 389–394. [CrossRef]
14. Sánchez-López, E.; Marina, M.L. Chapter 20-Neuroscience Applications of Capillary Electrophoretic Methods. In *Capillary Electromigration Separation Methods*; Poole, C.F., Ed.; Elsevier: Amsterdam, The Netherlands, 2018; pp. 481–510. [CrossRef]
15. Aravalli, R.N.; Shiao, M.; Lu, W.-C.; Xie, H.; Pearce, C.; Toman, N.G.; Danczyk, G.; Sipe, C.; Miller, Z.D.; Crane, A.; et al. Chapter 15-The Bioengineering of Exogenic Organs and/or Cells for Use in Regenerative Medicine. In *Engineering in Medicine*; Iaizzo, P.A., Ed.; Academic Press: Cambridge, MA, USA, 2019; pp. 381–415. [CrossRef]
16. Gherasim, D.N.; Gyorki, G.; Balasa, A.J.R.N. Single center experience and technical nuances in the treatment of distal anterior cerebral artery aneurysms. *Rom. Neurosurg.* **2017**, *31*, 17–24. [CrossRef]
17. Serafín, V.; Gamella, M.; Pedrero, M.; Montero-Calle, A.; Razzino, C.A.; Yáñez-Sedeño, P.; Barderas, R.; Campuzano, S.; Pingarrón, J.M. Enlightening the advancements in electrochemical bioanalysis for the diagnosis of Alzheimer's disease and other neurodegenerative disorders. *J. Pharm. Biomed. Anal.* **2020**, *189*, 113437. [CrossRef] [PubMed]

18. Brazaca, L.C.; Sampaio, I.; Zucolotto, V.; Janegitz, B.C. Applications of biosensors in Alzheimer's disease diagnosis. *Talanta* **2020**, *210*, 120644. [CrossRef]
19. Chávez-Gutiérrez, L.; Szaruga, M. Mechanisms of neurodegeneration—Insights from familial Alzheimer's disease. *Semin. Cell Dev. Biol.* **2020**, *105*, 75–85. [CrossRef] [PubMed]
20. Monajjemi, M. Molecular vibration of dopamine neurotransmitter: A relation between its normal modes and harmonic notes. *Biointerface Res. Appl. Chem.* **2019**, *9*, 3956–3962. [CrossRef]
21. Pham, T.T.; Monajjemi, M.; Dang, D.M.T.; Mollaamin, F.; Dang, C.M. Reaction of cell membrane bilayers "as a variable capacitor" with G-protein: A reason for neurotransmitter signaling. *Biointerface Res. Appl. Chem.* **2019**, *9*, 3874–3883. [CrossRef]
22. Gupta, J.; Fatima, M.T.; Islam, Z.; Khan, R.H.; Uversky, V.N.; Salahuddin, P. Nanoparticle formulations in the diagnosis and therapy of Alzheimer's disease. *Int. J. Biol. Macromol.* **2019**, *130*, 515–526. [CrossRef]
23. Yao, F.; Zhang, K.; Zhang, Y.; Guo, Y.; Li, A.; Xiao, S.; Liu, Q.; Shen, L.; Ni, J. Identification of Blood Biomarkers for Alzheimer's Disease Through Computational Prediction and Experimental Validation. *Front. Neurol.* **2019**, *9*, 1158. [CrossRef]
24. Adina, S.; Anca, M.; Zoltan, B.; Adrian, B. Guillain–Barré and Acute Transverse Myelitis Overlap Syndrome Following Obstetric Surgery. *J. Crit. Care Med.* **2020**, *6*, 74–79. [CrossRef]
25. Maier, S.; Motataianu, A.; Bajko, Z.; Romaniuc, A.; Balasa, A. Pontine cavernoma haemorrhage at 24 weeks of pregnancy that resulted in eight-and-a-half syndrome. *Acta Neurol. Belg.* **2019**, *119*, 471–474. [CrossRef]
26. Balasa, A.; Chinezu, R.; Gherasim, D.N.J.R.N. Surgical management of tuberculum sellae and planum sphenoidale meningiomas. *Rom. Neurosurg.* **2013**, *20*, 92–99.
27. Anca, M.; Laura Iulia, B.; Smaranda, M.; Adrian, B.; Adina, S. Cardiac Autonomic Neuropathy in Diabetes Mellitus Patients–Are We Aware of the Consequences? *Acta Marisiensis-Ser. Med.* **2020**, *66*, 3–8. [CrossRef]
28. Rossini, P.M.; Di Iorio, R.; Vecchio, F.; Anfossi, M.; Babiloni, C.; Bozzali, M.; Bruni, A.C.; Cappa, S.F.; Escudero, J.; Fraga, F.J.; et al. Early diagnosis of Alzheimer's disease: The role of biomarkers including advanced EEG signal analysis. Report from the IFCN-sponsored panel of experts. *Clin. Neurophysiol.* **2020**, *131*, 1287–1310. [CrossRef]
29. Atri, A. The Alzheimer's Disease Clinical Spectrum: Diagnosis and Management. *Med. Clin. N. Am.* **2019**, *103*, 263–293. [CrossRef]
30. Khoury, R.; Ghossoub, E. Diagnostic biomarkers of Alzheimer's disease: A state-of-the-art review. *Biomark. Neuropsychiatry* **2019**, *1*, 100005. [CrossRef]
31. Premi, E.; Calhoun, V.D.; Diano, M.; Gazzina, S.; Cosseddu, M.; Alberici, A.; Archetti, S.; Paternicò, D.; Gasparotti, R.; van Swieten, J.; et al. The inner fluctuations of the brain in pre-symptomatic Frontotemporal Dementia: The chronnectome fingerprint. *NeuroImage* **2019**, *189*, 645–654. [CrossRef]
32. Mobed, A.; Hasanzadeh, M. Biosensing: The best alternative for conventional methods in detection of Alzheimer's disease biomarkers. *Int. J. Biol. Macromol.* **2020**, *161*, 59–71. [CrossRef] [PubMed]
33. Kawata, K.; Tierney, R.; Langford, D. Blood and cerebrospinal fluid biomarkers. *Handb. Clin. Neurol.* **2018**, *158*, 217–233. [CrossRef] [PubMed]
34. Lewczuk, P.; Riederer, P.; O'Bryant, S.E.; Verbeek, M.M.; Dubois, B.; Visser, P.J.; Jellinger, K.A.; Engelborghs, S.; Ramirez, A.; Parnetti, L.; et al. Cerebrospinal fluid and blood biomarkers for neurodegenerative dementias: An update of the Consensus of the Task Force on Biological Markers in Psychiatry of the World Federation of Societies of Biological Psychiatry. *World J. Biol. Psychiatry* **2018**, *19*, 244–328. [CrossRef] [PubMed]
35. Lee, J.C.; Kim, S.J.; Hong, S.; Kim, Y. Diagnosis of Alzheimer's disease utilizing amyloid and tau as fluid biomarkers. *Exp. Mol. Med.* **2019**, *51*, 1–10. [CrossRef]
36. Rosenberg, G.A. Chapter 4-Cerebrospinal Fluid: Formation, Absorption, Markers, and Relationship to Blood–Brain Barrier. In *Primer on Cerebrovascular Diseases (Second Edition)*; Caplan, L.R., Biller, J., Leary, M.C., Lo, E.H., Thomas, A.J., Yenari, M., Zhang, J.H., Eds.; Academic Press: San Diego, CA, USA, 2017; pp. 25–31. [CrossRef]
37. Niemantsverdriet, E.; Valckx, S.; Bjerke, M.; Engelborghs, S. Alzheimer's disease CSF biomarkers: Clinical indications and rational use. *Acta Neurol. Belg.* **2017**, *117*, 591–602. [CrossRef]
38. Teunissen, C.E.; Verheul, C.; Willemse, E.A.J. Chapter 1-The use of cerebrospinal fluid in biomarker studies. In *Handbook of Clinical Neurology*; Deisenhammer, F., Teunissen, C.E., Tumani, H., Eds.; Elsevier: Amsterdam, The Netherlands, 2018; Volume 146, pp. 3–20.

39. Robey, T.T.; Panegyres, P.K. Cerebrospinal fluid biomarkers in neurodegenerative disorders. *Future Neurol.* **2019**, *14*, FNL6. [CrossRef]
40. Cognat, E.; Mouton Liger, F.; Troussière, A.-C.; Wallon, D.; Dumurgier, J.; Magnin, E.; Duron, E.; Gabelle, A.; Croisile, B.; de la Sayette, V.; et al. What is the clinical impact of cerebrospinal fluid biomarkers on final diagnosis and management in patients with mild cognitive impairment in clinical practice? Results from a nation-wide prospective survey in France. *BMJ Open* **2019**, *9*, e026380. [CrossRef] [PubMed]
41. Mounsey, A.L.; Zeitler, M.R. Cerebrospinal Fluid Biomarkers for Detection of Alzheimer Disease in Patients with Mild Cognitive Impairment. *Am. Fam. Physician* **2018**, *97*, 714–715.
42. Pawlowski, M.; Meuth, S.G.; Duning, T. Cerebrospinal Fluid Biomarkers in Alzheimer's Disease-From Brain Starch to Bench and Bedside. *Diagnostics* **2017**, *7*, 42. [CrossRef]
43. Boumenir, A.; Cognat, E.; Sabia, S.; Hourregue, C.; Lilamand, M.; Dugravot, A.; Bouaziz-Amar, E.; Laplanche, J.-L.; Hugon, J.; Singh-Manoux, A.; et al. CSF level of β-amyloid peptide predicts mortality in Alzheimer's disease. *Alzheimer's Res. Ther.* **2019**, *11*, 29. [CrossRef]
44. Hu, W.T.; Watts, K.D.; Shaw, L.M.; Howell, J.C.; Trojanowski, J.Q.; Basra, S.; Glass, J.D.; Lah, J.J.; Levey, A.I. CSF beta-amyloid 1-42-what are we measuring in Alzheimer's disease? *Ann. Clin. Transl. Neurol.* **2015**, *2*, 131–139. [CrossRef]
45. Biscetti, L.; Salvadori, N.; Farotti, L.; Cataldi, S.; Eusebi, P.; Paciotti, S.; Parnetti, L. The added value of Aβ42/Aβ40 in the CSF signature for routine diagnostics of Alzheimer's disease. *Clin. Chim. Acta* **2019**, *494*, 71–73. [CrossRef]
46. Milà-Alomà, M.; Suárez-Calvet, M.; Molinuevo, J.L. Latest advances in cerebrospinal fluid and blood biomarkers of Alzheimer's disease. *Ther. Adv. Neurol. Disord.* **2019**, *12*, 1756286419888819. [CrossRef]
47. Bjerke, M.; Engelborghs, S. Cerebrospinal Fluid Biomarkers for Early and Differential Alzheimer's Disease Diagnosis. *J. Alzheimers Dis.* **2018**, *62*, 1199–1209. [CrossRef]
48. Liu, T.C.; Zheng, T.; Duan, R.; Zhu, L.; Zhang, Q.G. On the Biomarkers of Alzheimer's Disease. *Adv. Exp. Med. Biol.* **2020**, *1232*, 409–414. [CrossRef]
49. Habib, A.; Sawmiller, D.; Tan, J. Restoring Soluble Amyloid Precursor Protein α Functions as a Potential Treatment for Alzheimer's Disease. *J. Neurosci. Res.* **2017**, *95*, 973–991. [CrossRef]
50. Araki, W.; Hattori, K.; Kanemaru, K.; Yokoi, Y.; Omachi, Y.; Takano, H.; Sakata, M.; Yoshida, S.; Tsukamoto, T.; Murata, M.; et al. Re-evaluation of soluble APP-α and APP-β in cerebrospinal fluid as potential biomarkers for early diagnosis of dementia disorders. *Biomark. Res.* **2017**, *5*, 28. [CrossRef]
51. Barbier, P.; Zejneli, O.; Martinho, M.; Lasorsa, A.; Belle, V.; Smet-Nocca, C.; Tsvetkov, P.O.; Devred, F.; Landrieu, I. Role of Tau as a Microtubule-Associated Protein: Structural and Functional Aspects. *Front. Aging Neurosci.* **2019**, *11*, 204. [CrossRef]
52. Hervy, J.; Bicout, D.J. Dynamical decoration of stabilized-microtubules by Tau-proteins. *Sci. Rep.* **2019**, *9*, 12473. [CrossRef]
53. Andone, S.; Petrutiu, S.; Bajko, Z.; Motataianu, A.; Maier, S.; Macavei, I.; Stoian, A.; Balasa, A.; Balasa, R.J.R.J.O.N. Sporadic Creutzfeldt-Jakob Disease: A Clinical Approach of A Small Case Series and Literature Review. *Rom. J. Neurol.* **2017**, *16*, 109–115.
54. Motataianu, A.; Barcutean, L.; Gherman, I.; Maier, S.; Bajko, Z.; Balasa, A.J.R.J.O.N. Cerebellar and brainstem infarction secondary to basilar artery dolichoectasia. *Rom. J. Neurol.* **2019**, *18*, 109–115.
55. Rares, C.; Hurghis, C.; Tamas, F.; Balasa, A.J.R.N. Our Experience with the Use of Oich Score in Intracerebral Haemorrhage. *Rom. J. Neurosurg.* **2019**, *33*, 41–43.
56. Vogel, J.W.; Iturria-Medina, Y.; Strandberg, O.T.; Smith, R.; Levitis, E.; Evans, A.C.; Hansson, O.; Weiner, M.; Aisen, P.; Petersen, R.; et al. Spread of pathological tau proteins through communicating neurons in human Alzheimer's disease. *Nat. Commun.* **2020**, *11*, 2612. [CrossRef]
57. Hansson, O.; Lehmann, S.; Otto, M.; Zetterberg, H.; Lewczuk, P. Advantages and disadvantages of the use of the CSF Amyloid β (Aβ) 42/40 ratio in the diagnosis of Alzheimer's Disease. *Alzheimer's Res. Ther.* **2019**, *11*, 34. [CrossRef]
58. Zetterberg, H.; Bendlin, B.B. Biomarkers for Alzheimer's disease-preparing for a new era of disease-modifying therapies. *Mol. Psychiatry* **2020**. [CrossRef]
59. Jin, M.; Cao, L.; Dai, Y.-P. Role of Neurofilament Light Chain as a Potential Biomarker for Alzheimer's Disease: A Correlative Meta-Analysis. *Front. Aging Neurosci.* **2019**, *11*, 254. [CrossRef] [PubMed]

60. Zetterberg, H.; Blennow, K. From Cerebrospinal Fluid to Blood: The Third Wave of Fluid Biomarkers for Alzheimer's Disease. *J. Alzheimer's Dis.* **2008**, *64*, S271–S279. [CrossRef]
61. Park, S.A.; Han, S.M.; Kim, C.E. New fluid biomarkers tracking non-amyloid-β and non-tau pathology in Alzheimer's disease. *Exp. Mol. Med.* **2020**, *52*, 556–568. [CrossRef] [PubMed]
62. Glushakova, O.Y.; Glushakov, A.V.; Mannix, R.; Miller, E.R.; Valadka, A.B.; Hayes, R.L. Chapter 8-The Use of Blood-Based Biomarkers to Improve the Design of Clinical Trials of Traumatic Brain Injury. In *Handbook of Neuroemergency Clinical Trials*, 2nd ed.; Skolnick, B.E., Alves, W.M., Eds.; Academic Press: Cambridge, MA, USA, 2018; pp. 139–166. [CrossRef]
63. Sillman, B.; Woldstad, C.; McMillan, J.; Gendelman, H.E. Chapter 3-Neuropathogenesis of human immunodeficiency virus infection. In *Handbook of Clinical Neurology*; Brew, B.J., Ed.; Elsevier: Amsterdam, The Netherlands, 2018; Volume 152, pp. 21–40.
64. Zetterberg, H.; Skillbäck, T.; Mattsson, N.; Trojanowski, J.Q.; Portelius, E.; Shaw, L.M.; Weiner, M.W.; Blennow, K.; Initiative, F.T.A.S.D.N. Association of Cerebrospinal Fluid Neurofilament Light Concentration With Alzheimer Disease Progression. *JAMA Neurol.* **2016**, *73*, 60–67. [CrossRef] [PubMed]
65. Didonna, A.; Opal, P. The role of neurofilament aggregation in neurodegeneration: Lessons from rare inherited neurological disorders. *Mol. Neurodegener.* **2019**, *14*, 19. [CrossRef] [PubMed]
66. Becker, B.; Nazir, F.H.; Brinkmalm, G.; Camporesi, E.; Kvartsberg, H.; Portelius, E.; Boström, M.; Kalm, M.; Höglund, K.; Olsson, M.; et al. Alzheimer-associated cerebrospinal fluid fragments of neurogranin are generated by Calpain-1 and prolyl endopeptidase. *Mol. Neurodegener.* **2018**, *13*, 47. [CrossRef]
67. Liu, W.; Lin, H.; He, X.; Chen, L.; Dai, Y.; Jia, W.; Xue, X.; Tao, J.; Chen, L. Neurogranin as a cognitive biomarker in cerebrospinal fluid and blood exosomes for Alzheimer's disease and mild cognitive impairment. *Transl. Psychiatry* **2020**, *10*, 125. [CrossRef]
68. Willemse, E.A.J.; De Vos, A.; Herries, E.M.; Andreasson, U.; Engelborghs, S.; van der Flier, W.M.; Scheltens, P.; Crimmins, D.; Ladenson, J.H.; Vanmechelen, E.; et al. Neurogranin as Cerebrospinal Fluid Biomarker for Alzheimer Disease: An Assay Comparison Study. *Clin. Chem.* **2018**, *64*, 927–937. [CrossRef]
69. Hampel, H.; Vassar, R.; De Strooper, B.; Hardy, J.; Willem, M.; Singh, N.; Zhou, J.; Yan, R.; Vanmechelen, E.; De Vos, A.; et al. The β-Secretase BACE1 in Alzheimer's Disease. *Biol. Psychiatry* **2020**. [CrossRef]
70. Schipke, C.G.; De Vos, A.; Fuentes, M.; Jacobs, D.; Vanmechelen, E.; Peters, O. Neurogranin and BACE1 in CSF as Potential Biomarkers Differentiating Depression with Cognitive Deficits from Early Alzheimer's Disease: A Pilot Study. *Dement. Geriatr. Cogn. Disord. Extra* **2018**, *8*, 277–289. [CrossRef]
71. Kellner, S.; Ferchichi, M.J.I.J.O.A.R. Diagnosis and monitoring of Alzheimer Disease with saliva biomarker BACE1. *Int. J. Aging Res.* **2018**, *1*, 21.
72. Das, B.; Yan, R. Role of BACE1 in Alzheimer's synaptic function. *Transl. Neurodegen.* **2017**, *6*, 23. [CrossRef] [PubMed]
73. Alexopoulos, P.; Thierjung, N.; Grimmer, T.; Ortner, M.; Economou, P.; Assimakopoulos, K.; Gourzis, P.; Politis, A.; Perneczky, R. Cerebrospinal Fluid BACE1 Activity and sAβPPβ as Biomarker Candidates of Alzheimer's Disease. *Dement. Geriatr. Cogn. Disord.* **2018**, *45*, 152–161. [CrossRef] [PubMed]
74. Wang, D.; Wang, P.; Bian, X.; Xu, S.; Zhou, Q.; Zhang, Y.; Ding, M.; Han, M.; Huang, L.; Bi, J.; et al. Elevated plasma levels of exosomal BACE1-AS combined with the volume and thickness of the right entorhinal cortex may serve as a biomarker for the detection of Alzheimer's disease. *Mol. Med. Rep.* **2020**, *22*, 227–238. [CrossRef]
75. Tam, J.M.; Josephson, L.; Pilozzi, A.R.; Huang, X. A Novel Dual Fluorochrome Near-Infrared Imaging Probe for Potential Alzheimer's Enzyme Biomarkers-BACE1 and Cathepsin D. *Molecules* **2020**, *25*, 274. [CrossRef] [PubMed]
76. Calderon-Garcidueñas, A.L.; Duyckaerts, C. Chapter 23-Alzheimer disease. In *Handbook of Clinical Neurology*; Kovacs, G.G., Alafuzoff, I., Eds.; Elsevier: Amsterdam, The Netherlands, 2018; Volume 145, pp. 325–337.
77. Belsare, K.; Wu, H.; DeGrado, W. Interaction of sTREM2 with Amyloid Beta: Implication on the Protective Role of sTREM2 in Alzheimer's Disease. *FASEB J.* **2020**, *34*, 1. [CrossRef]
78. Halaas, N.B.; Henjum, K.; Blennow, K.; Dakhil, S.; Idland, A.-V.; Nilsson, L.N.; Sederevicius, D.; Vidal-Piñeiro, D.; Walhovd, K.B.; Wyller, T.B.; et al. CSF sTREM2 and Tau Work Together in Predicting Increased Temporal Lobe Atrophy in Older Adults. *Cereb. Cortex* **2019**, *30*, 2295–2306. [CrossRef]

79. Suárez-Calvet, M.; Morenas-Rodríguez, E.; Kleinberger, G.; Schlepckow, K.; Araque Caballero, M.Á.; Franzmeier, N.; Capell, A.; Fellerer, K.; Nuscher, B.; Eren, E.; et al. Early increase of CSF sTREM2 in Alzheimer's disease is associated with tau related-neurodegeneration but not with amyloid-β pathology. *Mol. Neurodegener.* **2019**, *14*, 1. [CrossRef]
80. Falcon, C.; Monté-Rubio, G.C.; Grau-Rivera, O.; Suárez-Calvet, M.; Sánchez-Valle, R.; Rami, L.; Bosch, B.; Haass, C.; Gispert, J.D.; Molinuevo, J.L. CSF glial biomarkers YKL40 and sTREM2 are associated with longitudinal volume and diffusivity changes in cognitively unimpaired individuals. *Neuroimage Clin.* **2019**, *23*, 101801. [CrossRef]
81. Zhong, L.; Xu, Y.; Zhuo, R.; Wang, T.; Wang, K.; Huang, R.; Wang, D.; Gao, Y.; Zhu, Y.; Sheng, X.; et al. Soluble TREM2 ameliorates pathological phenotypes by modulating microglial functions in an Alzheimer's disease model. *Nat. Commun.* **2019**, *10*, 1365. [CrossRef]
82. Knapskog, A.-B.; Henjum, K.; Idland, A.-V.; Eldholm, R.S.; Persson, K.; Saltvedt, I.; Watne, L.O.; Engedal, K.; Nilsson, L.N.G. Cerebrospinal fluid sTREM2 in Alzheimer's disease: Comparisons between clinical presentation and AT classification. *Sci. Rep.* **2020**, *10*, 15886. [CrossRef] [PubMed]
83. Suárez-Calvet, M.; Kleinberger, G.; Araque Caballero, M.; Brendel, M.; Rominger, A.; Alcolea, D.; Fortea, J.; Lleó, A.; Blesa, R.; Gispert, J.D.; et al. sTREM2 cerebrospinal fluid levels are a potential biomarker for microglia activity in early-stage Alzheimer's disease and associate with neuronal injury markers. *EMBO Mol. Med.* **2016**, *8*, 466–476. [CrossRef] [PubMed]
84. Väänänen, T.; Vuolteenaho, K.; Kautiainen, H.; Nieminen, R.; Möttönen, T.; Hannonen, P.; Korpela, M.; Kauppi, M.J.; Laiho, K.; Kaipiainen-Seppänen, O.; et al. Glycoprotein YKL-40: A potential biomarker of disease activity in rheumatoid arthritis during intensive treatment with csDMARDs and infliximab. Evidence from the randomised controlled NEO-RACo trial. *PLoS ONE* **2017**, *12*, e0183294. [CrossRef]
85. Salomon, J.; Matusiak, Ł.; Nowicka-Suszko, D.; Szepietowski, J.C. Chitinase-3-Like Protein 1 (YKL-40) Is a New Biomarker of Inflammation in Psoriasis. *Mediat. Inflamm.* **2017**, *2017*, 9538451. [CrossRef]
86. Llorens, F.; Thüne, K.; Tahir, W.; Kanata, E.; Diaz-Lucena, D.; Xanthopoulos, K.; Kovatsi, E.; Pleschka, C.; Garcia-Esparcia, P.; Schmitz, M.; et al. YKL-40 in the brain and cerebrospinal fluid of neurodegenerative dementias. *Mol. Neurodegen.* **2017**, *12*, 83. [CrossRef]
87. Wang, L.; Gao, T.; Cai, T.; Li, K.; Zheng, P.; Liu, J. Cerebrospinal fluid levels of YKL-40 in prodromal Alzheimer's disease. *Neurosci. Lett.* **2020**, *715*, 134658. [CrossRef]
88. Schmitz, U.; Gupta, S.K.; Vera, J.; Wolkenhauer, O. Computational Approaches in microRNA Biology. In *Encyclopedia of Biomedical Engineering*; Narayan, R., Ed.; Elsevier: Oxford, UK, 2019; pp. 317–330. [CrossRef]
89. O'Brien, J.; Hayder, H.; Zayed, Y.; Peng, C. Overview of MicroRNA Biogenesis, Mechanisms of Actions, and Circulation. *Front. Endocrinol.* **2018**, *9*, 402. [CrossRef]
90. Jevšinek Skok, D.; Hauptman, N.; Boštjančič, E.; Zidar, N. The integrative knowledge base for miRNA-mRNA expression in colorectal cancer. *Sci. Rep.* **2019**, *9*, 18065. [CrossRef]
91. Swarbrick, S.; Wragg, N.; Ghosh, S.; Stolzing, A. Systematic Review of miRNA as Biomarkers in Alzheimer's Disease. *Mol. Neurobiol.* **2019**, *56*, 6156–6167. [CrossRef]
92. Wiedrick, J.T.; Phillips, J.I.; Lusardi, T.A.; McFarland, T.J.; Lind, B.; Sandau, U.S.; Harrington, C.A.; Lapidus, J.A.; Galasko, D.R.; Quinn, J.F.; et al. Validation of MicroRNA Biomarkers for Alzheimer's Disease in Human Cerebrospinal Fluid. *J. Alzheimers Dis.* **2019**, *67*, 875–891. [CrossRef]
93. Mushtaq, G.; Greig, N.H.; Anwar, F.; Zamzami, M.A.; Choudhry, H.; Shaik, M.M.; Tamargo, I.A.; Kamal, M.A. miRNAs as Circulating Biomarkers for Alzheimer's Disease and Parkinson's Disease. *Med. Chem.* **2016**, *12*, 217–225. [CrossRef] [PubMed]
94. Angelucci, F.; Cechova, K.; Valis, M.; Kuca, K.; Zhang, B.; Hort, J. MicroRNAs in Alzheimer's Disease: Diagnostic Markers or Therapeutic Agents? *Front. Pharm.* **2019**, *10*, 665. [CrossRef]
95. Wei, W.; Wang, Z.-Y.; Ma, L.-N.; Zhang, T.-T.; Cao, Y.; Li, H. MicroRNAs in Alzheimer's Disease: Function and Potential Applications as Diagnostic Biomarkers. *Front. Mol. Neurosci.* **2020**, *13*, 160. [CrossRef]
96. Zendjabil, M. Circulating microRNAs as novel biomarkers of Alzheimer's disease. *Clin. Chim. Acta* **2018**, *484*, 99–104. [CrossRef] [PubMed]
97. Tariciotti, L.; Casadei, M.; Honig, L.S.; Teich, A.F.; McKhann Ii, G.M.; Tosto, G.; Mayeux, R. Clinical Experience with Cerebrospinal Fluid Aβ42, Total and Phosphorylated Tau in the Evaluation of 1,016 Individuals for Suspected Dementia. *J. Alzheimers Dis.* **2018**, *65*, 1417–1425. [CrossRef]

98. Slaets, S.; Le Bastard, N.; Martin, J.J.; Sleegers, K.; Van Broeckhoven, C.; De Deyn, P.P.; Engelborghs, S. Cerebrospinal fluid Aβ1-40 improves differential dementia diagnosis in patients with intermediate P-tau181P levels. *J. Alzheimers Dis.* **2013**, *36*, 759–767. [CrossRef] [PubMed]

99. Spies, P.E.; Slats, D.; Sjögren, J.M.; Kremer, B.P.; Verhey, F.R.; Rikkert, M.G.; Verbeek, M.M. The cerebrospinal fluid amyloid beta42/40 ratio in the differentiation of Alzheimer's disease from non-Alzheimer's dementia. *Curr. Alzheimer Res.* **2010**, *7*, 470–476. [CrossRef]

100. Dhiman, K.; Gupta, V.B.; Villemagne, V.L.; Eratne, D.; Graham, P.L.; Fowler, C.; Bourgeat, P.; Li, Q.-X.; Collins, S.; Bush, A.I.; et al. Cerebrospinal fluid neurofilament light concentration predicts brain atrophy and cognition in Alzheimer's disease. *Alzheimer's Dement. Diagn. Assess. Dis. Monit.* **2020**, *12*, e12005. [CrossRef]

101. Janelidze, S.; Zetterberg, H.; Mattsson, N.; Palmqvist, S.; Vanderstichele, H.; Lindberg, O.; van Westen, D.; Stomrud, E.; Minthon, L.; Blennow, K.; et al. CSF Aβ42/Aβ40 and Aβ42/Aβ38 ratios: Better diagnostic markers of Alzheimer disease. *Ann. Clin. Transl. Neurol.* **2016**, *3*, 154–165. [CrossRef]

102. Wellington, H.; Paterson, R.W.; Portelius, E.; Törnqvist, U.; Magdalinou, N.; Fox, N.C.; Blennow, K.; Schott, J.M.; Zetterberg, H. Increased CSF neurogranin concentration is specific to Alzheimer disease. *Neurology* **2016**, *86*, 829–835. [CrossRef]

103. Mouton-Liger, F.; Dumurgier, J.; Cognat, E.; Hourregue, C.; Zetterberg, H.; Vanderstichele, H.; Vanmechelen, E.; Bouaziz-Amar, E.; Blennow, K.; Hugon, J.; et al. CSF levels of the BACE1 substrate NRG1 correlate with cognition in Alzheimer's disease. *Alzheimer's Res. Ther.* **2020**, *12*, 88. [CrossRef]

104. Antonell, A.; Mansilla, A.; Rami, L.; Lladó, A.; Iranzo, A.; Olives, J.; Balasa, M.; Sanchez-Valle, R.; Molinuevo, J. Cerebrospinal Fluid Level of YKL-40 Protein in Preclinical and Prodromal Alzheimer's Disease. *J. Alzheimers Dis.* **2014**, *42*, 901–908. [CrossRef]

105. Altuna-Azkargorta, M.; Mendioroz-Iriarte, M. Blood biomarkers in Alzheimer's disease. *Neurol. (Engl. Ed.)* **2020**. [CrossRef]

106. Hampel, H.; O'Bryant, S.E.; Molinuevo, J.L.; Zetterberg, H.; Masters, C.L.; Lista, S.; Kiddle, S.J.; Batrla, R.; Blennow, K. Blood-based biomarkers for Alzheimer disease: Mapping the road to the clinic. *Nat. Rev. Neurol.* **2018**, *14*, 639–652. [CrossRef] [PubMed]

107. Balasa, R.; Barcutean, L.; Balasa, A.; Motataianu, A.; Roman-Filip, C.; Manu, D. The action of TH17 cells on blood brain barrier in multiple sclerosis and experimental autoimmune encephalomyelitis. *Hum. Immunol.* **2020**, *81*, 237–243. [CrossRef]

108. Zetterberg, H. Blood-based biomarkers for Alzheimer's disease-An update. *J. Neurosci. Methods* **2018**, 319. [CrossRef]

109. Zetterberg, H.; Burnham, S.C. Blood-based molecular biomarkers for Alzheimer's disease. *Mol. Brain* **2019**, *12*, 26. [CrossRef] [PubMed]

110. Gabelli, C. Blood and cerebrospinal fluid biomarkers for Alzheimer's disease. *J. Lab. Precis. Med.* **2020**, 5. [CrossRef]

111. Toombs, J.; Zetterberg, H. In the blood: Biomarkers for amyloid pathology and neurodegeneration in Alzheimer's disease. *Brain Commun.* **2020**, *2*, fcaa054. [CrossRef] [PubMed]

112. Oeckl, P.; Otto, M. A Review on MS-Based Blood Biomarkers for Alzheimer's Disease. *Neurol. Ther.* **2019**, *8*, 113–127. [CrossRef] [PubMed]

113. O'Bryant, S.E. Blood Biomarkers for Use in Alzheimer Disease—Moving From "If" to "How?". *JAMA Neurol.* **2019**, *76*, 1009–1010. [CrossRef] [PubMed]

114. Liu, Z.; Chen, H.; Wold, E.A.; Zhou, J. 2.13-Small-Molecule Inhibitors of Protein–Protein Interactions. In *Comprehensive Medicinal Chemistry III*; Chackalamannil, S., Rotella, D., Ward, S.E., Eds.; Elsevier: Oxford, UK, 2017; pp. 329–353. [CrossRef]

115. Mercier, J.; Provins, L.; Hannestad, J. 7.02-Progress and Challenges in the Development of PET Ligands to Aid CNS Drug Discovery. In *Comprehensive Medicinal Chemistry III*; Chackalamannil, S., Rotella, D., Ward, S.E., Eds.; Elsevier: Oxford, UK, 2017; pp. 20–64. [CrossRef]

116. Patel, P.; Woodgett, J.R. Chapter Eight-Glycogen Synthase Kinase 3: A Kinase for All Pathways? In *Current Topics in Developmental Biology*; Jenny, A., Ed.; Academic Press: Cambridge, MA, USA, 2017; Volume 123, pp. 277–302.

117. Shi, X.-L.; Yan, N.; Cui, Y.-J.; Liu, Z.-P. A Unique GSK-3β inhibitor B10 Has a Direct Effect on Aβ, Targets Tau and Metal Dyshomeostasis, and Promotes Neuronal Neurite Outgrowth. *Cells* **2020**, *9*, 649. [CrossRef] [PubMed]

118. Hugon, J.; Mouton-Liger, F.; Cognat, E.; Dumurgier, J.; Paquet, C. Blood-Based Kinase Assessments in Alzheimer's Disease. *Front Aging Neurosci.* **2018**, *10*, 338. [CrossRef]
119. Paciorkowski, A.R.; Seltzer, L.E.; Neul, J.L. 32-Developmental Encephalopathies. In *Swaiman's Pediatric Neurology (Sixth Edition)*; Swaiman, K.F., Ashwal, S., Ferriero, D.M., Schor, N.F., Finkel, R.S., Gropman, A.L., Pearl, P.L., Shevell, M.I., Eds.; Elsevier: Amsterdam, The Netherlands, 2017; pp. 242–248. [CrossRef]
120. McNerney, M.W.; Mobley, W.C.; Salehi, A. Down Syndrome or Trisomy 21☆. In *Reference Module in Neuroscience and Biobehavioral Psychology*; Elsevier: Amsterdam, The Netherlands, 2017. [CrossRef]
121. Kaas, G.A.; Hawkins, K.E.; Sweatt, J.D. 4.19-Genetic Mechanisms of Memory Disorders (Excluding Alzheimer's Disease). In *Learning and Memory: A Comprehensive Reference*, 2nd ed.; Byrne, J.H., Ed.; Academic Press: Oxford, UK, 2017; pp. 371–401. [CrossRef]
122. Dowjat, K.; Adayev, T.; Wojda, U.; Brzozowska, K.; Barczak, A.; Gabryelewicz, T.; Hwang, Y.-W. Abnormalities of DYRK1A-Cytoskeleton Complexes in the Blood Cells as Potential Biomarkers of Alzheimer's Disease. *J. Alzheimers Dis.* **2019**, *72*, 1059–1075. [CrossRef] [PubMed]
123. Mattsson, N.; Cullen, N.C.; Andreasson, U.; Zetterberg, H.; Blennow, K. Association Between Longitudinal Plasma Neurofilament Light and Neurodegeneration in Patients With Alzheimer Disease. *JAMA Neurol.* **2019**, *76*, 791–799. [CrossRef] [PubMed]
124. van der Ende, E.L.; Meeter, L.H.; Poos, J.M.; Panman, J.L.; Jiskoot, L.C.; Dopper, E.G.P.; Papma, J.M.; de Jong, F.J.; Verberk, I.M.W.; Teunissen, C.; et al. Serum neurofilament light chain in genetic frontotemporal dementia: A longitudinal, multicentre cohort study. *Lancet Neurol.* **2019**, *18*, 1103–1111. [CrossRef]
125. Weston, P.S.J.; Poole, T.; Ryan, N.S.; Nair, A.; Liang, Y.; Macpherson, K.; Druyeh, R.; Malone, I.B.; Ahsan, R.L.; Pemberton, H.; et al. Serum neurofilament light in familial Alzheimer disease: A marker of early neurodegeneration. *Neurology* **2017**, *89*, 2167–2175. [CrossRef]
126. Kinney, J.W.; Bemiller, S.M.; Murtishaw, A.S.; Leisgang, A.M.; Salazar, A.M.; Lamb, B.T. Inflammation as a central mechanism in Alzheimer's disease. *Alzheimers Dement* **2018**, *4*, 575–590. [CrossRef]
127. Newcombe, E.A.; Camats-Perna, J.; Silva, M.L.; Valmas, N.; Huat, T.J.; Medeiros, R. Inflammation: The link between co-morbidities, genetics, and Alzheimer's disease. *J. Neuroinflamm.* **2018**, *15*, 276. [CrossRef]
128. Figueroa, D.M.; Gordon, E.M.; Yao, X.; Levine, S.J. Chapter 13-Apolipoproteins as context-dependent regulators of lung inflammation. In *Mechanisms and Manifestations of Obesity in Lung Disease*; Johnston, R.A., Suratt, B.T., Eds.; Academic Press: Cambridge, MA, USA, 2019; pp. 301–326. [CrossRef]
129. Bornhorst, J.A.; Mbughuni, M.M. Chapter 3-Alcohol Biomarkers: Clinical Issues and Analytical Methods. In *Critical Issues in Alcohol and Drugs of Abuse Testing*, 2nd ed.; Dasgupta, A., Ed.; Academic Press: Cambridge, MA, USA, 2019; pp. 25–42. [CrossRef]
130. Foster, E.M.; Dangla-Valls, A.; Lovestone, S.; Ribe, E.M.; Buckley, N.J. Clusterin in Alzheimer's Disease: Mechanisms, Genetics, and Lessons From Other Pathologies. *Front. Neurosci.* **2019**, *13*, 164. [CrossRef]
131. Wu, Z.-C.; Yu, J.-T.; Li, Y.; Tan, L. Chapter 5-Clusterin in Alzheimer's disease. In *Advances in Clinical Chemistry*; Makowski, G.S., Ed.; Elsevier: Amsterdam, The Netherlands, 2012; Volume 56, pp. 155–173.
132. Kaneko, N.; Nakamura, A.; Washimi, Y.; Kato, T.; Sakurai, T.; Arahata, Y.; Bundo, M.; Takeda, A.; Niida, S.; Ito, K.; et al. Novel plasma biomarker surrogating cerebral amyloid deposition. *Proc. Jpn. Acad. Ser. B Phys. Biol. Sci.* **2014**, *90*, 353–364. [CrossRef] [PubMed]
133. Janelidze, S.; Stomrud, E.; Palmqvist, S.; Zetterberg, H.; van Westen, D.; Jeromin, A.; Song, L.; Hanlon, D.; Tan Hehir, C.A.; Baker, D.; et al. Plasma β-amyloid in Alzheimer's disease and vascular disease. *Sci. Rep.* **2016**, *6*, 26801. [CrossRef] [PubMed]
134. Fossati, S.; Ramos Cejudo, J.; Debure, L.; Pirraglia, E.; Sone, J.Y.; Li, Y.; Chen, J.; Butler, T.; Zetterberg, H.; Blennow, K.; et al. Plasma tau complements CSF tau and P-tau in the diagnosis of Alzheimer's disease. *Alzheimer's Dement. Diagn. Assess. Dis. Monit.* **2019**, *11*, 483–492. [CrossRef] [PubMed]
135. Karikari, T.K.; Pascoal, T.A.; Ashton, N.J.; Janelidze, S.; Benedet, A.L.; Rodriguez, J.L.; Chamoun, M.; Savard, M.; Kang, M.S.; Therriault, J.J.T.L.N. Blood phosphorylated tau 181 as a biomarker for Alzheimer's disease: A diagnostic performance and prediction modelling study using data from four prospective cohorts. *Lancet Neurol.* **2020**, *19*, 422–433. [CrossRef]
136. Lewczuk, P.; Ermann, N.; Andreasson, U.; Schultheis, C.; Podhorna, J.; Spitzer, P.; Maler, J.M.; Kornhuber, J.; Blennow, K.; Zetterberg, H. Plasma neurofilament light as a potential biomarker of neurodegeneration in Alzheimer's disease. *Alzheimer's Res. Ther.* **2018**, *10*, 71. [CrossRef] [PubMed]

137. Vishnu, V.Y.; Modi, M.; Sharma, S.; Mohanty, M.; Goyal, M.K.; Lal, V.; Khandelwal, N.; Mittal, B.R.; Prabhakar, S. Role of Plasma Clusterin in Alzheimer's Disease-A Pilot Study in a Tertiary Hospital in Northern India. *PLoS ONE* **2016**, *11*, e0166369. [CrossRef]
138. Lorenzo-Pouso, A.I.; Pérez-Sayáns, M.; Bravo, S.B.; López-Jornet, P.; García-Vence, M.; Alonso-Sampedro, M.; Carballo, J.; García-García, A. Protein-Based Salivary Profiles as Novel Biomarkers for Oral Diseases. *Dis. Markers* **2018**, *2018*, 6141845. [CrossRef]
139. Farah, R.; Haraty, H.; Salame, Z.; Fares, Y.; Ojcius, D.M.; Said Sadier, N. Salivary biomarkers for the diagnosis and monitoring of neurological diseases. *Biomed. J.* **2018**, *41*, 63–87. [CrossRef]
140. Jasim, H.; Carlsson, A.; Hedenberg-Magnusson, B.; Ghafouri, B.; Ernberg, M. Saliva as a medium to detect and measure biomarkers related to pain. *Sci. Rep.* **2018**, *8*, 3220. [CrossRef]
141. Smith, R.; Chepisheva, M.; Cronin, T.; Seemungal, B.M. Chapter 16-Diagnostic Approaches Techniques in Concussion/Mild Traumatic Brain Injury: Where are we? In *Neurosensory Disorders in Mild Traumatic Brain Injury*; Hoffer, M.E., Balaban, C.D., Eds.; Academic Press: Cambridge, MA, USA, 2019; pp. 247–277. [CrossRef]
142. Güvenç, I.A. *Salivary Glands: New Approaches in Diagnostics and Treatment*; BoD–Books on Demand: Hamburg, Germany, 2019.
143. Engeland, C.G.; Bosch, J.A.; Rohleder, N.J.C.O.I.B.S. Salivary biomarkers in psychoneuroimmunology. *Curr. Opin. Behav. Sci.* **2019**, *28*, 58–65. [CrossRef]
144. Andrews, J.L.; Fernandez, F. Salivary biomarkers in Alzheimer's disease. In *Diagnosis and Management in Dementia*; Elsevier: Amsterdam, The Netherlands, 2020; pp. 239–254.
145. Rapado-González, Ó.; Martínez-Reglero, C.; Salgado-Barreira, Á.; Takkouche, B.; López-López, R.; Suárez-Cunqueiro, M.M.; Muinelo-Romay, L. Salivary biomarkers for cancer diagnosis: A meta-analysis. *Ann. Med.* **2020**, *52*, 131–144. [CrossRef] [PubMed]
146. Cristaldi, M.; Mauceri, R.; Di Fede, O.; Giuliana, G.; Campisi, G.; Panzarella, V. Salivary Biomarkers for Oral Squamous Cell Carcinoma Diagnosis and Follow-Up: Current Status and Perspectives. *Front. Physiol.* **2019**, *10*, 1476. [CrossRef] [PubMed]
147. Tvarijonaviciute, A.; Zamora, C.; Ceron, J.J.; Bravo-Cantero, A.F.; Pardo-Marin, L.; Valverde, S.; Lopez-Jornet, P. Salivary biomarkers in Alzheimer's disease. *Clin. Oral Investig.* **2020**. [CrossRef] [PubMed]
148. Ashton, N.J.; Ide, M.; Zetterberg, H.; Blennow, K. Salivary Biomarkers for Alzheimer's Disease and Related Disorders. *Neurol. Ther.* **2019**, *8*, 83–94. [CrossRef] [PubMed]
149. Sabbagh, M.N.; Shi, J.; Lee, M.; Arnold, L.; Al-Hasan, Y.; Heim, J.; McGeer, P. Salivary beta amyloid protein levels are detectable and differentiate patients with Alzheimer's disease dementia from normal controls: Preliminary findings. *BMC Neurol.* **2018**, *18*, 155. [CrossRef] [PubMed]
150. Lee, M.; Guo, J.-P.; Kennedy, K.; McGeer, E.; McGeer, P. A Method for Diagnosing Alzheimer's Disease Based on Salivary Amyloid-β Protein 42 Levels. *J. Alzheimer's Dis.* **2016**, *55*, 1–8. [CrossRef]
151. Liang, D.; Lu, H. Salivary biological biomarkers for Alzheimer's disease. *Arch. Oral Biol.* **2019**, *105*, 5–12. [CrossRef]
152. Gleerup, H.S.; Hasselbalch, S.G.; Simonsen, A.H. Biomarkers for Alzheimer's Disease in Saliva: A Systematic Review. *Dis. Markers* **2019**, *2019*, 4761054. [CrossRef]
153. Pekeles, H.; Qureshi, H.Y.; Paudel, H.K.; Schipper, H.M.; Gornistky, M.; Chertkow, H. Development and validation of a salivary tau biomarker in Alzheimer's disease. *Alzheimer's Dement. Diagn. Assess. Dis. Monit.* **2019**, *11*, 53–60. [CrossRef]
154. Ashton, N.J.; Ide, M.; Schöll, M.; Blennow, K.; Lovestone, S.; Hye, A.; Zetterberg, H. No association of salivary total tau concentration with Alzheimer's disease. *Neurobiol. Aging* **2018**, *70*, 125–127. [CrossRef]
155. Bittner, E.A.; Martyn, J.A.J. 21-Neuromuscular Physiology and Pharmacology. In *Pharmacology and Physiology for Anesthesia*, 2nd ed.; Hemmings, H.C., Egan, T.D., Eds.; Elsevier: Philadelphia, PA, USA, 2019; pp. 412–427. [CrossRef]
156. Trang, A.; Khandhar, P.B. Physiology, Acetylcholinesterase. In *StatPearls [Internet]*; StatPearls Publishing: St, Petersburd, FL, USA, 2019.
157. Lushchekina, S.V.; Masson, P. Slow-binding inhibitors of acetylcholinesterase of medical interest. *Neuropharmacology* **2020**, *177*, 108236. [CrossRef] [PubMed]

158. Reale, M.; Gonzales-Portillo, I.; Borlongan, C.V. Saliva, an easily accessible fluid as diagnostic tool and potent stem cell source for Alzheimer's Disease: Present and future applications. *Brain Res.* **2020**, *1727*, 146535. [CrossRef] [PubMed]
159. Sharma, R. Chapter 17-Whey Proteins in Functional Foods. In *Whey Proteins*; Deeth, H.C., Bansal, N., Eds.; Academic Press: Cambridge, MA, USA, 2019; pp. 637–663. [CrossRef]
160. Mudgil, D.; Barak, S. 3-Dairy-Based Functional Beverages. In *Milk-Based Beverages*; Grumezescu, A.M., Holban, A.M., Eds.; Woodhead Publishing Sawton: Cambridge, UK, 2019; pp. 67–93. [CrossRef]
161. Bourbon, A.I.; Martins, J.T.; Pinheiro, A.C.; Madalena, D.A.; Marques, A.; Nunes, R.; Vicente, A.A. 6-Nanoparticles of lactoferrin for encapsulation of food ingredients. In *Biopolymer Nanostructures for Food Encapsulation Purposes*; Jafari, S.M., Ed.; Academic Press: Cambridge, MA, USA, 2019; pp. 147–168. [CrossRef]
162. Mehmood, A.M.M.T.; Iyer, A.B.; Arif, S.; Junaid, M.; Khan, R.S.; Nazir, W.; Khalid, N. 5-Whey Protein-Based Functional Energy Drinks Formulation and Characterization. In *Sports and Energy Drinks*; Grumezescu, A.M., Holban, A.M., Eds.; Woodhead Publishing Sawton: Cambridge, UK, 2019; pp. 161–181. [CrossRef]
163. Karav, S. Chapter 22-Application of a Novel Endo-β-N-Acetylglucosaminidase to Isolate an Entirely New Class of Bioactive Compounds: N-Glycans. In *Enzymes in Food Biotechnology*; Kuddus, M., Ed.; Academic Press: Cambridge, MA, USA, 2019; pp. 389–404. [CrossRef]
164. González-Sánchez, M.; Bartolome, F.; Antequera, D.; Puertas-Martín, V.; González, P.; Gómez-Grande, A.; Llamas-Velasco, S.; San Martín, A.H.; Pérez-Martínez, D.; Villarejo-Galende, A. Decreased salivary lactoferrin levels are specific to Alzheimer's disease. *EBioMedicine* **2020**, *57*. [CrossRef] [PubMed]
165. Mohamed, W.A.; Salama, R.M.; Schaalan, M.F. A pilot study on the effect of lactoferrin on Alzheimer's disease pathological sequelae: Impact of the p-Akt/PTEN pathway. *Biomed. Pharmacother.* **2019**, *111*, 714–723. [CrossRef]
166. Paraskevaidi, M.; Allsop, D.; Karim, S.; Martin, F.L.; Crean, S. Diagnostic Biomarkers for Alzheimer's Disease Using Non-Invasive Specimens. *J. Clin. Med.* **2020**, *9*, 1673. [CrossRef]
167. Dupree, E.J.; Darie, C.C.J.E. Examination of a non-invasive biomarker for the diagnosis of prodromal Alzheimer's disease and Alzheimer's disease Dementia. *EBioMedicine* **2020**, *57*. [CrossRef]
168. Carro, E.; Bartolomé, F.; Bermejo-Pareja, F.; Villarejo-Galende, A.; Molina, J.A.; Ortiz, P.; Calero, M.; Rabano, A.; Cantero, J.L.; Orive, G. Early diagnosis of mild cognitive impairment and Alzheimer's disease based on salivary lactoferrin. *Alzheimer's Dement. Diagn. Assess. Dis. Monit.* **2017**, *8*, 131–138. [CrossRef]
169. Bermejo-Pareja, F.; Antequera, D.; Vargas, T.; Molina, J.A.; Carro, E. Saliva levels of Abeta1-42 as potential biomarker of Alzheimer's disease: A pilot study. *BMC Neurol.* **2010**, *10*, 108. [CrossRef]
170. Bakhtiari, S.; Moghadam, N.B.; Ehsani, M.; Mortazavi, H.; Sabour, S.; Bakhshi, M.J.J.O.C.; JCDR, D.R. Can salivary acetylcholinesterase be a diagnostic biomarker for Alzheimer? *J. Clin. Diagn. Res.* **2017**, *11*, ZC58. [CrossRef]
171. Hagan, S.; Martin, E.; Enríquez-de-Salamanca, A. Tear fluid biomarkers in ocular and systemic disease: Potential use for predictive, preventive and personalised medicine. *EPMA J.* **2016**, *7*, 15. [CrossRef]
172. Jing, J.; Gao, Y. Urine biomarkers in the early stages of diseases: Current status and perspective. *Discov. Med.* **2018**, *25*, 57–65.
173. Harpole, M.; Davis, J.; Espina, V. Current state of the art for enhancing urine biomarker discovery. *Expert Rev. Proteom.* **2016**, *13*, 609–626. [CrossRef]
174. Hrubešová, K.; Fousková, M.; Habartová, L.; Fišar, Z.; Jirák, R.; Raboch, J.; Setnička, V. Search for biomarkers of Alzheimer's disease: Recent insights, current challenges and future prospects. *Clin. Biochem.* **2019**, *72*, 39–51. [CrossRef]
175. Hartmann, S.; Kist, T.B.L. A review of biomarkers of Alzheimer's disease in non-invasive samples. *Biomark. Med.* **2018**, *12*, 677–690. [CrossRef] [PubMed]
176. García-Blanco, A.; Peña-Bautista, C.; Oger, C.; Vigor, C.; Galano, J.-M.; Durand, T.; Martín-Ibáñez, N.; Baquero, M.; Vento, M.; Cháfer-Pericás, C. Reliable determination of new lipid peroxidation compounds as potential early Alzheimer Disease biomarkers. *Talanta* **2018**, *184*, 193–201. [CrossRef] [PubMed]
177. Dunstan, R.H.; Sparkes, D.L.; Macdonald, M.M.; De Jonge, X.J.; Dascombe, B.J.; Gottfries, J.; Gottfries, C.G.; Roberts, T.K. Diverse characteristics of the urinary excretion of amino acids in humans and the use of amino acid supplementation to reduce fatigue and sub-health in adults. *Nutr. J.* **2017**, *16*, 19. [CrossRef]

178. Zengi, O.; Karakas, A.; Ergun, U.; Senes, M.; Inan, L.; Yucel, D. Urinary 8-hydroxy-2′-deoxyguanosine level and plasma paraoxonase 1 activity with Alzheimer's disease %J Clinical Chemistry and Laboratory Medicine (CCLM). *Clin. Chem. Lab. Med.* **2012**, *50*, 529. [CrossRef] [PubMed]
179. Tamhane, M.; Cabrera-Ghayouri, S.; Abelian, G.; Viswanath, V. Review of Biomarkers in Ocular Matrices: Challenges and Opportunities. *Pharm. Res.* **2019**, *36*, 40. [CrossRef]
180. Iyengar, M.F.; Soto, L.F.; Requena, D.; Ruiz-Alejos, A.O.; Huaylinos, Y.; Velasquez, R.; Bernabe-Ortiz, A.; Gilman, R.H. Tear biomarkers and corneal sensitivity as an indicator of neuropathy in type 2 diabetes. *Diabetes Res. Clin. Pract.* **2020**, *163*, 108143. [CrossRef]
181. Willcox, M.D. Tear film, contact lenses and tear biomarkers. *Clin. Exp. Optom.* **2019**, *102*, 350–363. [CrossRef]
182. Fong, P.Y.; Shih, K.C.; Lam, P.Y.; Chan, T.C.Y.; Jhanji, V.; Tong, L. Role of tear film biomarkers in the diagnosis and management of dry eye disease. *Taiwan J. Ophthalmol.* **2019**, *9*, 150–159. [CrossRef] [PubMed]
183. Lim, J.K.H.; Li, Q.-X.; He, Z.; Vingrys, A.J.; Wong, V.H.Y.; Currier, N.; Mullen, J.; Bui, B.V.; Nguyen, C.T.O. The Eye as a Biomarker for Alzheimer's Disease. *Front. Neurosci.* **2016**, *10*, 536. [CrossRef] [PubMed]
184. Wood, H. Could tear proteins be biomarkers for Alzheimer disease? *Nat. Rev. Neurol.* **2016**, *12*, 432. [CrossRef] [PubMed]
185. Kalló, G.; Emri, M.; Varga, Z.; Ujhelyi, B.; Tőzsér, J.; Csutak, A.; Csősz, É. Changes in the Chemical Barrier Composition of Tears in Alzheimer's Disease Reveal Potential Tear Diagnostic Biomarkers. *PLoS ONE* **2016**, *11*, e0158000. [CrossRef] [PubMed]
186. Gijs, M.; Nuijts, R.M.; Ramakers, I.; Verhey, F.; Webers, C.A.J.I.O.; Science, V. Differences in tear protein biomarkers between patients with Alzheimer's disease and controls. *Investig. Ophthalmol. Vis. Sci.* **2019**, *60*, 1744.
187. Kenny, A.; Jiménez-Mateos, E.M.; Zea-Sevilla, M.A.; Rábano, A.; Gili-Manzanaro, P.; Prehn, J.H.M.; Henshall, D.C.; Ávila, J.; Engel, T.; Hernández, F. Proteins and microRNAs are differentially expressed in tear fluid from patients with Alzheimer's disease. *Sci. Rep.* **2019**, *9*, 15437. [CrossRef]
188. François, M.; Bull, C.F.; Fenech, M.F.; Leifert, W.R.J.C.A.R. Current state of saliva biomarkers for aging and Alzheimer's disease. *Curr. Alzheimer Res.* **2019**, *16*, 56–66. [CrossRef]

Publisher's Note: MDPI stays neutral with regard to jurisdictional claims in published maps and institutional affiliations.

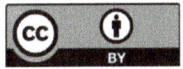

© 2020 by the authors. Licensee MDPI, Basel, Switzerland. This article is an open access article distributed under the terms and conditions of the Creative Commons Attribution (CC BY) license (http://creativecommons.org/licenses/by/4.0/).

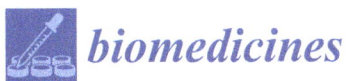

Review

NURR1 Alterations in Perinatal Stress: A First Step towards Late-Onset Diseases? A Narrative Review

Laura Bordoni [1], Irene Petracci [2], Jean Calleja-Agius [3], Joan G. Lalor [4] and Rosita Gabbianelli [1,*]

1. Unit of Molecular Biology and Nutrigenomics, School of Pharmacy, University of Camerino, 62032 Camerino, Italy; laura.bordoni@unicam.it
2. School of Advanced Studies, University of Camerino, 62032 Camerino, Italy; irene.petracci@unicam.it
3. Department of Anatomy, Faculty of Medicine and Surgery, University of Malta, MSD2080 Msida, Malta; jean.calleja-agius@um.edu.mt
4. School of Nursing and Midwifery, Trinity College Dublin, 24 D'Olier Street, Dublin 2, Ireland; j.lalor@tcd.ie
* Correspondence: rosita.gabbianelli@unicam.it; Tel.: +39-0737-634308

Received: 5 November 2020; Accepted: 7 December 2020; Published: 8 December 2020

Abstract: Perinatal life represents a delicate phase of development where stimuli of all sorts, coming to or from the mother, can influence the programming of the future baby's health. These stimuli may have consequences that persist throughout adulthood. Nuclear receptor related 1 protein (NURR1), a transcription factor with a critical role in the development of the dopaminergic neurons in the midbrain, mediates the response to stressful environmental stimuli in the perinatal period. During pregnancy, low-grade inflammation triggered by maternal obesity, hyperinsulinemia or vaginal infections alters NURR1 expression in human gestational tissues. A similar scenario is triggered by exposure to neurotoxic compounds, which are associated with *NURR1* epigenetic deregulation in the offspring, with potential intergenerational effects. Since these alterations have been associated with an increased risk of developing late-onset diseases in children, NURR1, alone, or in combination with other molecular markers, has been proposed as a new prognostic tool and a potential therapeutic target for several pathological conditions. This narrative review describes perinatal stress associated with *NURR1* gene deregulation, which is proposed here as a mediator of late-onset consequences of early life events.

Keywords: perinatal stress; NURR1; inflammation; late-onset diseases; early life

1. Introduction

Perinatal stress due to various environmental stimuli can have an impact on early fetal development, leading to long-term effects on cellular homeostasis [1–4]. Both prenatal and postnatal factors such as maternal nutrition, environmental pesticide exposure, stress, suboptimal antenatal care and neonatal trauma can cause epigenetic changes and impaired gene expression, especially at the neuronal level, with a consequent impact on fetal brain development and function [5].

According to the Barker hypothesis, in utero and postnatal stressors permanently program the structure and the physiology of the offspring, as a manifestation of the developmental plasticity to specific environmental stimuli [6]. This plasticity appears advantageous since it creates phenotypes that, once outside of the womb, are better matched to the environment that they are expected to enter into [6]. However, if in utero conditions do not match those following childbirth, this adaptive response could turn into a harmful mechanism. For instance, if the imprint left by a limited availability of nutrients during the prenatal stage is followed by overnutrition later in childhood, the risk of developing metabolic disorders increases, with consequent permanent changes in the metabolism of glucose-insulin established in the prenatal period [7]. The duration and timescale of exposure to various stimuli in early life are of key importance due to perinatal epigenetic plasticity. The interplay between environmental stimuli and genetic susceptibility in response to environmental stress is of a crucial importance in determining the final phenotype. Several genes play key roles in counterbalancing stress and maintaining cellular homeostasis. In the brain, the nuclear receptor related 1 protein (NURR1), a transcription factor able to modulate differentiation, survival and function of dopaminergic neurons, has been demonstrated to exert a neuroprotective role against neuropathological stress or insults. NURR1, as a glucocorticoid-responsive transcription factor, has an important endocrine regulatory role. It is a key factor in modulating the adaptive responses to stress by influencing the transcription of target genes in the hypothalamus-pituitary-adrenal axis (HPA), the major stress-responsive neuroendocrine system [8,9]. Changes in NURR1 expression have been observed in neurodegenerative conditions such as Parkinson's disease (PD) and Alzheimer's disease (AD), as well as in stroke and in multiple sclerosis [10,11]. NURR1 deregulation is also a causative factor for the onset of schizophrenia, through the modulation of genes associated with this pathology, particularly the dopamine D2 receptor co-expression gene set [12,13]. Considering epidemiological data on human cohorts [14–16] as well as the outcomes observed in PD animal models [17–21], it has been demonstrated that environmental stress during early life influences the programming of adult neuronal health. Thus, neonatal life represents the starting point during which the control of environmental stimuli can significantly drive the onset of neurodegeneration and other late-onset diseases.

This narrative review aims to describe the long-term effects of major environmental stressors occurring during the perinatal period and that affect NURR1 gene regulation. PubMed database was used for the search of peer-reviewed original research articles in English, published up to October 2020, without including electronic early-release publications. Search terms included "Nurr1" or "Nr4a2"and "disease" or "early-life" or "perinatal or prenatal" or "stress" or "trauma" or "inflammation" or "epigenetics" or "environmental exposure". The abstracts of retrieved citations were reviewed and prioritized by relevant content. Full articles were collected and secondary references from these articles were screened for inclusion.

This manuscript discusses how early determinants and maternal stress in perinatal life can modulate dopaminergic neuron homeostasis, as well as inflammatory and metabolic pathways, and affect health status later in life. The value of the early identification of risk factors lies in the fact that it may assist the introduction of prevention strategies aimed at reducing the burden of chronic diseases later in life. Consequently, it will assist policymakers to adopt appropriate clinical guidelines to prevent neuronal damage and inflammation-related diseases.

2. Early Determinants of Human Health

Increasing rates of prevalence of noncommunicable diseases (NCDs) (i.e., heart disease, diabetes, chronic respiratory diseases, cancer, PD, AD, mental illness, etc.) over recent decades, have been well-documented on a global scale. It is of particular concerning that the age of onset is reducing [22,23]. Major risk factors associated with the onset of NCDs are unhealthy diet, physical inactivity, alcohol consumption, smoking, air pollution and food xenobiotic exposure [24,25]. Considering the experimental, clinical and epidemiological evidence on the impact of early life on a wide range of NCDs, epigenetic processes occurring during the perinatal period have been identified as major mechanisms in the regulation of health later in life [26]. Human health can be programmed during prenatal and postnatal life as nutrition, life style, environment and genetics regulate gene expression and shape the phenotype. Starting from early prenatal life, parental exposure to healthy and unhealthy factors influence the child's epigenome, driving long-term effects on the adult health [27]. Paternal body weight, maternal caloric overload, junk food consumption and malnutrition exert their impact not only on child body weight at birth, but also on his/her inflammatory responses. A correlation between prenatal maternal depression and cytokine levels has been observed in postmortem fetal brains in response to the maternal condition, suggesting that proinflammatory cytokine genes can be expressed in specific fetal brain regions and may influence their development [28–30].

Furthermore, maternal education can influence the duration of breastfeeding, which impacts the infant's oral tolerance through immune modulation, the epithelial barrier function, the intestinal microbiome and body weight [31,32]. Shorter lengths of breastfeeding have been associated with increased proinflammatory responses, such as the production of interleukin 6 (IL-6) and C-reactive protein in the mother and in her offspring when reaching adulthood [33].

Social determinants of health, such as local neighborhood, social environment, exposure to chronic stress, education levels, socioeconomic status and access to health care, can cause epigenetic perturbations that influence disease susceptibility throughout life [34]. Social inequalities such as lower parental income/wealth, educational attainment, occupational social class, parental unemployment and lack of housing have been linked to unfavorable child health and development [35]. Poor housing conditions impact indoor air quality, leading, for example, to worsening asthma by epigenetic modulation [34]. Furthermore, in disadvantaged areas, the intake of healthy food is limited, with an excess of regular consumption of ultra-processed food, alcohol and tobacco, which contribute to the development of unhealthy phenotypes [34]. A low socioeconomical status, increased maternal weight and physical inactivity have been found to be related to children's weight and height [36,37]. A direct correlation between family income and child health also exists. In the United States of America, children aged <17 years living in poor families are at an increased risk of suffering from poor health [38]. All in all, the social determinants of health have been defined by the World Health Organization as "the conditions in which people are born, grow, live, work and age" and "the fundamental drivers of these conditions" can affect health-related behaviors. Levels of family income and education are strongly associated with a wide range of health outcomes. Life expectancy in men and women and infant mortality rate are directly related to educational attainment. Parental education has an impact on children's health because it influences dietary choices and exercise options early in life [38]. Finally, in addition to lifestyle-related determinants of health, traumatic events occurring in the perinatal life can also have a major impact on the child's future health.

3. Stressful Events that Might Occur in Perinatal Life

Several stressful events might occur during the perinatal life, thus impacting on the health status of children both in early and later life, in particular as they are related to the development of the central nervous system (CNS). Prenatal exposure to inflammatory insults has been shown to lead to neurodevelopmental disorders [39]. In particular, maternal infection has been associated with long-term neurological and neuro-psychiatric morbidity in the offspring [40]. Maternal immune activation in animal models induces transgenerational effects on the brain and behavior [41]. Maternal chorioamnionitis is associated with cerebral palsy in the offspring, independently of other factors such as preterm delivery and birthweight [42]. Prematurity is associated with perinatal neuroinflammation and injury [43], and maternal inflammation has been identified as a major risk factor for premature birth. After birth, premature infants often require supplemental oxygen for survival, and this exposure can lead to additional inflammatory responses. Adults born preterm are at an increased risk of suffering from long-term conditions as a consequence of the severe disruption of the normal developmental maturation of organ systems. These adverse health problems, which tend to appear earlier in the pre-term-born population, include neurological and mental health problems, hypertension, diabetes, cardiac dysfunction and obstructive lung disease [44]. Instead, the risk of developing asthma and allergic diseases in adult life is higher in babies born by caesarean section [45,46]. Babies born by caesarean section have a reduced diversity of gut microflora when compared to babies delivered vaginally, and this seems to be the most likely explanation for the increase in allergic diseases, given the impact of gastrointestinal flora on the neonate's immune system [47,48]. Maternal thyroid hormones are essential for normal neurodevelopment in the offspring, even after the onset of fetal thyroid function. This is particularly relevant for preterm infants who are deprived of maternal thyroid hormones following birth, who are at risk of suffering from hypothyroidism, and more likely to develop attention-deficit/hyperactivity disorder [49]. Rat models show that hypothyroid lactating females have a persistent low-quality milk, and both male and female hypothyroid offspring born of hypothyroid mothers gain less body mass with lower total adipose reserves and higher visceral reserves. The hypothyroid offspring also have higher levels of blood glucose, insulin and leptin, as well as dyslipidemia [50]. These long-term anthropometric effects have also been observed in humans [49]. Maternal diet has both short-term and long-term implications on fetal and child health. Maternal malnutrition can lead to micronutrient inadequacies and a suboptimal macronutrient balance [51–53]. For example, vitamin D deficiency together with maternal immune activation during development can induce schizophrenia-relevant dopaminergic abnormalities in the adult offspring of animal models [54]. Treating mothers with vitamin D could possibly lead to early neuroprotection to the fetus, since it has been shown to increase the number and the expression of mature Nurr1 mesencephalic dopaminergic neurons. Similar findings were observed in mothers with vitamin B deficiencies [55]. Bad eating habits can lead to maternal obesity with undesirable metabolism, which in turn influence the maternal health and, in the infant, lead to longer-term metabolic, neuropsychiatric and cognitive health consequences [56–58]. For instance, altered levels of plasma ceramides in the offspring of obese mothers have been implicated as early predictors of metabolic disease [59]. Maternal obesity has been implicated as being an independent risk factor of short- and long-term neuropsychiatric disorders in the offspring [60]. Low-grade inflammation is a central feature of pregnancies complicated by maternal obesity. This has also been observed in maternal type 2 diabetes, including gestational diabetes mellitus (GDM) [61]. Exposure in utero to maternal hyperglycemia, and consequent fetal hyperinsulinemia, carries not only several short-term consequences in the offspring, but also prompts metabolic imprinting that results in a greater risk of adverse long-term metabolic outcomes later in life. In particular, exposure in utero to maternal diabetes seems to influence long-term metabolic outcomes. The offspring of obese and/or mothers with diabetes carry a higher risk of obesity and type 2 diabetes, thus leading to a vicious cycle for future generations [62]. Exposure to toxins, including maternal smoking, is detrimental to the offspring. Animal models confirm that prenatal exposure to gestational nicotine before neurulation has a negative impact on the offspring's neurodevelopment [63]. Epidemiological studies show that in utero exposure to maternal active and passive smoking has long-term neurological effects on the children [64,65]. This has also been demonstrated for other environmental toxins, such as perchlorate [66]. Similarly, the safety of anesthetic agents has been questioned due to the occurrence of apoptotic neurodegeneration and permanent cognitive deficiencies in immature animals after exposure to anesthetic agents [67].

4. NURR1: An Orphan Nuclear Receptor at the Interface between Neural Development, Inflammation and the Environment

NURR1, also called NR4A2, is a nuclear receptor and a transcription factor that belongs to the NR4A subfamily of nuclear receptors, which also includes NOR-1 and NUR77. NURR1 shares structural similarities with the other NR4A family members. It consists of a modulator domain at the N-terminus, referred to as the activation function (AF)-1, a central double zinc finger DNA-binding domain (DBD), a ligand-binding domain (LBD) composed of 12 α-helices and its transactivation-dependent AF-2 at the C-terminus [68]. Similar to the other two members of this subfamily, NOR-1 and NUR77, NURR1 falls within the category of orphan receptors, since no specific ligand has yet been identified [69]. Because of the steric bulk of several hydrophobic residues, NURR1 (as well as other NR4A family members) does not have a LBD cavity, which explains the difficulty in finding proper ligands that can directly activate NURR1 through its LBD [70]. Instead, *NURR1* transcriptional activity seems to rely on the AF-1 domain [71]. However, residues 592, 593, and 577 in the NURR1 LBD can be the site of interaction with some regulatory compounds [72,73]. For example, omega-3 docosahexaenoic acid has recently been shown to have high affinity for the NURR1 LBD, modulating *NURR1* transactivation [74]. NURR1 exists as an active transcription factor in both its monomeric and homodimeric forms. As a monomer, NURR1 binds the nerve growth factor-inducible-β-binding response element (NBRE; 5'-AAAGGTCA-3'), while as a homodimer, it binds the nur-response element (NurRE; 5'-TGACCTTT-n6-AAAGGTCA-3'), resulting in the activation of several genes, including the tyrosine hydroxylase (*TH*) and the dopamine active transporter (*DAT*) genes [75]. Indeed, *NURR1* is widely expressed in the CNS where it has a crucial role in the differentiation of midbrain dopaminergic (DA) neurons. *NURR1* is expressed during DA neuron differentiation in limbic areas and in the ventral midbrain where it regulates dopamine synthesis through proteins such as TH, DAT, vesicular monoamine transporter 2 (VMAT2) and RET receptor tyrosine kinase. Deficient expression of *NURR1* in developing mesencephalic dopaminergic cells impairs them with regard to expressing TH [76,77]. NURR1 deficiency in embryonic ventral midbrain cells impairs their migration and their ability to innervate striatal target areas [78]. Given its well-established role in the CNS, altered functionality of NURR1 has been also associated with neurodegeneration (PD in particular), but also with attention-deficit/hyperactivity disorder [79], schizophrenia and manic-depressive disorders [80]. Moreover, a de novo deletion-induced haploinsufficiency of NR4A2 receptors is implicated in neurodevelopmental alterations, in particular language impairment [81]. The role of NURR1 at the interface with environmental stimuli in the management of stressful events has been demonstrated [82,83]. There is evidence that NURR1 transcription factor plays a prominent role in adaptive responses to stress, regulating the transcription of target genes in the HPA axis [71]. Moreover, NURR1 activity seems to be enhanced upon the interaction with the glucocorticoid receptor (GR) [84]. Rapid increase in NURR1 mRNA expression has been measured in limbic and cortical brain structures related to coping with depression-like behavior in mice [85,86], suggesting that an increase in *NURR1* expression might be a compensatory mechanism to counteract the changes in forebrain dopamine transmission while coping with acute stress. The direct relationship of NURR1 with the environment is also suggested by its association with circadian rhythms and catecholamine production [87]. Prenatal stress modulates NURR1 inducing different outcomes along the life span of the male offspring, leading to changes in the reproductive system and spermatogenesis after puberty [8]. Beyond its well-known role in the development, function and maintenance of midbrain dopaminergic neurons [88], NURR1 can also be found in non-neuronal tissues such as synovial tissues, bone, endothelial cells, adrenal gland, hepatocytes and macrophages [83,89], where it mediates essential physiological processes, including adaptive and innate immune cell differentiation, metabolism and inflammation [90]. Thus, the nuclear receptor superfamily has been proposed as key transcription factors capable of modulating both immune and metabolic pathways. Since the discovery that NURR1 is not only involved in neurodegenerative disorders but also in inflammatory processes, growing attention has been directed to explore the potential role of NURR1 alterations in several inflammation-related diseases (including obesity and diabetes, atherosclerosis, cancer) [91–95]. In fact, the NURR1 receptor can be rapidly induced by a range of cytokines, suggesting that this receptor acts as a potential transcriptional mediator of inflammatory signals [83,96]. It has shown an anti-inflammatory function [97], but the exact molecular mechanisms have not been clearly elucidated yet. Recently, NURR1 has been shown to be responsive to nonsteroidal anti-inflammatory drugs [98]. The pleiotropic effects of NURR1 and its interaction with environmental factors have contributed to the proposal of this transcription factor as a mediator of late-onset consequences of early life events [83,99–101]. Next, we review the current knowledge on NURR1 alterations in early life, especially in association with the previously mentioned perinatal stressful events, and the potential implications in premature prevention of late-onset diseases.

5. Perinatal Stress Modulates *NURR1* Expression: From Early-Life Stress to Late-Onset Diseases

Differential regulations of *NURR1* expression have been demonstrated in association with several environmental exposures, especially in early life. In relation to metabolic health, it must be considered that in human fetal membranes and myometrium, as well as other cells and tissues, *NURR1* expression is rapidly and transiently induced by a wide range of stimuli, including hormones, cellular stress and inflammatory signals. Among these, obesity and GDM are of particular concern during pregnancy as they trigger low-grade systemic inflammation [102,103]. High levels of activated macrophages in the intestinal stroma of the placenta and circulating proinflammatory cytokines, such as TNF-α, IL-1β and IL-6, are observed in overweight women or women with GDM. In particular, TNF-α is considered a predictor of insulin resistance during pregnancy and has been correlated with fetal adiposity [104]. Interestingly, it was found that proinflammatory stimuli from IL-1β and TNF-α upregulate *NURR1* expression (as well as NUR77) in the placenta of women with GDM compared to body mass index-matched normal glucose tolerant pregnant women, even though the exact mechanism has not been elucidated yet [105,106].

Upregulated levels of cytokines are also observed in case of maternal depression [28]. Depressive disorders, anxiety and post-traumatic stress disorders are associated with significantly elevated levels of circulating proinflammatory cytokines, such as IL-6, TNF-α and IL-1RA [29,107–109]. This may be due to the activation of central and peripheral immune cells releasing cytokines, and to the activation of the stress response system of the HPA axis by proinflammatory cytokines [110]. The directionality of the related cytokine-depressive behavior is still under investigation. Inflammation, which is accompanied by cytokine signaling, may play a role in the pathophysiology of psychiatric disorders [111]. Nevertheless, changes in cytokines levels could also follow as a consequence of the psychiatric disorder, for example, being induced by treatments with psychopharmacological agents or by weight changes that accompany acute episodes of the disorder [112].

No association was found between pre-existing maternal obesity and placental *NURR1* expression. However, a positive correlation was found previously in adipose tissue, suggesting a tissue-dependent modulation of obesity-induced NR4A receptor expression [113]. Moreover, Veum and co-workers measured a strong upregulation of the NR4As in extreme obesity and normalization after fat loss, showing an altered adipose tissue expression of the NR4As in obesity [92]. Therefore, these stress-responsive nuclear receptors may modulate pathogenic potential in humans, and early-life trauma might stimulate their deregulation. In addition, human gestational tissues express NR4A receptors, which regulate the processes of parturition at term through the modulation of cytokines and growth factors [114–116]. *NURR1* (and *NUR77*) knockdown on primary human trophoblast cells resulted in decreased TNF-α induced IL-6 and IL-8 expression and secretion, revealing a possible proinflammatory effect of NURR1 in human placenta [105]. Inflammation has a central role during labor and delivery, because cytokines stimulate uterine activation via the NF-kB pathway inducing the release of prostaglandins [117]. *NURR1* (and *NUR77*) expression is upregulated in human fetal membranes and myometrium as a consequence of spontaneous labor at term, which can explain the expression of proinflammatory and prolabor genes associated with fetal membrane rupture and myometrial contractions [118]. However, a similar effect is driven by bacterial infections, which are responsible for most spontaneous preterm births (before 32 weeks gestational age) [119] due to the inflammatory response triggered by bacterial products in human gestational tissues. In fetal membranes, *NURR1* expression was upregulated by bacterial lipopolysaccharide, fibroblast-stimulating lipopeptide and peptidoglycan muramyl dipeptide, whereas flagellin also increased *NURR1* expression in the myometrium. The upstream mechanisms behind *NURR1* upregulation are not clear yet; however, NF-kB activation seems to be involved [118]. By disrupting the normal developmental maturation of organ systems, preterm birth may result in long lasting adverse effects in adult age. Increased blood pressure, reduced insulin sensitivity, impaired vascular growth, chronic kidney disease (especially in the case of intrauterine growth restriction or neonatal acute kidney injury) and significant chronic airway obstruction are the most common adverse consequences connected to preterm birth that persist through adulthood [43]. Concerning CNS health, prenatal or early postnatal stress are considered risk factors for the development of psychiatric disorders, addiction and the ability to cope with stress. Prenatal stress strongly impacts fetal brain development in rats. Rats exposed to different types of stress during the last week of pregnancy give birth to offspring with anomalies in neuronal development and brain morphology which persist through adulthood [120,121]. The underlying mechanism has been thought to be most likely due to changes in D2-type dopamine (DA) neurotransmission induced by prenatal stress [122]. *NURR1* expression in dopaminergic neurons starts at embryonic day 10.5 before the appearance of the dopaminergic marker enzyme, TH (at embryonic day 11.5) and continues during adulthood [123]. A homeostatic function has been attributed to NURR1 in the case of stress. Levels of NURR1 were found to be increased in the ventral tegmental area of prenatally stressed adult offspring, most likely as a compensatory mechanism to counteract the reduction in dopamine levels observed as a consequence of prenatal stress [8,124]. A similar NURR1 increase was observed in cortical brain regions and the limbic system, including cornu ammonis-3 (CA3) of the hippocampus in mice, as a compensatory response to acute stress [85]. Montes et al. has shown that even if the hippocampus may be vulnerable to stress, it may also have enough plasticity to cope with stress. To test the resilience to stress of the hippocampus, NURR1 was downregulated in prenatally stressed (PS) and nonprenatally stressed (NPS) male rats, through the bilateral administration of NURR1 anti-sense oligodeoxynucleotide (ODN) into their hippocampal CA3 region. Then rats were exposed to an acute stressor (forced swimming test, FST) to analyze their behavioral responses. After the ODN treatment, NPS rats showed a depressive-like behavior manifested through immobility, while PS rats showed active behaviors (resilience). These findings suggest that prenatal stress might induce brain modifications that promote resilience to acute stress in adulthood [125]. Given the central role of NURR1 in the development of dopaminergic neurons, prenatal exposure to neurotoxic compounds, such as pesticides, could be implicated in its deregulation leading to the onset, later in life, of neurological disorders, such as PD. Exposure to atrazine (ATR), a volatile and water-soluble compound used as a herbicide worldwide, during pregnancy and lactation has been associated with decreased expression of NURR1 in offspring, together with changes in the expression of VMAT2, which controls the transport and reuptake of DA. The consequent decrease in DA levels in the striatum confirm that early-life exposure to ATR alters the dopaminergic system by modulating *NURR1* expression [126]. Additionally, early-life exposure to permethrin (PERM), a pyrethroid compound largely used for outdoor/indoor pest control and as anti-woodworm agent, induces dopaminergic neuronal disorders in adult life, through the alteration of Nurr1 expression levels [100,101,127]. Of note, early-life exposure to PERM seems to have intergenerational effects, most likely due to epigenetic mechanisms [128]. An increased DNA methylation at the promoter region of the dopamine-specifying factor, Nurr1, has been observed in the sperm of first-generation offspring of these mothers. In the ventral midbrain of second-generation offspring, the effect is further associated with reduced mRNA levels of Nurr1 [41]. The effects in the later life of early NURR1 perturbation are endorsed by a body of evidence. Remarkably, it has been demonstrated that maternal smoking and early postnatal exposure to nicotine alter children's behaviors and increase their propensity for drug abuse later in life, by altering the dopamine-mediated reward system [129]. This most likely occurs due to the nicotine-mediated circuit activation during development. In fact, studies on mice show that neonatal exposure to nicotine primes midbrain neurons to express NURR1; subsequent nicotine re-exposures in adulthood induce primed neurons to acquire the dopaminergic phenotype responsible for nicotine-mediated neurotransmitter plasticity [129]. In addition, prenatal exposure to infections is a known risk factor for the development of neuropsychiatric disorders, especially schizophrenia and autism [130,131]. However, it seems that other risk factors, in particular genetic factors, should be concomitant to developing severe neuronal disorders. Brain and behavioral consequences of prenatal infection-induced immune activation are exacerbated (synergistic effects) in offspring with genetic predisposition to dopaminergic abnormalities, in particular NURR1 deficiency [132]. NURR1 polymorphisms may also be implicated in the etiology of disorders characterized by altered dopaminergic signaling, such as attention-deficit/hyperactivity disorder, schizophrenia and PD. Thus, NURR1 may represent a future candidate gene to study the genetic predispositions to several neuropsychiatric disorders [79,130]. Furthermore, preclinical studies on rodents and nonhuman primates have questioned the safety of anesthetic agents used to relieve pain in the process of childbirth or surgical procedures. It emerged that under common clinical conditions, these chemical agents have a neurotoxic effect on the developing brain and can also induce long-term neurobehavioral abnormalities [133]. In particular, the use of sevoflurane in pregnant women seems to strongly impact fetal brain development. Sevoflurane impairs hippocampal CNS proliferation and differentiation through the upregulation of miR-183 and the downregulation of NURR1. The result is the progressive degeneration of the fetal brain, with long-term deficits in hippocampal-dependent learning and memory [133]. Finally, several studies also support the hypothesis of the intermediary role of inflammation and perinatal trauma underpinning the link between early-life exposure, NURR1 alterations, and CNS impairment later in life. Indeed, NURR1 expression may play a significant role in the modulation of brain development, especially in the case of a combination of maternal inflammation and premature birth. Premature infants often rely on supplemental oxygen for survival, which may represent an additional source of inflammation leading to neurodevelopmental impairment. Lallier et al. [134] found decreased numbers of oligodendrocytes and increased numbers of microglia in mice exposed to both maternal inflammation and neonatal hyperoxia. They hypothesized that alteration of NURR1 expression in the perinatal period could be responsible for the detrimental effects of the two combined sources of inflammation, bacterial infections and hypoxia [134]. Table 1 summarizes the main targets and modulators of NURR1.

Table 1. Main targets and modulators of Nuclear receptor related 1 protein (NURR1).

NURR1 Targets (T) and Modulators (M)	References
Hypothalamus-pituitary-adrenal axis (T)	[8,9,71]
Dopamine D2 receptor, tyrosine hydroxylase, dopamine active transporter, glucocorticoid receptor (T)	[12,13,75–77,84,85,122–126]
Environmental stress during early life (M)	[8,14–21,82,83,99–101,129–134]
Circadian rhythm and catecholamine production (T)	[87]
Micronutrient intake (M)	[55–58]
Omega-3 docosahexaenoic acid (M)	[74]
Adaptive and innate immune cell differentiation, metabolism and inflammation in various cells (T)	[83,90–98,105,135]
IL-1β and TNF-α (M)	[29,104–110]
Obesity (M)	[92,113]
Human gestational tissues (T)	[114–116,118]
Permethrin (M)	[41,100,101,127,128]

6. NURR1: An Early Biomarker and Novel Target for Prevention of Chronic Diseases?

Given the expression of NURR1 not only in the CNS but also in other tissues, such as adipose tissue, liver, skeletal muscles and heart tissues, a perturbation of its functionality can have a broad spectrum of consequences for human health, from neurological and psychiatric disorders to metabolic diseases. NURR1 is mainly known for its primary role in the development of dopaminergic neurons; however, it has been shown to be a significant dual actor in the inflammation process. While there is evidence of the anti-inflammatory behavior of NURR1 [135], other findings have associated NURR1 expression levels with increased proinflammatory cytokines, in particular in pathologies such as PD and type 2 diabetes, suggesting a potential of NURR1 in the etiology of these conditions [11,93]. Even though further research to clarify the mechanistic effects of NURR1 is needed, the usage of NURR1 expression as a biomarker has been proposed, at least for those conditions in which NURR1 deregulation has been established. The assessment of NURR1 levels in blood gave good results in aiding in the diagnosis of PD and monitoring disease progression when measured in association with mir-132 or cytokines [136,137]. Other findings also suggest NURR1 as a biomarker for early diagnosis or diseases' progression [93,138]. Additional studies investigating the role of NURR1 in predicting long-term effects of perinatal stress are warranted in order to extend the usage of NURR1 as a biomarker for other relevant clinical conditions.

In addition, NURR1 has been suggested as a potential pharmacological target for diseases characterized by its deregulation [139,140]. As an example, it has been demonstrated that the GR can act as a transcriptional regulator of NURR1, suggesting that glucocorticoids might be used to regulate NURR1 expression [87]. At present, a significant number of research projects aimed at identifying new NURR1 ligands for drug development are underway [141–143].

Moreover, knowledge that NURR1 expression can be regulated by modifiable factors (i.e., nutritional status) might pave the way for potential applications of nutrigenomics [144] in the early prevention of the previously mentioned conditions through strategies aimed to improve nutrition in the perinatal period and in early childhood.

7. Conclusions

The interactions between NURR1 and environmental factors, especially during early fetal development, are well-documented and are implicated in a variety of late-onset consequences for human health [99]. When considering that an intergenerational transmission of NURR1-mediated effects has been hypothesized [41,128], the ability of external stressors to control of NURR1 expression gains even more importance. This is of particular significance in the context of the prenatal and early neonatal periods. Further investigations to explore the role of NURR1 either alone or in combination with other molecular markers as a noninvasive biomarker, aiding in the prevention, diagnosis and evaluation of disease severity or response to treatments for several pathological conditions, should be considered.

Author Contributions: Conceptualization, R.G., L.B., J.C.-A.; writing—original draft preparation, L.B., R.G., I.P., J.C.-A.; writing—review and editing, R.G., L.B., J.C.-A. and J.G.L.; funding acquisition, J.G.L. All authors have read and agreed to the published version of the manuscript.

Funding: The publication of this manuscript was funded by COST Action CA18211:DEVoTION:Perinatal Mental Health and Birth-Related Trauma: Maximizing best practice and optimal outcomes (European Cooperation in Science and Technology).

Acknowledgments: This publication emerged from the EU funded COST action CA18211:DEVoTION: Perinatal Mental Health and Birth-Related Trauma: Maximizing best practice and optimal outcomes. R.G., J.C.A. and J.G.L. are authors, R.G., J.C.A. are Action management committee members and J.G.L. is the Action Chair.

Conflicts of Interest: The authors declare no conflict of interest.

References

1. Lähdepuro, A.; Savolainen, K.; Lahti-Pulkkinen, M.; Eriksson, J.G.; Lahti, J.; Tuovinen, S.; Kajantie, E.; Pesonen, A.-K.; Heinonen, K.; Räikkönen, K. The Impact of Early Life Stress on Anxiety Symptoms in Late Adulthood. *Sci. Rep.* **2019**, *9*, 4395. [CrossRef] [PubMed]
2. Hori, H.; Kim, Y. Inflammation and post-traumatic stress disorder. *Psychiatry Clin. Neurosci.* **2019**, *73*, 143–153. [CrossRef] [PubMed]
3. Merrill, D.A.; Masliah, E.; Roberts, J.A.; McKay, H.; Kordower, J.H.; Mufson, E.J.; Tuszynski, M.H. Association of early experience with neurodegeneration in aged primates. *Neurobiol. Aging* **2011**, *32*, 151–156. [CrossRef] [PubMed]
4. Carroll, J.C.; Iba, M.; Bangasser, D.A.; Valentino, R.J.; James, M.J.; Brunden, K.R.; Lee, V.M.-Y.; Trojanowski, J.Q. Chronic stress exacerbates tau pathology, neurodegeneration, and cognitive performance through a corticotropin-releasing factor receptor-dependent mechanism in a transgenic mouse model of tauopathy. *J. Neurosci.* **2011**, *31*, 14436–14449. [CrossRef]
5. Gabbianelli, R.; Damiani, E. Epigenetics and neurodegeneration: Role of early-life nutrition. *J. Nutr. Biochem.* **2018**, *57*, 1–13. [CrossRef]
6. Barker, D.J.P. The origins of the developmental origins theory. *J. Intern. Med.* **2007**, *261*, 412–417. [CrossRef]
7. Hales, C.N.; Barker, D.J.P. The thrifty phenotype hypothesis: Type 2 diabetes. *Br. Med. Bull.* **2001**, *60*, 5–20. [CrossRef]
8. Pallarés, M.E.; Antonelli, M.C. Hormonal modulation of catecholaminergic neurotransmission in a prenatal stress model. *Adv. Neurobiol.* **2015**, *10*, 45–59.
9. Murphy, E.P.; Conneely, O.M. Neuroendocrine regulation of the hypothalamic pituitary adrenal axis by the nurr1/nur77 subfamily of nuclear receptors. *Mol. Endocrinol.* **1997**, *11*, 39–47. [CrossRef]
10. Jeon, S.G.; Yoo, A.; Chun, D.W.; Hong, S.B.; Chung, H.; Kim, J.-I.; Moon, M. The Critical Role of Nurr1 as a Mediator and Therapeutic Target in Alzheimer's Disease-related Pathogenesis. *Aging Dis.* **2020**, *11*, 705–724. [CrossRef]

11. Li, T.; Yang, Z.; Li, S.; Cheng, C.; Shen, B.; Le, W. Alterations of NURR1 and Cytokines in the Peripheral Blood Mononuclear Cells: Combined Biomarkers for Parkinson's Disease. *Front. Aging Neurosci.* **2018**, *10*, 392. [CrossRef] [PubMed]
12. Torretta, S.; Rampino, A.; Basso, M.; Pergola, G.; Di Carlo, P.; Shin, J.H.; Kleinman, J.E.; Hyde, T.M.; Weinberger, D.R.; Masellis, R.; et al. NURR1 and ERR1 Modulate the Expression of Genes of a DRD2 Coexpression Network Enriched for Schizophrenia Risk. *J. Neurosci.* **2020**, *40*, 932–941. [CrossRef] [PubMed]
13. Corley, S.M.; Tsai, S.-Y.; Wilkins, M.R.; Shannon Weickert, C. Transcriptomic Analysis Shows Decreased Cortical Expression of NR4A1, NR4A2 and RXRB in Schizophrenia and Provides Evidence for Nuclear Receptor Dysregulation. *PLoS ONE* **2016**, *11*, e0166944. [CrossRef] [PubMed]
14. Holmes, L.J.; Shutman, E.; Chinaka, C.; Deepika, K.; Pelaez, L.; Dabney, K.W. Aberrant Epigenomic Modulation of Glucocorticoid Receptor Gene (NR3C1) in Early Life Stress and Major Depressive Disorder Correlation: Systematic Review and Quantitative Evidence Synthesis. *Int. J. Environ. Res. Public Health* **2019**, *16*, 4280. [CrossRef]
15. Luby, J.L.; Baram, T.Z.; Rogers, C.E.; Barch, D.M. Neurodevelopmental Optimization after Early-Life Adversity: Cross-Species Studies to Elucidate Sensitive Periods and Brain Mechanisms to Inform Early Intervention. *Trends Neurosci.* **2020**, *43*, 744–751. [CrossRef] [PubMed]
16. Hambrick, E.P.; Brawner, T.W.; Perry, B.D.; Brandt, K.; Hofmeister, C.; Collins, J.O. Beyond the ACE score: Examining relationships between timing of developmental adversity, relational health and developmental outcomes in children. *Arch. Psychiatr. Nurs.* **2019**, *33*, 238–247. [CrossRef]
17. Nasuti, C.; Brunori, G.; Eusepi, P.; Marinelli, L.; Ciccocioppo, R.; Gabbianelli, R. Early life exposure to permethrin: A progressive animal model of Parkinson's disease. *J. Pharmacol. Toxicol. Methods* **2017**, *83*, 80–86. [CrossRef]
18. Bordoni, L.; Nasuti, C.; Fedeli, D.; Galeazzi, R.; Laudadio, E.; Massaccesi, L.; López-Rodas, G.; Gabbianelli, R. Early impairment of epigenetic pattern in neurodegeneration: Additional mechanisms behind pyrethroid toxicity. *Exp. Gerontol.* **2019**, *124*, 110629. [CrossRef]
19. Nasuti, C.; Fattoretti, P.; Carloni, M.; Fedeli, D.; Ubaldi, M.; Ciccocioppo, R.; Gabbianelli, R. Neonatal exposure to permethrin pesticide causes lifelong fear and spatial learning deficits and alters hippocampal morphology of synapses. *J. Neurodev. Disord.* **2014**, *6*, 7. [CrossRef]
20. Bordoni, L.; Nasuti, C.; Di Stefano, A.; Marinelli, L.; Gabbianelli, R. Epigenetic Memory of Early-Life Parental Perturbation: Dopamine Decrease and DNA Methylation Changes in Offspring. *Oxid. Med. Cell. Longev.* **2019**, *2019*, 1472623. [CrossRef]
21. Bordoni, L.; Gabbianelli, R.; Fedeli, D.; Fiorini, D.; Bergheim, I.; Jin, C.J.; Marinelli, L.; Di Stefano, A.; Nasuti, C. Positive effect of an electrolyzed reduced water on gut permeability, fecal microbiota and liver in an animal model of Parkinson's disease. *PLoS ONE* **2019**, *14*, e0223238. [CrossRef]
22. Allen, L. Are we facing a noncommunicable disease pandemic? *J. Epidemiol. Glob. Health* **2017**, *7*, 5–9. [CrossRef]
23. Choo, C.C.; Chew, P.K.H.; Ho, R.C. Controlling Noncommunicable Diseases in Transitional Economies: Mental Illness in Suicide Attempters in Singapore-An Exploratory Analysis. *Biomed Res. Int.* **2019**, *2019*, 4652846. [CrossRef] [PubMed]
24. Reddy, K.S. Measuring mortality from non-communicable diseases: Broadening the band. *Lancet Glob. Health* **2020**, *8*, e456–e457. [CrossRef]
25. Bordoni, L.; Gabbianelli, R. Chapter 67—Nutrigenomics of Food Pesticides. In *Principles of Nutrigenetics and Nutrigenomics*; Caterina, R.D.E., Martinez, J.A., Kohlmeier, M., Eds.; Academic Press: Salt Lake City, UT, USA, 2020; pp. 513–518. ISBN 978-0-12-804572-5.
26. Hanson, M.A.; Gluckman, P.D. Developmental origins of health and disease—Global public health implications. *Best Pract. Res. Clin. Obstet. Gynaecol.* **2015**, *29*, 24–31. [CrossRef] [PubMed]
27. Gabbianelli, R. Modulation of the Epigenome by Nutrition and Xenobiotics during Early Life and across the Life Span: The Key Role of Lifestyle. *Lifestyle Genom.* **2018**, *11*, 9–12. [CrossRef] [PubMed]
28. Wu, Y.; Zhang, H.; Wang, C.; Broekman, B.F.P.; Chong, Y.-S.; Shek, L.P.; Gluckman, P.D.; Meaney, M.J.; Fortier, M.V.; Qiu, A. Inflammatory modulation of the associations between prenatal maternal depression and neonatal brain. *Neuropsychopharmacology* **2020**. [CrossRef] [PubMed]
29. McQuaid, R.J.; Gabrys, R.L.; McInnis, O.A.; Anisman, H.; Matheson, K. Understanding the Relation Between Early-Life Adversity and Depression Symptoms: The Moderating Role of Sex and an Interleukin-1β Gene Variant. *Front. Psychiatry* **2019**, *10*, 151. [CrossRef]

30. Dowlati, Y.; Herrmann, N.; Swardfager, W.; Liu, H.; Sham, L.; Reim, E.K.; Lanctôt, K.L. A meta-analysis of cytokines in major depression. *Biol. Psychiatry* **2010**, *67*, 446–457. [CrossRef]
31. Sarki, M.; Parlesak, A.; Robertson, A. Comparison of national cross-sectional breast-feeding surveys by maternal education in Europe (2006–2016). *Public Health Nutr.* **2019**, *22*, 848–861. [CrossRef]
32. Ortega-García, J.A.; Kloosterman, N.; Alvarez, L.; Tobarra-Sánchez, E.; Cárceles-Álvarez, A.; Pastor-Valero, R.; López-Hernández, F.A.; Sánchez-Solis, M.; Claudio, L. Full Breastfeeding and Obesity in Children: A Prospective Study from Birth to 6 Years. *Child. Obes.* **2018**, *14*, 327–337. [CrossRef] [PubMed]
33. Gabbianelli, R.; Bordoni, L.; Morano, S.; Calleja-Agius, J.; Lalor, J.G. Nutri-Epigenetics and Gut Microbiota: How Birth Care, Bonding and Breastfeeding Can Influence and Be Influenced? *Int. J. Mol. Sci.* **2020**, *21*, 5032. [CrossRef] [PubMed]
34. Mancilla, V.J.; Peeri, N.C.; Silzer, T.; Basha, R.; Felini, M.; Jones, H.P.; Phillips, N.; Tao, M.-H.; Thyagarajan, S.; Vishwanatha, J.K. Understanding the Interplay Between Health Disparities and Epigenomics. *Front. Genet.* **2020**, *11*, 903. [CrossRef] [PubMed]
35. Pillas, D.; Marmot, M.; Naicker, K.; Goldblatt, P.; Morrison, J.; Pikhart, H. Social inequalities in early childhood health and development: A European-wide systematic review. *Pediatr. Res.* **2014**, *76*, 418–424. [CrossRef]
36. Bann, D.; Johnson, W.; Li, L.; Kuh, D.; Hardy, R. Socioeconomic inequalities in childhood and adolescent body-mass index, weight, and height from 1953 to 2015: An analysis of four longitudinal, observational, British birth cohort studies. *Lancet Public Health* **2018**, *3*, e194–e203. [CrossRef]
37. Bann, D.; Fitzsimons, E.; Johnson, W. Determinants of the population health distribution: An illustration examining body mass index. *Int. J. Epidemiol.* **2020**, *49*, 731–737. [CrossRef]
38. Braveman, P.; Gottlieb, L. The social determinants of health: It's time to consider the causes of the causes. *Public Health Rep.* **2014**, *129* (Suppl. 2), 19–31. [CrossRef]
39. Nazzari, S.; Frigerio, A. The programming role of maternal antenatal inflammation on infants' early neurodevelopment: A review of human studies: Special Section on "Translational and Neuroscience Studies in Affective Disorders" Section Editor, Maria Nobile MD, PhD. *J. Affect. Disord.* **2020**, *263*, 739–746. [CrossRef]
40. Al-Haddad, B.J.S.; Jacobsson, B.; Chabra, S.; Modzelewska, D.; Olson, E.M.; Bernier, R.; Enquobahrie, D.A.; Hagberg, H.; Östling, S.; Rajagopal, L.; et al. Long-term Risk of Neuropsychiatric Disease After Exposure to Infection In Utero. *JAMA Psychiatry* **2019**, *76*, 594–602. [CrossRef]
41. Weber-Stadlbauer, U.; Richetto, J.; Zwamborn, R.A.J.; Slieker, R.C.; Meyer, U. Transgenerational modification of dopaminergic dysfunctions induced by maternal immune activation. *Neuropsychopharmacology* **2020**. [CrossRef]
42. Freud, A.; Wainstock, T.; Sheiner, E.; Beloosesky, R.; Fischer, L.; Landau, D.; Walfisch, A. Maternal chorioamnionitis & long-term neurological morbidity in the offspring. *Eur. J. Paediatr. Neurol.* **2019**, *23*, 484–490. [PubMed]
43. Luu, T.M.; Rehman Mian, M.O.; Nuyt, A.M. Long-Term Impact of Preterm Birth: Neurodevelopmental and Physical Health Outcomes. *Clin. Perinatol.* **2017**, *44*, 305–314. [CrossRef] [PubMed]
44. Raju, T.N.K.; Buist, A.S.; Blaisdell, C.J.; Moxey-Mims, M.; Saigal, S. Adults born preterm: A review of general health and system-specific outcomes. *Acta Paediatr.* **2017**, *106*, 1409–1437. [CrossRef]
45. Xu, B.; Pekkanen, J.; Hartikainen, A.L.; Järvelin, M.R. Caesarean section and risk of asthma and allergy in adulthood. *J. Allergy Clin. Immunol.* **2001**, *107*, 732–733. [CrossRef] [PubMed]
46. Thavagnanam, S.; Fleming, J.; Bromley, A.; Shields, M.D.; Cardwell, C.R. A meta-analysis of the association between Caesarean section and childhood asthma. *Clin. Exp. Allergy* **2008**, *38*, 629–633. [CrossRef] [PubMed]
47. Biasucci, G.; Rubini, M.; Riboni, S.; Morelli, L.; Bessi, E.; Retetangos, C. Mode of delivery affects the bacterial community in the newborn gut. *Early Hum. Dev.* **2010**, *86* (Suppl. 1), 13–15. [CrossRef]
48. Siggers, R.H.; Siggers, J.; Thymann, T.; Boye, M.; Sangild, P.T. Nutritional modulation of the gut microbiota and immune system in preterm neonates susceptible to necrotizing enterocolitis. *J. Nutr. Biochem.* **2011**, *22*, 511–521. [CrossRef]
49. Tapia-Martínez, J.; Torres-Manzo, A.P.; Franco-Colín, M.; Pineda-Reynoso, M.; Cano-Europa, E. Maternal Thyroid Hormone Deficiency During Gestation and Lactation Alters Metabolic and Thyroid Programming of the Offspring in the Adult Stage. *Horm. Metab. Res.* **2019**, *51*, 381–388. [CrossRef]
50. Muller, I.; Taylor, P.N.; Daniel, R.M.; Hales, C.; Scholz, A.; Candler, T.; Pettit, R.J.; Evans, W.D.; Shillabeer, D.; Draman, M.S.; et al. CATS II Long-term Anthropometric and Metabolic Effects of Maternal Sub-optimal Thyroid Function in Offspring and Mothers. *J. Clin. Endocrinol. Metab.* **2020**, *105*. [CrossRef]

51. Rees, W.D. Interactions between nutrients in the maternal diet and the implications for the long-term health of the offspring. *Proc. Nutr. Soc.* **2019**, *78*, 88–96. [CrossRef]
52. Srugo, S.A.; Bloise, E.; Nguyen, T.T.-T.N.; Connor, K.L. Impact of Maternal Malnutrition on Gut Barrier Defense: Implications for Pregnancy Health and Fetal Development. *Nutrients* **2019**, *11*, 1375. [CrossRef] [PubMed]
53. Chong, M.F.-F.; Godfrey, K.M.; Gluckman, P.; Tan, K.H.; Shek, L.P.-C.; Meaney, M.; Chan, J.K.Y.; Yap, F.; Lee, Y.S.; Chong, Y.-S. Influences of the perinatal diet on maternal and child health: Insights from the GUSTO study. *Proc. Nutr. Soc.* **2020**, 1–6. [CrossRef] [PubMed]
54. Luan, W.; Hammond, L.A.; Vuillermot, S.; Meyer, U.; Eyles, D.W. Maternal Vitamin D Prevents Abnormal Dopaminergic Development and Function in a Mouse Model of Prenatal Immune Activation. *Sci. Rep.* **2018**, *8*, 9741. [CrossRef]
55. Lai, J.S.; Mohamad Ayob, M.N.; Cai, S.; Quah, P.L.; Gluckman, P.D.; Shek, L.P.; Yap, F.; Tan, K.H.; Chong, Y.S.; Godfrey, K.M.; et al. Maternal plasma vitamin B12 concentrations during pregnancy and infant cognitive outcomes at 2 years of age. *Br. J. Nutr.* **2019**, *121*, 1303–1312. [CrossRef] [PubMed]
56. Godfrey, K.M.; Reynolds, R.M.; Prescott, S.L.; Nyirenda, M.; Jaddoe, V.W.V.; Eriksson, J.G.; Broekman, B.F.P. Influence of maternal obesity on the long-term health of offspring. *Lancet Diabetes Endocrinol.* **2017**, *5*, 53–64. [CrossRef]
57. Gaillard, R. Maternal obesity during pregnancy and cardiovascular development and disease in the offspring. *Eur. J. Epidemiol.* **2015**, *30*, 1141–1152. [CrossRef]
58. Gutvirtz, G.; Wainstock, T.; Landau, D.; Sheiner, E. Maternal Obesity and Offspring Long-Term Infectious Morbidity. *J. Clin. Med.* **2019**, *8*, 1466. [CrossRef]
59. León-Aguilar, L.F.; Croyal, M.; Ferchaud-Roucher, V.; Huang, F.; Marchat, L.A.; Barraza-Villarreal, A.; Romieu, I.; Ramakrishnan, U.; Krempf, M.; Ouguerram, K.; et al. Maternal obesity leads to long-term altered levels of plasma ceramides in the offspring as revealed by a longitudinal lipidomic study in children. *Int. J. Obes. (Lond.)* **2019**, *43*, 1231–1243. [CrossRef]
60. Neuhaus, Z.F.; Gutvirtz, G.; Pariente, G.; Wainstock, T.; Landau, D.; Sheiner, E. Maternal obesity and long-term neuropsychiatric morbidity of the offspring. *Arch. Gynecol. Obstet.* **2020**, *301*, 143–149. [CrossRef]
61. Farahvar, S.; Walfisch, A.; Sheiner, E. Gestational diabetes risk factors and long-term consequences for both mother and offspring: A literature review. *Expert Rev. Endocrinol. Metab.* **2019**, *14*, 63–74. [CrossRef]
62. Burlina, S.; Dalfrà, M.G.; Lapolla, A. Short- and long-term consequences for offspring exposed to maternal diabetes: A review. *J. Matern. Neonatal Med.* **2019**, *32*, 687–694. [CrossRef] [PubMed]
63. Omotoso, G.O.; Kadir, R.E.; Sulaimon, F.A.; Jaji-Sulaimon, R.; Gbadamosi, I.T. Prenatal Exposure to Gestational Nicotine before Neurulation is Detrimental to Neurodevelopment of Wistar Rats' Offspring. *Malays. J. Med. Sci.* **2018**, *25*, 35–47. [CrossRef] [PubMed]
64. Moore, B.F.; Starling, A.P.; Magzamen, S.; Harrod, C.S.; Allshouse, W.B.; Adgate, J.L.; Ringham, B.M.; Glueck, D.H.; Dabelea, D. Fetal exposure to maternal active and secondhand smoking with offspring early-life growth in the Healthy Start study. *Int. J. Obes. (Lond.)* **2019**, *43*, 652–662. [CrossRef] [PubMed]
65. Gutvirtz, G.; Wainstock, T.; Landau, D.; Sheiner, E. Maternal smoking during pregnancy and long-term neurological morbidity of the offspring. *Addict. Behav.* **2019**, *88*, 86–91. [CrossRef] [PubMed]
66. Rubin, R.; Pearl, M.; Kharrazi, M.; Blount, B.C.; Miller, M.D.; Pearce, E.N.; Valentin-Blasini, L.; DeLorenze, G.; Liaw, J.; Hoofnagle, A.N.; et al. Maternal perchlorate exposure in pregnancy and altered birth outcomes. *Environ. Res.* **2017**, *158*, 72–81. [CrossRef] [PubMed]
67. Jiang, J.; Li, S.; Wang, Y.; Xiao, X.; Jin, Y.; Wang, Y.; Yang, Z.; Yan, S.; Li, Y. Potential neurotoxicity of prenatal exposure to sevoflurane on offspring: Metabolomics investigation on neurodevelopment and underlying mechanism. *Int. J. Dev. Neurosci.* **2017**, *62*, 46–53. [CrossRef] [PubMed]
68. Ichinose, H.; Ohye, T.; Suzuki, T.; Sumi-Ichinose, C.; Nomura, T.; Hagino, Y.; Nagatsu, T. Molecular cloning of the human Nurr1 gene: Characterization of the human gene and cDNAs. *Gene* **1999**, *230*, 233–239. [CrossRef]
69. Germain, P.; Staels, B.; Dacquet, C.; Spedding, M.; Laudet, V. Overview of nomenclature of nuclear receptors. *Pharmacol. Rev.* **2006**, *58*, 685–704. [CrossRef]
70. Wang, Z.; Benoit, G.; Liu, J.; Prasad, S.; Aarnisalo, P.; Liu, X.; Xu, H.; Walker, N.P.C.; Perlmann, T. Structure and function of Nurr1 identifies a class of ligand-independent nuclear receptors. *Nature* **2003**, *423*, 555–560. [CrossRef]

71. Maira, M.; Martens, C.; Batsché, E.; Gauthier, Y.; Drouin, J. Dimer-specific potentiation of NGFI-B (Nur77) transcriptional activity by the protein kinase A pathway and AF-1-dependent coactivator recruitment. *Mol. Cell. Biol.* **2003**, *23*, 763–776. [CrossRef]
72. Volakakis, N.; Malewicz, M.; Kadkhodai, B.; Perlmann, T.; Benoit, G. Characterization of the Nurr1 ligand-binding domain co-activator interaction surface. *J. Mol. Endocrinol.* **2006**, *37*, 317–326. [CrossRef] [PubMed]
73. Codina, A.; Benoit, G.; Gooch, J.T.; Neuhaus, D.; Perlmann, T.; Schwabe, J.W.R. Identification of a novel co-regulator interaction surface on the ligand binding domain of Nurr1 using NMR footprinting. *J. Biol. Chem.* **2004**, *279*, 53338–53345. [CrossRef] [PubMed]
74. de Vera, I.M.S.; Giri, P.K.; Munoz-Tello, P.; Brust, R.; Fuhrmann, J.; Matta-Camacho, E.; Shang, J.; Campbell, S.; Wilson, H.D.; Granados, J.; et al. Identification of a Binding Site for Unsaturated Fatty Acids in the Orphan Nuclear Receptor Nurr1. *ACS Chem. Biol.* **2016**, *11*, 1795–1799. [CrossRef] [PubMed]
75. Maira, M.; Martens, C.; Philips, A.; Drouin, J. Heterodimerization between members of the Nur subfamily of orphan nuclear receptors as a novel mechanism for gene activation. *Mol. Cell. Biol.* **1999**, *19*, 7549–7557. [CrossRef] [PubMed]
76. Giguère, V. Orphan nuclear receptors: From gene to function. *Endocr. Rev.* **1999**, *20*, 689–725. [CrossRef]
77. Kim, K.-S.; Kim, C.-H.; Hwang, D.-Y.; Seo, H.; Chung, S.; Hong, S.J.; Lim, J.-K.; Anderson, T.; Isacson, O. Orphan nuclear receptor Nurr1 directly transactivates the promoter activity of the tyrosine hydroxylase gene in a cell-specific manner. *J. Neurochem.* **2003**, *85*, 622–634. [CrossRef]
78. Wallén A, A.; Castro, D.S.; Zetterström, R.H.; Karlén, M.; Olson, L.; Ericson, J.; Perlmann, T. Orphan nuclear receptor Nurr1 is essential for Ret expression in midbrain dopamine neurons and in the brain stem. *Mol. Cell. Neurosci.* **2001**, *18*, 649–663. [CrossRef]
79. Smith, K.M.; Bauer, L.; Fischer, M.; Barkley, R.; Navia, B.A. Identification and characterization of human NR4A2 polymorphisms in attention deficit hyperactivity disorder. *Am. J. Med. Genet. Part B* **2005**, *133B*, 57–63. [CrossRef]
80. Buervenich, S.; Carmine, A.; Arvidsson, M.; Xiang, F.; Zhang, Z.; Sydow, O.; Jönsson, E.G.; Sedvall, G.C.; Leonard, S.; Ross, R.G.; et al. NURR1 mutations in cases of schizophrenia and manic-depressive disorder. *Am. J. Med. Genet.* **2000**, *96*, 808–813. [CrossRef]
81. Reuter, M.S.; Krumbiegel, M.; Schlüter, G.; Ekici, A.B.; Reis, A.; Zweier, C. Haploinsufficiency of NR4A2 is associated with a neurodevelopmental phenotype with prominent language impairment. *Am. J. Med. Genet. Part A* **2017**, *173*, 2231–2234. [CrossRef]
82. Campos-Melo, D.; Galleguillos, D.; Sánchez, N.; Gysling, K.; Andrés, M.E. Nur transcription factors in stress and addiction. *Front. Mol. Neurosci.* **2013**, *6*, 44. [CrossRef] [PubMed]
83. Fedeli, D.; Montani, M.; Carloni, M.; Nasuti, C.; Amici, A.; Gabbianelli, R. Leukocyte Nurr1 as peripheral biomarker of early-life environmental exposure to permethrin insecticide. *Biomarkers* **2012**, *17*, 604–609. [CrossRef] [PubMed]
84. Martens, C.; Bilodeau, S.; Maira, M.; Gauthier, Y.; Drouin, J. Protein-protein interactions and transcriptional antagonism between the subfamily of NGFI-B/Nur77 orphan nuclear receptors and glucocorticoid receptor. *Mol. Endocrinol.* **2005**, *19*, 885–897. [CrossRef] [PubMed]
85. Rojas, P.; Joodmardi, E.; Perlmann, T.; Ogren, S.O. Rapid increase of Nurr1 mRNA expression in limbic and cortical brain structures related to coping with depression-like behavior in mice. *J. Neurosci. Res.* **2010**, *88*, 2284–2293. [CrossRef]
86. Bensinger, S.J.; Tontonoz, P. A Nurr1 Pathway for Neuroprotection. *Cell* **2009**, *137*, 26–28. [CrossRef]
87. Carpentier, R.; Sacchetti, P.; Ségard, P.; Staels, B.; Lefebvre, P. The glucocorticoid receptor is a co-regulator of the orphan nuclear receptor Nurr1. *J. Neurochem.* **2008**, *104*, 777–789. [CrossRef]
88. Luo, Y. The function and mechanisms of Nurr1 action in midbrain dopaminergic neurons, from development and maintenance to survival. *Int. Rev. Neurobiol.* **2012**, *102*, 1–22.
89. Fan, X.; Luo, G.; Ming, M.; Pu, P.; Li, L.; Yang, D.; Le, W. Nurr1 expression and its modulation in microglia. *Neuroimmunomodulation* **2009**, *16*, 162–170. [CrossRef]
90. Kurakula, K.; Koenis, D.S.; van Tiel, C.M.; de Vries, C.J.M. NR4A nuclear receptors are orphans but not lonesome. *Biochim. Biophys. Acta* **2014**, *1843*, 2543–2555. [CrossRef]
91. Wan, P.K.; Siu, M.K.; Leung, T.H.; Mo, X.-T.; Chan, K.K.; Ngan, H.Y. Role of Nurr1 in Carcinogenesis and Tumor Immunology: A State of the Art Review. *Cancers* **2020**, *12*, 3044. [CrossRef]

92. Veum, V.L.; Dankel, S.N.; Gjerde, J.; Nielsen, H.J.; Solsvik, M.H.; Haugen, C.; Christensen, B.J.; Hoang, T.; Fadnes, D.J.; Busch, C.; et al. The nuclear receptors NUR77, NURR1 and NOR1 in obesity and during fat loss. *Int. J. Obes. (Lond.)* **2012**, *36*, 1195–1202. [CrossRef] [PubMed]

93. Xu, Y.; Huang, Q.; Zhang, W.; Wang, Y.; Zeng, Q.; He, C.; Xue, J.; Chen, J.; Hu, X.; Xu, Y. Decreased expression levels of Nurr1 are associated with chronic inflammation in patients with type 2 diabetes. *Mol. Med. Rep.* **2015**, *12*, 5487–5493. [CrossRef] [PubMed]

94. Ranhotra, H.S. The NR4A orphan nuclear receptors: Mediators in metabolism and diseases. *J. Recept. Signal Transduct.* **2015**, *35*, 184–188. [CrossRef]

95. Bonta, P.I.; van Tiel, C.M.; Mariska, V.; Pols, T.W.H.; van Thienen, J.V.; Valérie, F.; Karin, A.E.; Jurgen, S.; Arnold, S.C.; van der Poll, T.; et al. Nuclear Receptors Nur77, Nurr1, and NOR-1 Expressed in Atherosclerotic Lesion Macrophages Reduce Lipid Loading and Inflammatory Responses. *Arterioscler. Thromb. Vasc. Biol.* **2006**, *26*, 2288–2294. [CrossRef] [PubMed]

96. McMorrow, J.P.; Murphy, E.P. Inflammation: A role for NR4A orphan nuclear receptors? *Biochem. Soc. Trans.* **2011**, *39*, 688–693. [CrossRef] [PubMed]

97. Oh, M.; Kim, S.Y.; Gil, J.-E.; Byun, J.-S.; Cha, D.-W.; Ku, B.; Lee, W.; Kim, W.-K.; Oh, K.-J.; Lee, E.-W.; et al. Nurr1 performs its anti-inflammatory function by regulating RasGRP1 expression in neuro-inflammation. *Sci. Rep.* **2020**, *10*, 10755. [CrossRef] [PubMed]

98. Willems, S.; Kilu, W.; Ni, X.; Chaikuad, A.; Knapp, S.; Heering, J.; Merk, D. The orphan nuclear receptor Nurr1 is responsive to non-steroidal anti-inflammatory drugs. *Commun. Chem.* **2020**, *3*, 85. [CrossRef]

99. Fedeli, D.; Montani, M.; Bordoni, L.; Galeazzi, R.; Nasuti, C.; Correia-Sá, L.; Domingues, V.F.; Jayant, M.; Brahmachari, V.; Massaccesi, L.; et al. In vivo and in silico studies to identify mechanisms associated with Nurr1 modulation following early life exposure to permethrin in rats. *Neuroscience* **2017**, *340*, 411–423. [CrossRef]

100. Bordoni, L.; Fedeli, D.; Nasuti, C.; Capitani, M.; Fiorini, D.; Gabbianelli, R. Permethrin pesticide induces NURR1 up-regulation in dopaminergic cell line: Is the pro-oxidant effect involved in toxicant-neuronal damage? *Comp. Biochem. Physiol. C Toxicol. Pharmacol.* **2017**, *201*, 51–57. [CrossRef]

101. Carloni, M.; Nasuti, C.; Fedeli, D.; Montani, M.; Vadhana, M.S.D.; Amici, A.; Gabbianelli, R. Early life permethrin exposure induces long-term brain changes in Nurr1, NF-kB and Nrf-2. *Brain Res.* **2013**, *1515*, 19–28. [CrossRef]

102. Aye, I.L.M.H.; Lager, S.; Ramirez, V.I.; Gaccioli, F.; Dudley, D.J.; Jansson, T.; Powell, T.L. Increasing maternal body mass index is associated with systemic inflammation in the mother and the activation of distinct placental inflammatory pathways. *Biol. Reprod.* **2014**, *90*, 129. [CrossRef] [PubMed]

103. Challier, J.C.; Basu, S.; Bintein, T.; Minium, J.; Hotmire, K.; Catalano, P.M.; Hauguel-de Mouzon, S. Obesity in pregnancy stimulates macrophage accumulation and inflammation in the placenta. *Placenta* **2008**, *29*, 274–281. [CrossRef] [PubMed]

104. Kirwan, J.P.; Hauguel-De Mouzon, S.; Lepercq, J.; Challier, J.-C.; Huston-Presley, L.; Friedman, J.E.; Kalhan, S.C.; Catalano, P.M. TNF-alpha is a predictor of insulin resistance in human pregnancy. *Diabetes* **2002**, *51*, 2207–2213. [CrossRef] [PubMed]

105. Lappas, M. The NR4A receptors Nurr1 and Nur77 are increased in human placenta from women with gestational diabetes. *Placenta* **2014**, *35*, 866–875. [CrossRef]

106. Radaelli, T.; Varastehpour, A.; Catalano, P.; Hauguel-de Mouzon, S. Gestational diabetes induces placental genes for chronic stress and inflammatory pathways. *Diabetes* **2003**, *52*, 2951–2958. [CrossRef] [PubMed]

107. Anisman, H.; Merali, Z. Cytokines, stress, and depressive illness. *Brain. Behav. Immun.* **2002**, *16*, 513–524. [CrossRef]

108. Irwin, M.R.; Miller, A.H. Depressive disorders and immunity: 20 years of progress and discovery. *Brain. Behav. Immun.* **2007**, *21*, 374–383. [CrossRef]

109. Goldsmith, D.R.; Rapaport, M.H.; Miller, B.J. A meta-analysis of blood cytokine network alterations in psychiatric patients: Comparisons between schizophrenia, bipolar disorder and depression. *Mol. Psychiatry* **2016**, *21*, 1696–1709. [CrossRef]

110. Irwin, M.R.; Cole, S.W. Reciprocal regulation of the neural and innate immune systems. *Nat. Rev. Immunol.* **2011**, *11*, 625–632. [CrossRef]

111. Himmerich, H.; Patsalos, O.; Lichtblau, N.; Ibrahim, M.A.A.; Dalton, B. Cytokine Research in Depression: Principles, Challenges, and Open Questions. *Front. Psychiatry* **2019**, *10*, 30. [CrossRef]

112. Himmerich, H.; Minkwitz, J.; Kirkby, K.C. Weight Gain and Metabolic Changes During Treatment with Antipsychotics and Antidepressants. *Endocr. Metab. Immune Disord. Drug Targets* **2015**, *15*, 252–260. [CrossRef] [PubMed]
113. Pearen, M.A.; Muscat, G.E.O. Minireview: Nuclear hormone receptor 4A signaling: Implications for metabolic disease. *Mol. Endocrinol.* **2010**, *24*, 1891–1903. [CrossRef] [PubMed]
114. Holdsworth-Carson, S.J.; Permezel, M.; Riley, C.; Rice, G.E.; Lappas, M. Peroxisome proliferator-activated receptors and retinoid X receptor-alpha in term human gestational tissues: Tissue specific and labour-associated changes. *Placenta* **2009**, *30*, 176–186. [CrossRef] [PubMed]
115. Holdsworth-Carson, S.J.; Lim, R.; Mitton, A.; Whitehead, C.; Rice, G.E.; Permezel, M.; Lappas, M. Peroxisome proliferator-activated receptors are altered in pathologies of the human placenta: Gestational diabetes mellitus, intrauterine growth restriction and preeclampsia. *Placenta* **2010**, *31*, 222–229. [CrossRef] [PubMed]
116. Holdsworth-Carson, S.J.; Permezel, M.; Rice, G.E.; Lappas, M. Preterm and infection-driven preterm labor: The role of peroxisome proliferator-activated receptors and retinoid X receptor. *Reproduction* **2009**, *137*, 1007–1015. [CrossRef]
117. Christiaens, I.; Zaragoza, D.B.; Guilbert, L.; Robertson, S.A.; Mitchell, B.F.; Olson, D.M. Inflammatory processes in preterm and term parturition. *J. Reprod. Immunol.* **2008**, *79*, 50–57. [CrossRef]
118. Lappas, M. Effect of spontaneous term labour on the expression of the NR4A receptors nuclear receptor related 1 protein (Nurr1), neuron-derived clone 77 (Nur77) and neuron-derived orphan receptor 1 (NOR1) in human fetal membranes and myometrium. *Reprod. Fertil. Dev.* **2016**, *28*, 893–906. [CrossRef]
119. Romero, R.; Espinoza, J.; Kusanovic, J.P.; Gotsch, F.; Hassan, S.; Erez, O.; Chaiworapongsa, T.; Mazor, M. The preterm parturition syndrome. *BJOG* **2006**, *113* (Suppl. 3), 17–42. [CrossRef]
120. Weinstock, M. Alterations induced by gestational stress in brain morphology and behaviour of the offspring. *Prog. Neurobiol.* **2001**, *65*, 427–451. [CrossRef]
121. Weinstock, M. Can the behaviour abnormalities induced by gestational stress in rats be prevented or reversed? *Stress* **2002**, *5*, 167–176. [CrossRef]
122. Huizink, A.C.; Mulder, E.J.H.; Buitelaar, J.K. Prenatal stress and risk for psychopathology: Specific effects or induction of general susceptibility? *Psychol. Bull.* **2004**, *130*, 115–142. [CrossRef] [PubMed]
123. Saucedo-Cardenas, O.; Quintana-Hau, J.D.; Le, W.D.; Smidt, M.P.; Cox, J.J.; De Mayo, F.; Burbach, J.P.; Conneely, O.M. Nurr1 is essential for the induction of the dopaminergic phenotype and the survival of ventral mesencephalic late dopaminergic precursor neurons. *Proc. Natl. Acad. Sci. USA* **1998**, *95*, 4013–4018. [CrossRef] [PubMed]
124. Katunar, M.R.; Saez, T.; Brusco, A.; Antonelli, M.C. Immunocytochemical expression of dopamine-related transcription factors Pitx3 and Nurr1 in prenatally stressed adult rats. *J. Neurosci. Res.* **2009**, *87*, 1014–1022. [CrossRef] [PubMed]
125. Montes, P.; Ruiz-Sánchez, E.; Calvillo, M.; Rojas, P. Active coping of prenatally stressed rats in the forced swimming test: Involvement of the Nurr1 gene. *Stress* **2016**, *19*, 506–515. [CrossRef] [PubMed]
126. Sun, Y.; Li, Y.-S.; Yang, J.-W.; Yu, J.; Wu, Y.-P.; Li, B.-X. Exposure to atrazine during gestation and lactation periods: Toxicity effects on dopaminergic neurons in offspring by downregulation of Nurr1 and VMAT2. *Int. J. Mol. Sci.* **2014**, *15*, 2811–2825. [CrossRef]
127. Patel, V.P.; Chu, C.T. Nuclear transport, oxidative stress, and neurodegeneration. *Int. J. Clin. Exp. Pathol.* **2011**, *4*, 215–229.
128. Bordoni, L.; Nasuti, C.; Mirto, M.; Caradonna, F.; Gabbianelli, R. Intergenerational Effect of Early Life Exposure to Permethrin: Changes in Global DNA Methylation and in Nurr1 Gene Expression. *Toxics* **2015**, *3*, 451–461. [CrossRef]
129. Romoli, B.; Lozada, A.F.; Sandoval, I.M.; Manfredsson, F.P.; Hnasko, T.S.; Berg, D.K.; Dulcis, D. Neonatal Nicotine Exposure Primes Midbrain Neurons to a Dopaminergic Phenotype and Increases Adult Drug Consumption. *Biol. Psychiatry* **2019**, *86*, 344–355. [CrossRef]
130. Brown, A.S.; Derkits, E.J. Prenatal infection and schizophrenia: A review of epidemiologic and translational studies. *Am. J. Psychiatry* **2010**, *167*, 261–280. [CrossRef]
131. Brown, A.S.; Meyer, U. Maternal Immune Activation and Neuropsychiatric Illness: A Translational Research Perspective. *Am. J. Psychiatry* **2018**, *175*, 1073–1083. [CrossRef]

132. Vuillermot, S.; Joodmardi, E.; Perlmann, T.; Ögren, S.O.; Feldon, J.; Meyer, U. Prenatal immune activation interacts with genetic Nurr1 deficiency in the development of attentional impairments. *J. Neurosci.* **2012**, *32*, 436–451. [CrossRef] [PubMed]
133. Shao, C.-Z.; Xia, K.-P. Sevoflurane anesthesia represses neurogenesis of hippocampus neural stem cells via regulating microRNA-183-mediated NR4A2 in newborn rats. *J. Cell. Physiol.* **2019**, *234*, 3864–3873. [CrossRef] [PubMed]
134. Lallier, S.W.; Graf, A.E.; Waidyarante, G.R.; Rogers, L.K. Nurr1 expression is modified by inflammation in microglia. *Neuroreport* **2016**, *27*, 1120–1127. [CrossRef] [PubMed]
135. Popichak, K.A.; Hammond, S.L.; Moreno, J.A.; Afzali, M.F.; Backos, D.S.; Slayden, R.D.; Safe, S.; Tjalkens, R.B. Compensatory Expression of Nur77 and Nurr1 Regulates NF-κB-Dependent Inflammatory Signaling in Astrocytes. *Mol. Pharmacol.* **2018**, *94*, 1174–1186. [CrossRef]
136. Lungu, G.; Stoica, G.; Ambrus, A. MicroRNA profiling and the role of microRNA-132 in neurodegeneration using a rat model. *Neurosci. Lett.* **2013**, *553*, 153–158. [CrossRef] [PubMed]
137. Yang, Z.; Li, T.; Li, S.; Wei, M.; Qi, H.; Shen, B.; Chang, R.C.-C.; Le, W.; Piao, F. Altered Expression Levels of MicroRNA-132 and Nurr1 in Peripheral Blood of Parkinson's Disease: Potential Disease Biomarkers. *ACS Chem. Neurosci.* **2019**, *10*, 2243–2249. [CrossRef]
138. Valsecchi, V.; Boido, M.; Montarolo, F.; Guglielmotto, M.; Perga, S.; Martire, S.; Cutrupi, S.; Iannello, A.; Gionchiglia, N.; Signorino, E.; et al. The transcription factor Nurr1 is upregulated in amyotrophic lateral sclerosis patients and SOD1-G93A mice. *Dis. Model. Mech.* **2020**, *13*. [CrossRef]
139. Jakaria, M.; Haque, M.E.; Cho, D.-Y.; Azam, S.; Kim, I.-S.; Choi, D.-K. Molecular Insights into NR4A2(Nurr1): An Emerging Target for Neuroprotective Therapy Against Neuroinflammation and Neuronal Cell Death. *Mol. Neurobiol.* **2019**, *56*, 5799–5814. [CrossRef]
140. Moon, H.; Jeon, S.G.; Kim, J.-I.; Kim, H.S.; Lee, S.; Kim, D.; Park, S.; Moon, M.; Chung, H. Pharmacological Stimulation of Nurr1 Promotes Cell Cycle Progression in Adult Hippocampal Neural Stem Cells. *Int. J. Mol. Sci.* **2019**, *21*, 4. [CrossRef]
141. Munoz-Tello, P.; Lin, H.; Khan, P.; de Vera, I.M.S.; Kamenecka, T.M.; Kojetin, D.J. Assessment of NR4A Ligands that Directly Bind and Modulate the Orphan Nuclear Receptor Nurr1. *bioRxiv* **2020**. [CrossRef]
142. de Vera, I.M.S.; Munoz-Tello, P.; Zheng, J.; Dharmarajan, V.; Marciano, D.P.; Matta-Camacho, E.; Giri, P.K.; Shang, J.; Hughes, T.S.; Rance, M.; et al. Defining a Canonical Ligand-Binding Pocket in the Orphan Nuclear Receptor Nurr1. *Structure* **2019**, *27*, 66–77.e5. [CrossRef] [PubMed]
143. Bruning, J.M.; Wang, Y.; Oltrabella, F.; Tian, B.; Kholodar, S.A.; Liu, H.; Bhattacharya, P.; Guo, S.; Holton, J.M.; Fletterick, R.J.; et al. Covalent Modification and Regulation of the Nuclear Receptor Nurr1 by a Dopamine Metabolite. *Cell Chem. Biol.* **2019**, *26*, 674–685.e6. [CrossRef] [PubMed]
144. Bordoni, L.; Gabbianelli, R. Primers on nutrigenetics and nutri(epi)genomics: Origins and development of precision nutrition. *Biochimie* **2019**, *160*, 156–171. [CrossRef] [PubMed]

Publisher's Note: MDPI stays neutral with regard to jurisdictional claims in published maps and institutional affiliations.

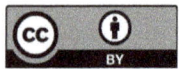

© 2020 by the authors. Licensee MDPI, Basel, Switzerland. This article is an open access article distributed under the terms and conditions of the Creative Commons Attribution (CC BY) license (http://creativecommons.org/licenses/by/4.0/).

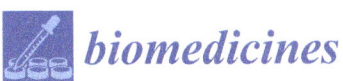

Article

Using Artificial Neural Network to Discriminate Parkinson's Disease from Other Parkinsonisms by Focusing on Putamen of Dopamine Transporter SPECT Images

Chung-Yao Chien [1,2], Szu-Wei Hsu [3], Tsung-Lin Lee [2], Pi-Shan Sung [2] and Chou-Ching Lin [1,2,*]

[1] Department of Biomedical Engineering, National Cheng Kung University, Tainan 704, Taiwan; p88041075@ncku.edu.tw

[2] Department of Neurology, National Cheng Kung University Hospital, College of Medicine, National Cheng Kung University, Tainan 704, Taiwan; c2481023@hotmail.com (T.-L.L.); pishansung@gmail.com (P.-S.S.)

[3] Department of Nuclear Medicine, National Cheng Kung University Hospital, College of Medicine, National Cheng Kung University, Tainan 704, Taiwan; i54921514@gmail.com

* Correspondence: cxl45@mail.ncku.edu.tw; Tel.: +886-6-235-3535 (ext. 2692)

Abstract: Background: The challenge of differentiating, at an early stage, Parkinson's disease from parkinsonism caused by other disorders remains unsolved. We proposed using an artificial neural network (ANN) to process images of dopamine transporter single-photon emission computed tomography (DAT-SPECT). Methods: Abnormal DAT-SPECT images of subjects with Parkinson's disease and parkinsonism caused by other disorders were divided into training and test sets. Striatal regions of the images were segmented by using an active contour model and were used as the data to perform transfer learning on a pre-trained ANN to discriminate Parkinson's disease from parkinsonism caused by other disorders. A support vector machine trained using parameters of semi-quantitative measurements including specific binding ratio and asymmetry index was used for comparison. Results: The predictive accuracy of the ANN classifier (86%) was higher than that of the support vector machine classifier (68%). The sensitivity and specificity of the ANN classifier in predicting Parkinson's disease were 81.8% and 88.6%, respectively. Conclusions: The ANN classifier outperformed classical biomarkers in differentiating Parkinson's disease from parkinsonism caused by other disorders. This classifier can be readily included into standalone computer software for clinical application.

Keywords: artificial neural network; deep learning; Parkinson's disease; atypical parkinsonian syndrome; dopamine transporter SPECT

1. Introduction

Disease-modifying therapies including target therapy are under development to treat Parkinson's disease (PD). According to the targeted pathogenesis, some treatment strategies focus on the very initial phase of the disease [1,2]. However, early in the disease progress, PD and parkinsonism caused by other disorders, including atypical parkinsonian syndromes share similar clinical features because the hallmarks of PD or other parkinsonism may not have emerged [3,4]. To date, the diagnosis of PD is solely based on clinical diagnostic criteria and gene tests. However, it takes time to fulfil these clinical diagnostic criteria, and only less than 5% of all PD patients have known causative genes [1,5]. Therefore, new diagnostic tools aiding efficient screening are required to address this unmet need.

Clinicopathological studies based on brain bank material have shown that clinicians diagnose PD incorrectly in about 25% of patients. One of the most common reasons for misdiagnosis was atypical parkinsonian syndromes [6]. To differentiate PD from other forms of parkinsonism, the guidelines of the European Federation of Neurological Societies suggest transcranial sonography of the mesencephalic brainstem. In clinical practice, proper evaluation of the substantial nigra depends on experienced technicians and investigators, and also on the quality of the temporal bone window. Structural magnetic resonance imaging (MRI) reveals typical signs of Parkinson-plus syndromes only in the middle or later course of the diseases. Many types of advanced MRI techniques such as voxel-wise analysis [7], diffusion [8,9], susceptibility [10,11], neuromelanin [12], and functional imaging have been evaluated, however their overall sensitivity and specificity have been insufficient to meet the clinical demand. 18F-fluorodeoxyglucose positron emission tomography (FDG-PET) is an imaging modality that has a prediction accuracy above 90% [13,14]. Due to the long procedure time, the influence of the subject's blood glucose status, cost-effectiveness, and usage of diagnostic template images, to date, FDG-PET has not been recommended in clinical practice. Moreover, other clinical diagnostic modalities such as 123I-metaiodobenzylguanidine (MIBG) myocardial scintigraphy and olfactory testing have been reported to achieve a higher specificity of up to 80% when compared with gold-standard clinical or clinicopathologic diagnoses in differentiating PD from other parkinsonisms [3]. However, several olfactory test studies have reported a sensitivity ranging from 61–77% [3,5,15,16], and when MIBG myocardial scintigraphy was used prospectively in general parkinsonian cases, the accuracy was somewhat limited [17].

An abnormal dopamine transporter single-photon emission computed tomography (DAT-SPECT) image reflects the dysfunction of striatal neurons, and its discrimination of PD or not PD relies on clinical information and other structural images. However, in daily clinical scenarios discriminative information is not always obtainable. To classify parkinsonism based on DAT-SPECT images, advanced engineering techniques with semi-quantitative analysis have been applied [18]. In addition, images or signals from striatal regions (SRs) alone can provide adequate differentiating information [19]. One research group differentiated degenerative parkinsonism using a computer-aided automatic algorithm and SR and whole-brain uptake patterns. Both were shown to have adequate specificity (84–90%), however the whole-brain uptake pattern demonstrated lower sensitivity [20]. Another study group discovered that in voxel-based analysis of DAT-SPECT images, SR alone could differentiate PD from dementia with Lewy bodies (DLB), while regions outside SRs were not contributory [21].

Machine learning and artificial neural networks (ANNs) have developed rapidly and been applied in clinical settings [22]. Recently, Vaccaro et al. demonstrated that a careful analysis of neuropsychological deficits through a machine-learning approach successfully discriminated PD and progressive supranuclear palsy [23]. An ANN application on DAT-SPECT images reported a classification accuracy of up to 90% in identifying PD with a mean Hoehn and Yahr (H&Y) stage of 1.6 from healthy controls [24], a great leap from the 80% achieved with conventional or semi-quantitative analysis [24,25]. Thus, in this study, we combined appropriate segmentation of SR images derived from DAT-SPECT with a widely-used pre-trained neural network for computer-vision to investigate the efficiency of this integrated method in identification of PD from parkinsonism caused by other disorders.

2. Material and Methods
2.1. Subjects

Ethical review and approval were waived for this study, due to collection, analysis and publication of the retrospectively obtained and anonymized data for this non-interventional study. As a retrospective study evaluating SPECT images performed in the diagnostic setting without disclosing any personal information of the patients, the need for written consent was waived.

2.1.1. First Set of Images for ANN Training and Validation

Medical charts of subjects with parkinsonian syndromes (ICD-9 coded 332.0 and 332.1) who received DAT-SPECT imaging (99mTc-TRODAT-1-SPECT) from 2017 to 2019 at the outpatient clinic performed by three neurologists specializing in movement disorders were retrospectively reviewed. The initial number of collected subjects was 518. The images reported as normal or aging-related were firstly excluded. The remaining 379 patients (234 subjects with clinically-favored idiopathic PD and 145 subjects with clinically-favored non-PD) were then assigned into two groups: those with PD and those with parkinsonism caused by other disorders (non-PDs), according to the following criteria. In the PD group, in order to establish higher sensitivity and specificity (>90%) of "ground truth" images, we followed the Queen Square Brain Bank (QSBB) criteria to exclude those with a history of stroke or exposure to neuroleptic agents. Finally, 105 cases who had been regularly followed up for more than three years were classified into the PD group. In the non-PD group, cases with drug-induced parkinsonism were excluded, and 100 cases with a diagnosis of possible or probable Parkinson-plus syndromes (such as multiple system atrophy or progressive supranuclear palsy), DLB, vascular parkinsonism, or other causes of parkinsonism characterized by parkinsonian syndromes with symmetrical features and unresponsive to L-dopa treatment were selected (Figure 1). Finally, a total of 205 images were used to train the ANN as a classifier through randomly splitting these images into 90% for training and 10% for validation.

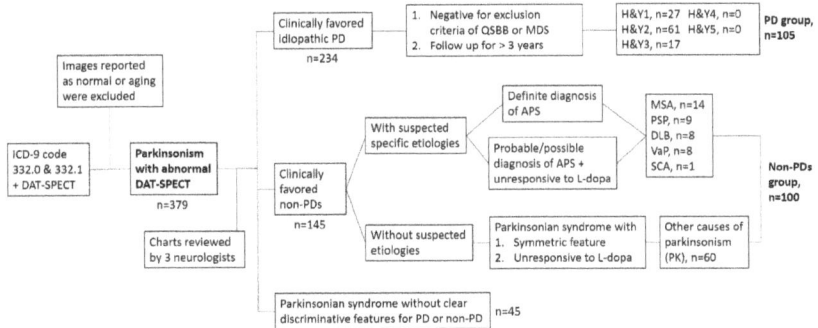

Figure 1. The flow chart of subject selection for artificial neural network (ANN)-classifier training. The cases with drug-induced parkinsonism which reported as normal DAT-SPECT were excluded. ICD, international classification diagnosis; DAT-SPECT, dopamine transporter single-photon emission computed tomography; PD, Parkinson's disease; APS, atypical parkinsonian syndrome; QSBB, Queen Square Brain Bank; MDS, movement disorder society; H&Y, Hoehn and Yahr stage; MSA, multiple system atrophy; PSP, progressive supranuclear palsy; DLB, dementia with Lewy bodies; VaP, vascular parkinsonism; SCA, spinocerebellar ataxia.

2.1.2. Second Set of Images for Testing the ANN Classifier

To test the performance of the trained ANN classifier, a second dataset of DAT-SPECT images performed from January to March 2020 of cases with a diagnosis of parkinsonian syndrome (n = 57) was obtained. Cases with a history of unilateral onset of parkinsonian symptoms and adequate responsiveness to levodopa treatment, but who did not meet the QSBB exclusion criteria were defined as having PD. Those with prominent red flags such as bilateral onset of symptoms and unresponsive to levodopa treatment, or who met the QSBB exclusion criteria such as early cognitive impairment, cerebellar signs, or with structural imaging suggesting vascular parkinsonism or hydrocephalus were defined as having parkinsonism caused by other disorders (non-PDs).

2.2. Image Processing

2.2.1. Image Pre-Processing

First, a mask to remove scalp uptake was applied to all images. The intensity of images was then normalized by contrast stretching. To select the region of interest (ROI), i.e., the SR, an active contour model was applied [26]. The physician first selected an ROI using the same procedure as in the conventional method for calculating striatal/occipital ratio, and the active contour model automatically adjusted the outline of the ROI [27] to minimize the summarized values contributed by both inside and outside of the ROI, and a fitted ROI was then segmented out for the next step. This method also minimized selection bias and physician inconsistency. We also kept the images before segmentation for further comparison.

2.2.2. Binary Classification by ANN

The segmented SR images were fed into the ANN training process for classification. We applied the method of transfer learning to a pretrained network from an open source. AlexNet is a standard model for image classification through deep learning that has been widely applied to medical images. It is composed of five convolutional layers and three fully-connected layers. We froze the parameters of convolutional layers for basic feature extraction. In the last three fully-connected layers, we replaced the label space with our image categories. This trained ANN classifier was first validated using the validation data targeting an accuracy > 90%, and then re-confirmed using the independent test dataset. The results of training/validation and test dataset were presented by calculating the area under the receiver operating characteristic curve (AUROC). For comparison, we also trained another ANN classifier using images of the whole brain without segmentation (Figure 2).

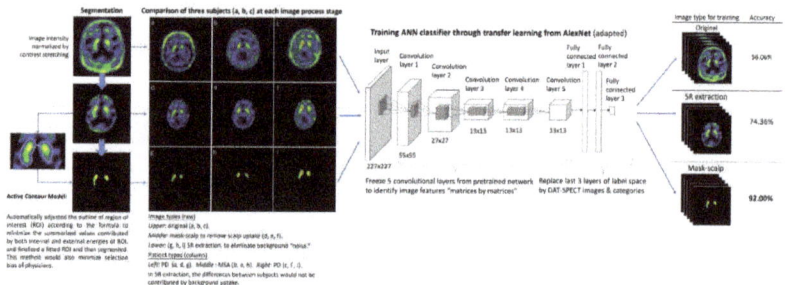

Figure 2. Workflow of image preprocessing, SR segmentation, and ANN classifier training. The ANN classifier was trained by different types of images (original, whole brain, and segmented SR). The SR segmentation demonstrated higher accuracy than the other two types of images.

2.2.3. Semi-Quantitative Measurements and Machine-Learning Classification

Two indicators were evaluated—specific binding ratio (SBR), which was calculated as ((SR-occipital)/occipital) and asymmetry index (ASI), which was calculated as ((2 |SRleft − SRright|)/(SRleft + SRright)). Classification of the PD and non-PD groups was attempted using SBR and ASI with machine-learning approaches including linear discrimination, support vector machine (SVM) with quadratic, cubic, and Gaussian kernel methods, with or without primary component analysis (PCA) from the classification learner toolbox of Matlab 2018b (MathWorks, Natick, Massachusetts). The SVM handled both linear and nonlinear classification. In linear models, the SVM attempted to define the largest margin between the points on either side of the decision line, whereas in non-linear models, a hyperplane approach was applied for binary classification of the dataset.

Details of the DAT-SPECT scanning protocol and imaging data acquisition are described in Appendix A. Statistical analyses were performed using SPSS software (SPSS Statistics for Windows, version 17.0, SPSS Inc., Chicago, IL, USA).

2.2.4. Class-Activation Mapping to Visually Explain the ANN Classifier

Computer-vision examines images in matrices using a matrix method and convolutes them into complicated features which are usually meaningless to the human eye. These features are not regarded as being biomarkers and are hardly correlated to clinical facts. One way to visualize computer-vision is through class-activation mapping (CAM), which produces "visual explanations" from an ANN using parts of the image that weigh most while performing classification. CAM has been widely applied in deep learning methods of medical imaging [28], and we used it in this study to visually explain the results from the ANN classifier.

All image processing and ANN procedures were implemented in Matlab 2018b (MathWorks, Natick, MA, USA).

3. Results

3.1. Demographic Characteristics

The clinical characteristics of the patient groups are summarized in Table 1. There were no significant differences in age or gender (for training/validation set, $p = 0.44$ and for test set, $p = 0.91$). For the training/validation dataset, there were 105 subjects in the PD group with an average H&Y stage of 1.93 (median H&Y stage 2). The non-PD group (100 subjects) included 23 cases with Parkinson-plus syndrome, 8 cases with DLB, 8 cases with vascular parkinsonism, 1 case with spinocerebellar ataxia, and 60 cases with other forms of parkinsonism. For the test dataset, there were 22 subjects in the PD group, with an average H&Y stage of 1.95 (median H&Y stage 2), and 35 subjects in the non-PD group, including 6 cases with Parkinson-plus syndrome, 8 cases with DLB and 21 cases with other forms of parkinsonism.

Table 1. Demographic characteristics of the subjects.

Data	Training/Validation Set (n = 205)			Test Set (n = 57)		
Group	PD	Non-PD	p Value	PD	Non-PD	p Value
Age (years) (mean ± SD)	65.4 ± 10.2	66.6 ± 12.8	0.44	70.3 ± 9.8	70.6 ± 13.4	0.93
Gender (F/M)	52/53	45/55	0.51	8/14	12/23	0.87
Mean disease duration (years) (IQR)	2.32 (2)	1.89 (1)	0.27	2.57 (2.5)	3.56 (3)	0.34

PD, Parkinson's disease; SD, standard deviation; IQR, interquartile range.

3.2. Comparisons of Semi-Quantitative Measurements and ANN Classifier

The performances of classifying the test dataset using semi-quantitative measurements and ANN classifier were compared. The distributions of both SBR and ASI of the test dataset were found to be normal according to the Shapiro–Wilk test. The unpaired t tests between the PD and non-PD groups were $p = 0.003$ for SBR and $p = 0.083$ for ASI. The test datasets were classified using SBR and ASI, respectively. According to the boxplot, the distributions of SBR and ASI values between groups greatly overlapped (Figure 3A,B). Classification by SVM using features from the combination of SBR and ASI revealed that moderate Gaussian kernel through PCA feature extraction resulted in the best result among the methods of machine learning (Figure 3C). There were still several remarkable errors within each classification region. The classification accuracy was 68.4% with sensitivity and specificity of 31.8% and 91.4%, respectively, in predicting PD. For the ANN classifier, an accuracy of 92% was obtained through repetitively fine-tuning and validating the training dataset. Classification of the test dataset through best parameters (feature maps) from computer-vision with ANN revealed an accuracy of 86% with sensitivity and specificity of 81.8% and 88.6%, respectively, in predicting PD (Table 2). The performance of this classifier was favorable (Table 3). The AUROC was 0.94 for the training/validation dataset and 0.76 for the test dataset (Figure 4A). Another ANN classifier trained and tested using whole-brain images (without segmentation) from the same groups of subjects had lower accuracy, sensitivity, and specificity (Table 2).

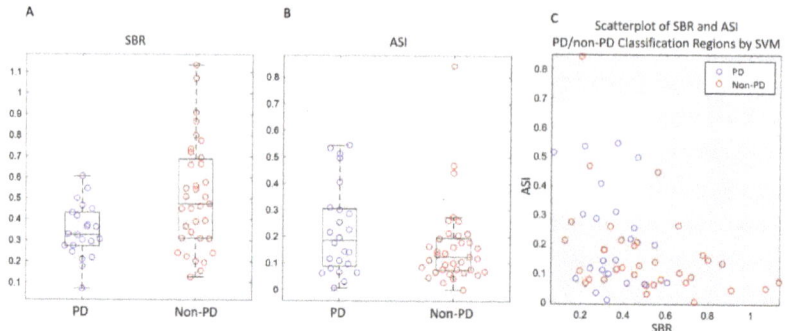

Figure 3. Distribution of indicators derived from semi-quantitative methods (SBR and ASI) in the test dataset (n = 57). (**A**) Dot diagram overlaid whisker-boxplot of SBR showed a wider range of distribution in the non-PD group. The range of the PD group almost totally overlapped with that of the non-PD group. (**B**) Dot diagram overlaid whisker-boxplot of ASI showed a wider range of distribution in the PD group. The range of the non-PD group almost totally overlapped with that of the PD group. (**C**) Scatterplot of SBR and ASI of both groups showing the classification results of median Gaussian kernel SVM with PCA. In the PD (lighter) region only one non-PD point was included, while there were 12 PD points in the non-PD's (darker) region. The overall accuracy was 68.4% using this machine-learning method.

Table 2. Comparisons of the prediction accuracy of the test dataset with different classifiers.

Classifier	SVM	ANN	
Learning Method	Machine Learning	Deep Learning	
Input data	SBR & ASI	Whole-brain image	SR image
Accuracy	68.4%	68.4%	86.0%
Sensitivity	31.8%	81.8%	81.8%
Specificity	91.4%	60.0%	88.6%

SVM, support vector machine; ANN, artificial neural network; SBR, specific binding ratio; ASI, asymmetry index; SR, striatal region.

3.3. Visualization of Computer-Vision through CAM

Class-activation mapping revealed the most discriminative parts of the images, and the results showed that computer-vision focused on the most informative regions of both sides of the putamen (tail of comma) (Figure 4B) to classify PD and non-PD. However, which of the intensity, shape, curvature, or convexity of contour was the most characteristic feature was not available for further analysis.

Table 3. Confusion matrix of ANN classifier for predicting PD.

	Predicted Positive (Classified as PD)	Predicted Negative (Classified as non-PD)	
Actual positive (PDs = 22)	TP 18	FN 4	Sensitivity (recall) 0.818
Actual negative (non-PDs = 35)	FP 4	TN 31	Specificity 0.886
	Precision 0.818	Negative Predictive value 0.886	Accuracy 0.860
	F1 score: 2 × (precision × recall)/(precision + recall) = **0.818**		

PD, Parkinson's disease; TP, true positive; FP, false positive; FN, false negative; TN, true positive.

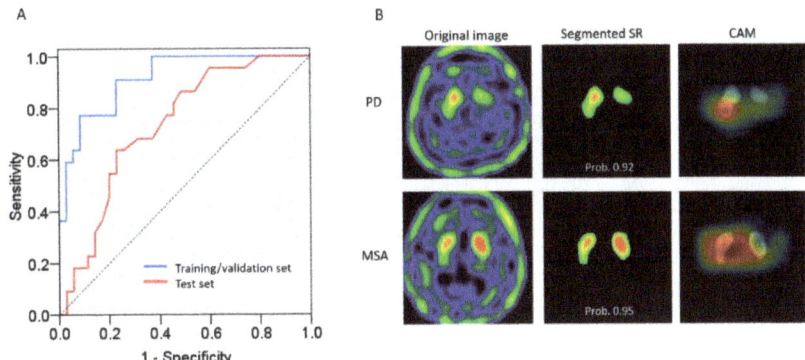

Figure 4. Classification of the test dataset using the ANN classifier. (**A**) The area under the receiver operating characteristic curve (AUROC) was 0.94 in the training/validation dataset (blue line) and 0.76 in the test dataset (red line). (**B**) Examples of classification using the ANN classifier for each group. Upper row is an example of PD and the lower row non-PDs. Left column: the images before scalp-mask and segmentation. Middle column: the images of segmented SR using the active contour model. Right column: the CAM represented with a heat map. The computer-vision weighted more on areas with a warmer color when examining the images. Overlaying on SR images showed that the computer focused most on the putamen. This PD subject was a 58-year-old male with symptoms of resting tremors in his right hand for 2 years and H&Y stage 2 when DAT-SPECT was obtained. Another example case of multiple system atrophy was a 69-year-old male who had symptoms of urinary incontinence, orthostatic hypotension, and cerebellar features of dysmetria and parkinsonism. The disease duration before DAT-SPECT was obtained was 2 years. Prob., probability of class.

4. Discussion

The accuracy of differentiating parkinsonian syndromes through visually rating DAT-SPECT images has been reported to be quite low [29]. Although the semi-quantitative measurements revealed statistical differences between the PD and non-PD groups in testing data in this study, the individual values overlapped greatly between groups (Figure 3). The ANN classifier provided a higher specificity in prediction using "computer-vision parameters". Our results showed acceptable accuracy in differentiating PD from parkinsonism caused by other disorders using only DAT-SPECT images without additional information. The performance of the ANN classifier, with sensitivity and specificity both above 80%, was comparable to that of quantitative olfactory examinations and MIBG myocardiac scintigraphy suggested by diagnostic guidelines. Furthermore, this method is promising because of several advantages: (1) as the sample size of the dataset increases, training results can be further improved; (2) with an adequate number of images taken during the earlier phase of disease (PD or atypical parkinsonian syndromes), the ANN classifier may be trained to identify PD at an early phase [24] or even possibly at a preclinical phase; (3) medical centers and hospitals can train a site-specific ANN classifier using SPECT images based on their own existing dataset without developing new diagnostic modalities or purchasing expensive machines, especially for places where MIBG is not available; (4) SPECT is more widely available, so that when the diagnosis is not straightforward, physicians tend to order SPECT imaging first to confirm striatal neuron loss, such as to differentiate essential tremors from PD, but not MIBG myocardial scintigraphy before proving a neurodegenerative disease in the early phase; and (5) PD can be differentiated from many disease types of parkinsonism, not just a few Parkinson-plus syndromes or other Lewy body diseases [19,30]. Therefore, this classifier is more applicable when facing uncertain types of parkinsonism in clinical practice. In addition, we chose easily-accessible methods and basic application programs, including an active contour model for segmentation and AlexNet for learning and classification. These two tools are widely utilized and can be obtain from online resources. All the processing in this paper were done by a PhD student with entry-level graphics processing unit (GPU, NVIDIA GeForce GTX 1060) in a personal computer. This avoided the need for complicated image processing procedures, experienced engineers, or high-performance computer equipment.

For a feasible classifier, the discriminative parameters do not necessarily need to be clinically correlated, such as extracted features from component analysis [25] or shape/morphological fitting characteristics [18]. Even though SPECT is an imaging technique with a lower resolution than MRI, ANN analyzes an image by decomposing hundreds of thousands of pixels into hundreds of pixeled "matrices" to extract local features. Computer-vision sees patterns of relationships between decomposed pixels of matrices, even if the images do not represent actual anatomical structure in fine detail. However, the excessive number of parameters is also a pitfall of ANN. When training the neural network with SPECT images of whole-brain uptake, the accuracy was lower. This might be because the ANN automatically counted differences in intra- and extra-striatal uptake or background noise equally. Unlike computer-vision, when humans examine DAT-SPECT images they spontaneously focus on the uptake in the SR much more than in extra-striatal regions. This has been shown in previous studies in which better classification accuracy was achieved by looking only at the SR rather than at the whole brain [20]. It could be argued that comparing only the SR may result in the loss of too much information. For example, PD, multiple system atrophy, and DLB are all associated with the same fibrillar α-synuclein protein, but the differences are the sites in which it accumulates in the brain. Although it may be reasonable to compare different patterns of the whole brain, according to prior studies, only the SR was sufficient to differentiate PD from multiple-system atrophy or DLB [21,31].

In order to feed the ANN with segmented images, an active contour model is not only a feasible tool to select the ROI of the SR as with human vision, but also a highly-reproducible method to diminish inter-individual errors in ROI contour outlining. The successful classification using a combination of active contour method and ANN was supported by CAM. The most informative area to differentiate PD from parkinsonism caused by other disorders was the putamen. The region on which computer-vision focused most in this study has also been reported in previous studies using semi-quantitative measurements and other imaging modalities such as diffusion MRI.

We proposed a feasible method to develop a diagnostic tool capable of differentiating PD from parkinsonism caused by other disorders at an early stage through DAT-SPECT images. However, there are some limitations: (1) As a general rule, a bigger dataset is better for training an ANN. A test dataset with more cases with a confirmed diagnosis or even a prospective study is needed to prove and improve the accuracy. Unfortunately, the number of medical images is usually limited. In this study, we used learning from a well-pretrained network to address this limitation. To develop customized and appropriate layers of a neural network is another solution [24,28] to avoiding overfitting during training. (2) Using images from multi-centers to recruit a larger amount of data may result in compatibility problems among different reconstruction algorithms and different machines. Although ANNs may accommodate discrepancies resulting from different reconstruction algorithms by using more parameters, the accuracy may be lower. To consider raw image information such as a "probability map" before reconstruction, appropriate normalization protocols may also be able to solve this issue [25]. (3) In the clinical scenario, the really difficult cases are those that did not fit any diagnostic criteria, the so called gray cases. Although this ANN classifier was trained by images from subjects with discriminative features, it had the potential to study the diagnostic accuracy in gray cases. However, the exact diagnosis of these gray cases is the main obstacle and may depend on pathology. (4) The basis for the diagnosis in this study was purely clinical without underlying pathology. (5) AlexNet is not the most up-to-date tool. To further explore the methodology of applying a pretrained neural network, advanced ANN with more convincing validation algorithms should be considered. (6) Differential diagnosis based only on images could be limited. To promote diagnostic accuracy, a combination of clinical, neuroimaging, and neuropsychology may provide better discrimination between parkinsonisms [23].

5. Conclusions

In this study, an ANN classifier focusing on the putamen region of DAT-SPECT images outperformed the classical biomarkers to differentiate PD from parkinsonism caused by other disorders, with an accuracy of 86% (sensitivity of 81.8% and sensitivity of 88.6%). This method is easily accessible and clinically applicable and provides opportunities to develop an early diagnostic tool to allow for the appropriate application of disease-modifying therapies, in clinical trials and even possibly for bedside treatment in the future.

Author Contributions: Conceptualization, C.-Y.C. and C.-C.L.; methodology, C.-Y.C. and C.-C.L.; software, C.-Y.C.; validation, P.-S.S. and C.-C.L.; formal analysis, C.-Y.C. and S.-W.H., investigation, C.-Y.C. and T.-L.L.; resources, C.-Y.C. and S.-W.H..; data curation, C.-Y.C.; S.-W.H., and T.-L.L.; writing—original draft preparation, C.-Y.C.; writing—review and editing, C.-Y.C., P.-S.S., and C.-C.L.; visualization, C.-Y.C., P.-S.S., and C.-C.L.; supervision, C.-C.L.; project administration, C.-Y.C., S.-W.H., and T.-L.L.; funding acquisition, C.-Y.C. All authors have read and agreed to the published version of the manuscript.

Funding: This research was funded by the National Cheng Kung University Hospital (Project number: NCKUH-10904004).

Institutional Review Board Statement: Ethical review and approval were waived for this study, due to collection, analysis and publication of the retrospectively obtained and anonymized data for this non-interventional study.

Informed Consent Statement: As a retrospective study evaluating SPECT images performed in the diagnostic setting without disclosing any personal information of the patients, the need for written consent was waived.

Data Availability Statement: Data sharing not applicable.

Acknowledgments: This work was partly supported by the National Cheng Kung University Hospital (Project number: NCKUH-10904004).

Conflicts of Interest: The authors declare no conflict of interest.

Appendix A

DAT-SPECT Scan and Reconstruction Protocol

Subjects were intravenously administered with 740 MBq (20 mCi) (99mTc) TRODAT-1 (a radiolabeled form of a tropan derivative for the selective labeling of DAT) in a quiet environment about 10 min after insertion of an intravenous line. The SPECT data were obtained using an energy window of 15% centered on 140 keV for (99mTc). Imaging of (99mTc) TRODAT-1 was initiated approximately 240 min after injection, and SPECT images were acquired over a circular 360° rotation in 120 steps, 50 s per step, in a 128 × 128 × 16 matrix. The images were then reconstructed using Butterworth and Ramp filters (cutoff frequency = 0.3 Nyquist, and power factor = 7) with attenuations according to Chang's method [1], and the reconstructed transverse images were realigned parallel to the canthomeatal line. The slice thickness of each transverse image was 2.89 mm [1]. Chang LT. A method for attenuation correction in radionuclide computed tomography. IEEE Trans Nucl Sci. (25) (1978) 638-43.

References

1. Sardi, S.P.; Simuni, T. New Era in disease modification in Parkinson's disease: Review of genetically targeted therapeutics. *Parkinsonism Relat. Disord.* **2019**, *59*, 32–38. [CrossRef] [PubMed]
2. Lang, A.E.; Espay, A.J. Disease Modification in Parkinson's Disease: Current Approaches, Challenges, and Future Considerations. *Mov. Disord.* **2018**, *33*, 660–677. [CrossRef] [PubMed]
3. Postuma, R.B.; Berg, D.; Stern, M.; Poewe, W.; Olanow, C.W.; Oertel, W.; Obeso, J.; Marek, K.; Litvan, I.; Lang, A.E.; et al. MDS clinical diagnostic criteria for Parkinson's disease. *Mov. Disord.* **2015**, *30*, 1591–1601. [CrossRef] [PubMed]
4. Marshall, V.L.; Reininger, C.B.; Marquardt, M.; Patterson, J.; Hadley, D.M.; Oertel, W.H.; Benamer, H.T.S.; Kemp, P.; Burn, D.; Tolosa, E.; et al. Parkinson's disease is overdiagnosed clinically at baseline in diagnostically uncertain cases: A 3-year European multicenter study with repeat [123I]FP-CIT SPECT. *Mov. Disord.* **2009**. [CrossRef]
5. Berardelli, A.; Wenning, G.K.; Antonini, A.; Berg, D.; Bloem, B.R.; Bonifati, V.; Brooks, D.; Burn, D.J.; Colosimo, C.; Fanciulli, A.; et al. EFNS/MDS-ES/ENS [corrected] recommendations for the diagnosis of Parkinson's disease. *Eur. J. Neurol.* **2013**, *20*, 16–34. [CrossRef]
6. Tolosa, E.; Wenning, G.; Poewe, W. The diagnosis of Parkinson's disease. *Lancet Neurol.* **2006**, *5*, 75–86. [CrossRef]
7. Huppertz, H.J.; Möller, L.; Südmeyer, M.; Hilker, R.; Hattingen, E.; Egger, K.; Amtage, F.; Respondek, G.; Stamelou, M.; Schnitzler, A.; et al. Differentiation of neurodegenerative parkinsonian syndromes by volumetric magnetic resonance imaging analysis and support vector machine classification. *Mov. Disord.* **2016**. [CrossRef]
8. Yang, J.; Archer, D.B.; Burciu, R.G.; Muller, M.; Roy, A.; Ofori, E.; Bohnen, N.I.; Albin, R.L.; Vaillancourt, D.E. Multimodal dopaminergic and free-water imaging in Parkinson's disease. *Parkinsonism Relat. Disord.* **2019**, *62*, 10–15. [CrossRef]
9. Paviour, D.C.; Thornton, J.S.; Lees, A.J.; Jager, H.R. Diffusion-weighted magnetic resonance imaging differentiates Parkinsonian variant of multiple-system atrophy from progressive supranuclear palsy. *Mov. Disord.* **2007**, *22*, 68–74. [CrossRef]
10. Sjostrom, H.; Granberg, T.; Westman, E.; Svenningsson, P. Quantitative susceptibility mapping differentiates between parkinsonian disorders. *Parkinsonism Relat. Disord.* **2017**, *44*, 51–57. [CrossRef]
11. Cheng, Z.; He, N.; Huang, P.; Li, Y.; Tang, R.; Sethi, S.K.; Ghassaban, K.; Yerramsetty, K.K.; Palutla, V.K.; Chen, S.; et al. Imaging the Nigrosome 1 in the substantia nigra using susceptibility weighted imaging and quantitative susceptibility mapping: An application to Parkinson's disease. *NeuroImage Clin.* **2020**. [CrossRef] [PubMed]
12. Shinto, A.; Vijayan, K.; Antony, J.; Kamaleshwaran, K.; Kameshwaran, M.; Korde, A.; Samuel, G.; Selvan, A. Correlative 99m Tc-labeled tropane derivative single photon emission computer tomography and clinical assessment in the staging of parkinson disease. *World J. Nucl. Med.* **2014**. [CrossRef] [PubMed]
13. Eckert, T.; Barnes, A.; Dhawan, V.; Frucht, S.; Gordon, M.F.; Feigin, A.S.; Eidelberg, D. FDG PET in the differential diagnosis of parkinsonian disorders. *Neuroimage* 2005, *26*, 912–921. [CrossRef] [PubMed]
14. Garraux, G.; Phillips, C.; Schrouff, J.; Kreisler, A.; Lemaire, C.; Degueldre, C.; Delcour, C.; Hustinx, R.; Luxen, A.; Destée, A.; et al. Multiclass classification of FDG PET scans for the distinction between Parkinson's disease and atypical parkinsonian syndromes. *NeuroImage Clin.* **2013**. [CrossRef] [PubMed]
15. Wenning, G.K.; Shephard, B.; Hawkes, C.; Petruckevitch, A.; Lees, A.; Quinn, N. Olfactory function in atypical parkinsonian syndromes. *Acta Neurol. Scand.* **1995**, *91*, 247–250. [CrossRef]
16. Goldstein, D.S.; Holmes, C.; Bentho, O.; Sato, T.; Moak, J.; Sharabi, Y.; Imrich, R.; Conant, S.; Eldadah, B.A. Biomarkers to detect central dopamine deficiency and distinguish Parkinson disease from multiple system atrophy. *Parkinsonism Relat. Disord.* **2008**, *14*, 600–607. [CrossRef]
17. Skowronek, C.; Zange, L.; Lipp, A. Cardiac 123I-MIBG Scintigraphy in Neurodegenerative Parkinson Syndromes: Performance and Pitfalls in Clinical Practice. *Front. Neurol.* **2019**, *10*, 152. [CrossRef]
18. Augimeri, A.; Cherubini, A.; Cascini, G.L.; Galea, D.; Caligiuri, M.E.; Barbagallo, G.; Arabia, G.; Quattrone, A. CADA—computer-aided DaTSCAN analysis. *EJNMMI Phys.* **2016**. [CrossRef]
19. Nicastro, N.; Wegrzyk, J.; Preti, M.G.; Fleury, V.; Van de Ville, D.; Garibotto, V.; Burkhard, P.R. Classification of degenerative parkinsonism subtypes by support-vector-machine analysis and striatal (123)I-FP-CIT indices. *J. Neurol.* **2019**, *266*, 1771–1781. [CrossRef]
20. Badoud, S.; Van De Ville, D.; Nicastro, N.; Garibotto, V.; Burkhard, P.R.; Haller, S. Discriminating among degenerative parkinsonisms using advanced 123I-ioflupane SPECT analyses. *NeuroImage Clin.* **2016**. [CrossRef]
21. Joling, M.; Vriend, C.; van der Zande, J.J.; Lemstra, A.W.; van den Heuvel, O.A.; Booij, J.; Berendse, H.W. Lower 123I-FP-CIT binding to the striatal dopamine transporter, but not to the extrastriatal serotonin transporter, in Parkinson's disease compared with dementia with Lewy bodies. *NeuroImage Clin.* **2018**. [CrossRef] [PubMed]

22. Litjens, G.; Kooi, T.; Bejnordi, B.E.; Setio, A.A.A.; Ciompi, F.; Ghafoorian, M.; van der Laak, J.; van Ginneken, B.; Sanchez, C.I. A survey on deep learning in medical image analysis. *Med. Image Anal.* **2017**, *42*, 60–88. [CrossRef] [PubMed]
23. Vaccaro, M.G.; Sarica, A.; Quattrone, A.; Chiriaco, C.; Salsone, M.; Morelli, M.; Quattrone, A. Neuropsychological assessment could distinguish among different clinical phenotypes of progressive supranuclear palsy: A Machine Learning approach. *J. Neuropsychol.* **2020**. [CrossRef]
24. Choi, H.; Ha, S.; Im, H.J.; Paek, S.H.; Lee, D.S. Refining diagnosis of Parkinson's disease with deep learning-based interpretation of dopamine transporter imaging. *NeuroImage Clin.* **2017**, *16*, 586–594. [CrossRef]
25. Taylor, J.C.; Fenner, J.W. Comparison of machine learning and semi-quantification algorithms for (I123)FP-CIT classification: The beginning of the end for semi-quantification? *EJNMMI Phys.* **2017**. [CrossRef] [PubMed]
26. Yushkevich, P.A.; Piven, J.; Hazlett, H.C.; Smith, R.G.; Ho, S.; Gee, J.C.; Gerig, G. User-guided 3D active contour segmentation of anatomical structures: Significantly improved efficiency and reliability. *NeuroImage* **2006**, *31*, 1116–1128. [CrossRef] [PubMed]
27. Chan, T.F.; Vese, L.A. Active contours without edges. *IEEE Trans. Image Process.* **2001**, *10*, 266–277. [CrossRef]
28. Iizuka, T.; Fukasawa, M.; Kameyama, M. Deep-learning-based imaging-classification identified cingulate island sign in dementia with Lewy bodies. *Sci. Rep.* **2019**, *9*, 8944. [CrossRef]
29. Vlaar, A.M.; van Kroonenburgh, M.J.; Kessels, A.G.; Weber, W.E. Meta-analysis of the literature on diagnostic accuracy of SPECT in parkinsonian syndromes. *BMC Neurol.* **2007**, *7*, 27. [CrossRef] [PubMed]
30. Joling, M.; Vriend, C.; Raijmakers, P.G.H.M.; van der Zande, J.J.; Lemstra, A.W.; Berendse, H.W.; Booij, J.; van den Heuvel, O.A. Striatal DAT and extrastriatal SERT binding in early-stage Parkinson's disease and dementia with Lewy bodies, compared with healthy controls: An 123 I-FP-CIT SPECT study. *NeuroImage Clin.* **2019**. [CrossRef]
31. Swanson, R.L.; Newberg, A.B.; Acton, P.D.; Siderowf, A.; Wintering, N.; Alavi, A.; Mozley, P.D.; Plossl, K.; Udeshi, M.; Hurtig, H. Differences in [99mTc]TRODAT-1 SPECT binding to dopamine transporters in patients with multiple system atrophy and Parkinson's disease. *Eur. J. Nucl. Med. Mol. Imaging* **2005**, *32*, 302–307. [CrossRef] [PubMed]

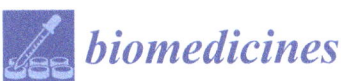

Article

Somatostatin Ameliorates β-Amyloid-Induced Cytotoxicity via the Regulation of CRMP2 Phosphorylation and Calcium Homeostasis in SH-SY5Y Cells

Seungil Paik [†], Rishi K. Somvanshi [†], Helen A. Oliveira, Shenglong Zou and Ujendra Kumar *

Faculty of Pharmaceutical Sciences, The University of British Columbia, Vancouver, BC V6T 1Z3, Canada; paikseungil@gmail.com (S.P.); rishiks@mail.ubc.ca (R.K.S.); aophelen@gmail.com (H.A.O.); zoe.s.long@gmail.com (S.Z.)
* Correspondence: ujkumar@mail.ubc.ca; Tel.: +1-604-827-3660; Fax: +1-604-822-3035
† These authors contributed equally to this work.

Abstract: Somatostatin is involved in the regulation of multiple signaling pathways and affords neuroprotection in response to neurotoxins. In the present study, we investigated the role of Somatostatin-14 (SST) in cell viability and the regulation of phosphorylation of Collapsin Response Mediator Protein 2 (CRMP2) (Ser522) via the blockade of Ca^{2+} accumulation, along with the inhibition of cyclin-dependent kinase 5 (CDK5) and Calpain activation in differentiated SH-SY5Y cells. Cell Viability and Caspase 3/7 assays suggest that the presence of SST ameliorates mitochondrial stability and cell survival pathways while augmenting pro-apoptotic pathways activated by Aβ. SST inhibits the phosphorylation of CRMP2 at Ser522 site, which is primarily activated by CDK5. Furthermore, SST effectively regulates Ca^{2+} influx in the presence of Aβ, directly affecting the activity of calpain in differentiated SH-SY5Y cells. We also demonstrated that SSTR2 mediates the protective effects of SST. In conclusion, our results highlight the regulatory role of SST in intracellular Ca^{2+} homeostasis. The neuroprotective role of SST via axonal regeneration and synaptic integrity is corroborated by regulating changes in CRMP2; however, SST-mediated changes in the blockade of Ca^{2+} influx, calpain expression, and toxicity did not correlate with CDK5 expression and p35/25 accumulation. To summarize, our findings suggest two independent mechanisms by which SST mediates neuroprotection and confirms the therapeutic implications of SST in AD as well as in other neurodegenerative diseases where the effective regulation of calcium homeostasis is required for a better prognosis.

Keywords: β-Amyloid; calpain; Collapsin Response Mediator Protein-2; human-neuroblastoma SH-SY5Y cells; Somatostatin-14; somatostatin receptor

Citation: Paik, S.; Somvanshi, R.K.; Oliveira, H.A.; Zou, S.; Kumar, U. Somatostatin Ameliorates β-Amyloid-Induced Cytotoxicity via the Regulation of CRMP2 Phosphorylation and Calcium Homeostasis in SH-SY5Y Cells. Biomedicines 2021, 9, 27. https://doi.org/10.3390/biomedicines9010027

Received: 2 December 2020
Accepted: 25 December 2020
Published: 2 January 2021

Publisher's Note: MDPI stays neutral with regard to jurisdictional claims in published maps and institutional affiliations.

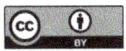

Copyright: © 2021 by the authors. Licensee MDPI, Basel, Switzerland. This article is an open access article distributed under the terms and conditions of the Creative Commons Attribution (CC BY) license (https://creativecommons.org/licenses/by/4.0/).

1. Introduction

Alzheimer's disease (AD) is a progressive neurodegenerative disorder and the most common form of dementia in the elderly population. Standard clinical features of the disease include memory loss, abnormal social behavior, and deterioration of cognitive function [1–3]. AD is characterized by the formation of amyloid plaques, composed of abnormally truncated fragments of the amyloid precursor protein called β-amyloid (Aβ), and intracellular neurofibrillary tangles (NFT), consisting of hyperphosphorylated Tau protein [4,5]. The complex pathophysiology observed in AD is associated with the accumulation of plaques and the formation of NFTs, along with other pathological changes, resulting in synaptic dysfunction, excitotoxicity, dendritic spine loss and overall destabilization of the neural network [6,7]. The overaccumulation of Aβ is considered as the prominent cause of disease severity and neuronal cell death; however, the precise mechanism of interconnecting AD onset and progression is not fully understood, despite the identification of signaling pathways that exert determinant roles [8,9]. One such crucial signaling molecule that may represent a critical determinant is collapse response mediator

2 (CRMP2). Initially identified as a signaling molecule of a repulsive axon growth and guidance molecule Semaphorin3A, CRMP2 has since been identified as a critical marker of synapse formation, the establishment of neuronal cell polarity, dendritic patterning, learning, and memory [10,11]. In particular, CRMP2 regulates neuronal microtubule dynamics by binding to the tubulin heterodimers, leading to polymerization, in addition to colocalization and binding to actin [12–15]. Furthermore, CRMP2 also plays a critical role in the transportation of soluble tubulin and vesicles by acting as a cargo adaptor protein [16,17].

Like many other microtubule-binding proteins, such as Tau or microtubule-associated proteins (MAP), CRMP2 is phosphorylated by cyclin-dependent kinase (CDK5) and glycogen synthase kinase-3β (GSK-3β) near its C-terminus. Specifically, CDK5-mediated phosphorylation of CRMP2 at Ser522 primes the subsequent phosphorylation by GSK-3β at sites Ser518, Thr514 and Thr509 [18–21]. In addition to Cdk5 and GSK-3β, Rho/Rho-associated protein kinase has also been identified to phosphorylate CRMP2 at Thr555 [11]. Taken together, the phosphorylation of CRMP2 at these sites is associated with the regulation of neurite outgrowth, possibly due to the modifications of microtubule dynamics [19,21]. Several previous studies have reported hyperphosphorylation of CRMP2 in AD patients when compared to the age-matched control [2,19,20]. However, the exact mechanism of CRMP2 phosphorylation during the progression of AD remains elusive. Although controversy exists, it is well established that the hyperphosphorylation of CRMP2 occurs before the onset of pathology in the AD mouse model, implicating CRMP2 hyperphosphorylation as an early indicator of AD [2].

CDK5 is the primary kinase responsible for the CRMP2 phosphorylation at Ser522 [22,23]. CDK5 plays a critical role in the CNS, including neuronal migration, synapse formation, plasticity, and neurogenesis [24–29]. In contrast to other members of the CDK family that are regulated by p21 and p27, CDK5 activity is mainly regulated by p35 [30,31]. Moreover, while the activation of CDK5 by p35 in the physiological condition is essential for normal neuronal development, synaptic activity, and axonal transport, the abnormal activation of CDK5 leads to cell death and neurodegeneration [24,26,32–37]. In AD, the abnormal increase in CDK5 activation leading to hyperphosphorylation of various tubulin-associated proteins, including Tau and CRMP2, is associated with the accumulation of truncated fragments of p35 called p25, which induces the constitutive activation and mislocalization of CDK5 in vivo [37]. In this regard, the same study has also determined that calpain mediates the cleavage of p35 into p25 [37]. Calpain is a crucial enzyme involved in calcium-mediated neurodegeneration [38]. In AD, the accumulation of Aβ leads to the increase in intracellular Ca^{2+} levels, mitochondrial Ca^{2+} overload, production of pro-apoptotic proteins such as cytochrome c, and generation of superoxide radicals, eventually resulting in cell death and neurodegeneration [39]. We have previously demonstrated the effect of SST in promoting the retinoic acid (RA)-induced differentiation of SH-SY5Y cells [40]. We hypothesize that the identification of a molecule capable of downregulating the hyperphosphorylation of CRMP2 via the blockade of Ca^{2+} accumulation in AD may serve as a novel therapeutic agent.

We recently demonstrated that Somatostatin-14 (SST) mediates the promotion of the overall neurite length in RA-differentiated SH-SY5Y cells, with specific effects on microtubule-associated proteins such as MAP2 and Tau [40]. CRMP2 is a microtubule-associated protein and exhibits a close resemblance with MAP2 and Tau, with significant changes during the progression of AD. Taking this into consideration, we hypothesize that SST might be involved in the regulation of CRMP2 during the differentiation of SH-SY5Y cells. Among the various phosphorylation sites of CRMP2, we have focused on the Ser522 site due to its dual role, first as a phosphorylation site and second as the requirement in phosphorylation of a subsequent site, Thr514. Accordingly, in the present study, we sought to determine the role of SST and a possible mechanism involving the phosphorylation of Ser522 in the presence of $Aβ_{1-42}$-induced toxicity in SH-SY5Y cells as an in-vitro model of AD. Our results revealed SST as a novel molecule capable of inhibiting the Aβ-induced hyper-influx of Ca^{2+}, leading to the inhibition of calpain activity. Furthermore, SST inhibits the p35/p25-induced hyper-activation of CDK5 and the subsequent hyper-phosphorylation of CRMP2.

2. Experimental Section

2.1. SH-SY5Y Cell Culture

Human SH-SY5Y neuroblastoma cells were kindly obtained from Dr. Neil Cashman, University of British Columbia, BC, Canada, and grown as described earlier [40]. Briefly, the cells were grown on a 75 cm² culture flask coated with Matrigel (10 mg/mL, BD Bioscience, San Jose, CA, USA). The culture medium comprised Dulbecco's Modified Eagles Medium (DMEM; Invitrogen, Burlington, ON, Canada) supplemented with 10% fetal bovine serum (FBS), penicillin (100 U/mL) and streptomycin (100 µg/mL) in a 5% CO_2 humidified incubator at 37 °C. For neuronal differentiation, the cells were treated with all-trans-retinoic acid (RA, 10 µM, Sigma, St. Louis, MO, USA) for 5–7 days as previously described [41]. All experiments were performed on cells differentiated for 5–7 days unless otherwise stated. Treatments with $A\beta_{1-42}$ (Anaspec, Fremont, CA, USA) or SST-14 (Bachem, Torrance, CA, USA) were performed as described in the methods.

2.2. MTT Cell Viability Assay

To determine cell viability in response to $A\beta$, SH-SY5Y cells were processed for the MTT (3-(4,5-dimethylthiazol-2-yl)-2,5-diphenyl tetrazolium bromide) assay, as previously described [42]. Briefly, differentiated SH-SY5Y cells were treated with increasing concentrations of $A\beta_{1-42}$ (0, 1, 5, 10 and 20 µM) or SST (0.4, 2 and 10 µM) alone, and with the combination of $A\beta_{1-42}$ (5 and 20 µM) and SST (10 µM) for 24 h. Post-treatment, the cells were washed with phosphate-buffered saline (PBS) and incubated for 2 h at 37 °C in the presence of 300 µg/mL of methyl-thiazolyl diphenyl-tetrazolium bromide solution (Sigma) prepared in serum-free DMEM. The cells were subsequently washed in PBS, and the resulting formazan formed in the cells was dissolved in 200 µL of isopropanol for 15 min on a rotating shaker. The changes in color were analyzed using a spectrophotometer at a wavelength of 570 nm, with the background absorbance measured at 650 nm. The results are presented as percentage changes between the treated versus the control group.

2.3. Caspase/Apoptosis Activity Assay

The $A\beta_{1-42}$ induced apoptosis in differentiated SH-SY5Y cells was analyzed using the Caspase-3/7 Green Apoptosis Assay kit (Essen Bioscience, Ann Arbor, MI, USA) following the manufacturer's instructions. Briefly, SH-SY5Y cells were treated with $A\beta_{1-42}$ (5 µM) alone or in combination with an increasing concentration of SST (0.4, 2, 10 µM) in the presence of a DNA intercalating dye NucView™ 488 (Essen Bioscience). The resulting fluorescence was analyzed in the IncuCyte™ live-cell imaging system (Essen Bioscience), and the Caspase-3/7 activity was assessed as an index of cells undergoing apoptosis using an IncuCyte basic analyzer (Essen Bioscience).

2.4. Live/Dead Cell Assay

The $A\beta_{1-42}$-induced toxicity in the presence or absence of SST was also analyzed using a LIVE/DEAD Cell Vitality Assay (Thermo Fisher Scientific, Waltham, MA, USA), following the manufacturer's instructions. The differentiated SH-SY5Y cells were treated with $A\beta_{1-42}$ (5 µM) or SST (10 µM) alone or in combination for 24 h. Post-treatment, the cells were washed with PBS and collected in 0.05% trypsin-EDTA (Thermo Fisher Scientific). The cells were then re-suspended in 100 µL of PBS in the presence of C_{12}-resazurin (20 ng/µL) and SYTOX dye (1 µM) and incubated for 15 min at 37 °C. Following incubation, the cells were immediately assessed on LSR II (BD Bioscience, San Jose, CA, USA) with excitation at 488 nm and emission at 530 and 570 nm, and analyzed using FlowJo workstation (BD Bioscience).

2.5. Western Blot Analysis

For the Western blot analysis, post-differentiation, control and treated SH-SY5Y cells were harvested using a lysis buffer (Cat# 9803; Cell Signaling) [40]. The total protein content of the cell lysate was determined using a Bradford assay, and whole-cell lysates (15 µg protein) were subjected to 10% SDS-polyacrylamide gel electrophoresis followed by transfer to nitrocellulose membrane. The membranes were blocked with 5% skim milk in TBS-T (Tris-buffered saline with 0.05% Tween-20) for 1 h at room temperature (RT) and immunoblotted overnight in the presence of respective rabbit polyclonal primary antibodies: C-terminal CRMP2 (1:1000; Cat # CP2161; ECM Bioscience, Versailles, KY, USA), Thr514-CRMP2 (1:1000; Cat# ab62478; Abcam, Cambridge, UK), Ser522-CRMP2 (1:1000, Cat# CP2191; ECM Bioscience), Thr555-CRMP2 (1:1000; Cat# CP2251; ECM Bioscience), SSTR2 (1:500; Cat# sc-25676; Santa Cruz Biotechnologies, Santa Cruz, CA, USA), SSTR4 (1:500, Cat# sc-25678; Santa Cruz Biotechnologies), Calpain I (1:500; Cat# 2556; Cell Signaling). Other antibodies used were mouse monoclonal CDK5 (1:2000; Cat# 05-364; Millipore) and rabbit monoclonal p35/25 (1:250; Cat# 64310; Cell Signaling). After incubation with the primary antibodies overnight, the membranes were washed in TBST and incubated for 1 h at RT with either horseradish peroxidase (HRP)-conjugated goat anti-mouse (1:2000) or goat anti-rabbit secondary antibodies (1:2000) (Jackson Lab). The membranes were washed in TBST and developed using a chemiluminescence detection kit (Millipore, Billerica, MA, USA) on Alpha Innotech FluorChem 8800. β-actin was used as a loading control. A densitometric analysis of protein expression levels was performed using ImageJ software.

2.6. Immunofluorescence Immunocytochemistry

The control and treated cells were fixed with 4% paraformaldehyde for 20 min and permeabilized with 0.1% Triton-X100 in PBS for 15 min at RT. Following three washes in PBS, the cells were blocked with 5% Normal Goat Serum (NGS) for 1 h at RT. The cells were then incubated with rabbit polyclonal primary antibody Ser522-CRMP2 (Cat# CP2191; ECM Bioscience) and mouse monoclonal βIII Tubulin (Cat# 801202; BioLegend) in 5% NGS overnight at 4 °C. Following the overnight incubation with the primary antibodies, the cells were washed with PBS and incubated with Alexa-conjugated secondary antibodies for 1 h at RT (1:200; Invitrogen). For nucleus visualization, the cells were incubated with Hoechst dye 33258 (0.5 µg/mL, Calbiochem, La Jolla, CA, USA) for 10 min at RT. The coverslips were then mounted onto the slides and photographed using a Zeiss LSM700 confocal microscope (Carl Zeiss, Oberkochen, Germany). Image panels were constructed using Carl Zeiss Zen software.

2.7. Agonist Treatment

SSTR2 and 4 specific non-peptide agonists (L-779976 and L-803087) were kindly provided by Dr S.P. Rohrer, Merck. Briefly, the differentiated SH-SY5Y cells were treated with SSTR specific agonists (3, 10, 30 nM) with or without Aβ for 24 h. Following treatment, the whole cell lysate prepared was processed to determine the expression levels and the activity of proteins of interest using Western blot analysis.

2.8. Fluo-4 Calcium Assay

The intracellular calcium levels were assessed using the Fluo-4 Direct^{TM} calcium assay kit (Invitrogen) following the manufacturer's instructions. Briefly, the SH-SY5Y cells were plated onto a 96-well plate coated with Matrigel and differentiated with RA for up to 5 days. Following differentiation, the cells were incubated with an equal volume of 2 X Fluo-4 Direct^{TM} calcium reagents (including probenecid) at 37 °C for 60 min. Following the loading of the dye, the cells were treated with $A\beta_{1-42}$ (5 or 20 µM) or SST (10 µM) alone and in a combination. The changes in the fluorescence intensity were measured (excitation at 494 nm and emission at 516 nm) in a spectrophotometer in a time-dependent manner for 50 cycles (20 s each). Untreated cells were used as internal control. The changes in absorbance are presented as a fold-difference between the treatment versus control ($n = 3$; each experiment represents an average of 3–6 independent readings).

2.9. Statistical Analysis

All results are presented as mean ± SD of a minimum of three independent experiments, as indicated. All statistical analyses have been performed in Graph Prism5.0. Student's t-test, or one-way analysis of variance (ANOVA) was used as indicated. * $p < 0.05$ against control or $A\beta_{1-42}$ treatment was taken into consideration as significant.

3. Results

3.1. SST Inhibits $A\beta_{1-42}$-Induced Toxicity in Differentiated SH-SY5Y Cells

To determine the cell viability of SH-SY5Y cells in response to $A\beta_{1-42}$-induced toxicity, multiple approaches were applied. Initially, the overall cell metabolism was assessed using MTT assay as recently described [43]. As shown in Figure 1A, in response to increasing the concentration of $A\beta_{1-42}$ (1, 5, 10 and 20 µM), differentiated SH-SY5Y cells exhibited dose-dependent toxicity in comparison to controls. At lower doses, SST displayed no significant effect on cell viability, whereas, at the higher dose (10 µM), SST produced a cytotoxic effect post 24 hr treatment (Figure 1B). However, differentiated cells treated with $A\beta_{1-42}$ (5 and 20 µM) in combination with SST (10 µM) display enhanced cell viability when compared to $A\beta_{1-42}$ alone (Figure 1C).

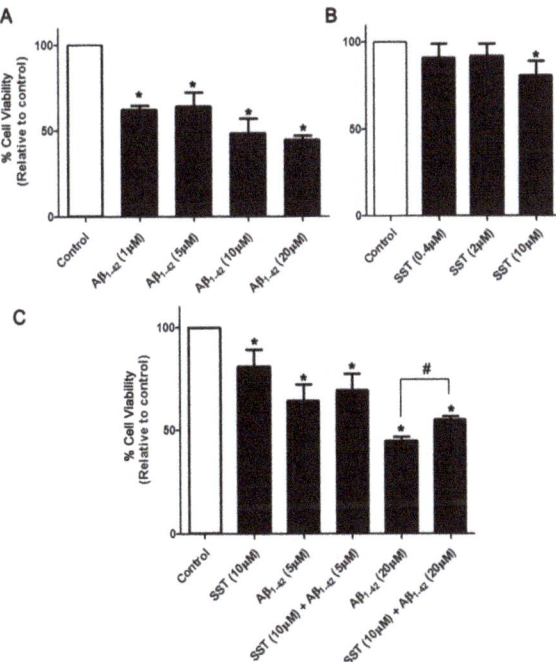

Figure 1. SST inhibits Aβ-induced cytotoxicity. Changes in cell survival following treatment with increasing concentrations of Aβ and SST alone or in combination were assessed by the MTT assay. (**A**) $A\beta_{1-42}$ induced dose-dependent toxicity in differentiated SH-SY5Y cells with maximal toxicity observed at 20 µM of $A\beta_{1-42}$. In contrast, SST displayed a marginal cytotoxic effect at higher doses only, without any significant effect at the lower concentrations (**B**). Cells treated with $A\beta_{1-42}$ (5 and 20 µM) in combination with SST (10 µM) displayed enhanced cell viability when compared to $A\beta_{1-42}$ alone (**C**). The data represent the mean ± SD of three independent experiments. * $p < 0.05$ against control; # against $A\beta_{1-42}$ (20 µM).

Next, we assessed the effect of Aβ$_{1-42}$ on cell viability by evaluating the activity level of caspase-3/7 as an index of apoptosis. As shown in Figure 2A, the SH-SY5Y cells treated with Aβ$_{1-42}$ displayed an increase in basal caspase-3/7 activity that was significantly different when compared to the control. In contrast, the cells treated with SST alone displayed inhibition of caspase-3/7 activity. As shown in Figure 2A, SST in combination with Aβ$_{1-42}$ displayed time- and concentration-dependent inhibition of caspase-3/7 activity when compared to the cells treated with Aβ$_{1-42}$ alone. These results suggest that SST mediates the inhibition of Aβ-induced apoptosis in differentiated SH-SY5Y cells.

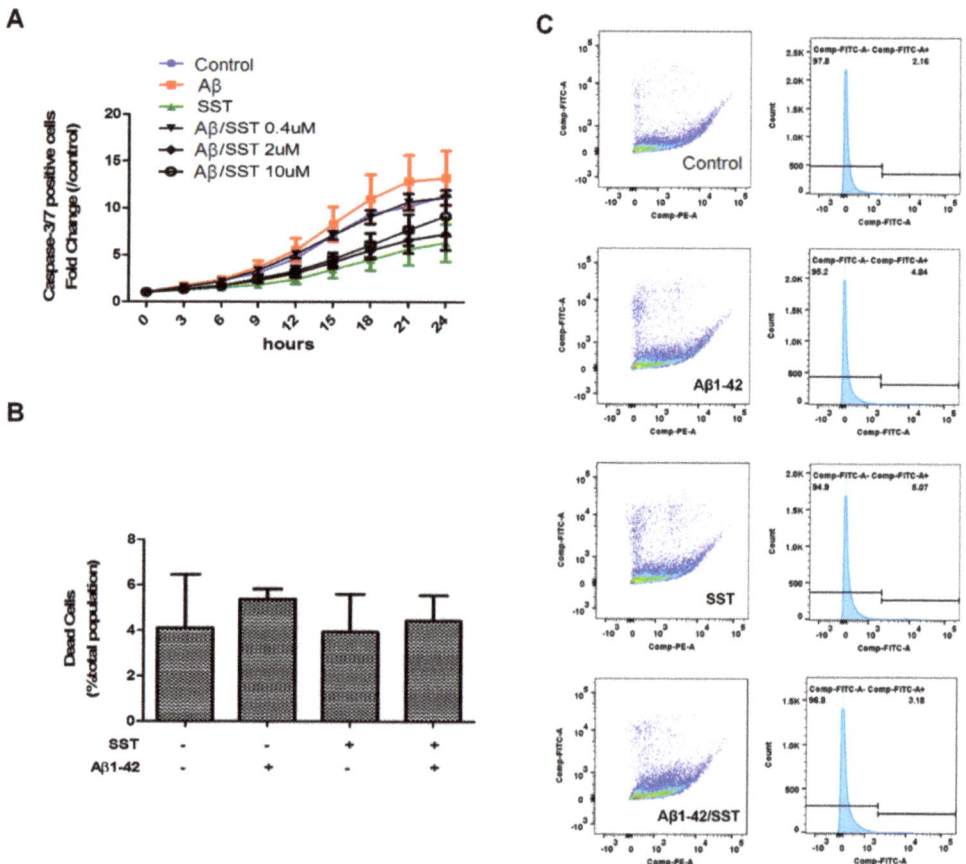

Figure 2. SST inhibits the Aβ-induced activation of apoptosis. (**A**) Apoptosis induction was assessed by measuring caspase-3/7 activity. Cells treated with Aβ (5 µM) alone displayed an elevation of caspase-3/7 activity, while cells treated with SST alone (10 µM) exhibited the lowest caspase-3/7 activity. Co-treatment of Aβ$_{1-42}$ (5 µM) and SST resulted in reduced caspase-3/7 activity compared to the cells treated with Aβ$_{1-42}$ alone. Data are shown as a fold-change against 0 h time point. (**B**) Cell viability assessed by a live/dead assay using metabolic activity and cell permeability as an index following treatment with Aβ (5 µM) and SST (10 µM) alone or in combination (**C**). Representative FACS data of C$_{12}$-resazurin and SYTOX fluorescence intensity (dot plot) and FITC intensity distribution (histogram) displaying the distribution of cells based on viability. The cells were treated with Aβ (5 µM) and SST (10 µM) alone or in combination. The data represent the mean ± SD of three independent experiments.

To determine the changes in metabolism as well as cell membrane integrity in response to the Aβ$_{1-42}$-induced toxicity, a Live/Dead cell assay was performed in SH-SY5Y cells. Interestingly, the Live/Dead assay did not show significant changes in metabolic activity, which may be due to the metabolic demand of cells undergoing apoptosis (Figure 2B,C). However, when assessed strictly for the cell membrane integrity, the Live/Dead cell assay showed an increasing trend in cell permeability upon treatment with $A\beta_{1-42}$ alone, albeit insignificantly, indicative of the toxic effect of $A\beta$ (Figure 2B).

3.2. Somatostatin Downregulates the Phosphorylation of CRMP2 at the Ser522 Site

Previous studies have demonstrated that SST, when used in combination with neurite-promoting drugs, including nerve growth factor (NGF), brain-derived nerve growth factor (BDNF), or RA, increases the neurite outgrowth and promotes the differentiation of various cells, including SH-SY5Y cells [40,44]. It is well known that CRMP2 plays a critical role in mediating tubulin stability and neurite outgrowth [45]. However, whether SST-mediated neurite growth and elongation is directly associated with the suppression of CRMP2 phosphorylation in $A\beta_{1-42}$-induced toxicity model is not well understood. Accordingly, we sought to examine whether SST attenuates the $A\beta_{1-42}$-induced hyperphosphorylation of CRMP2 using Western blot analysis. Differentiated SH-SY5Y cells were treated with increasing concentrations of SST (0.4, 2 and 10 µM) in the presence of $A\beta_{1-42}$ (5 µM). Vehicle treated cells or the cells treated with scrambled $A\beta_{42-1}$ were considered as controls.

Furthermore, to determine changes in site-specific phosphorylation, three phosphorylation sites of CRMP2 that have been previously reported to be hyperphosphorylated in AD patients were selected (Thr514, Ser522 and Thr555) [46]. As shown in Figure 3, the phosphorylation levels of Thr514- or Thr555-CRMP2 did not show a dose-dependent response to any of the concentrations of SST in combination with $A\beta_{1-42}$ (Figure 3, panels A, B, and D). Although the level of CRMP2 phosphorylation at site Ser522 was not relatively altered by $A\beta_{1-42}$ alone, it was significantly downregulated in the presence of SST in a dose-dependent manner, with a maximal reduction in the presence of SST at 10 µM (Figure 3, panels A and C). Therefore, based on the cell viability assay and site-specific Thr522-CRMP2 phosphorylation, all subsequent experiments were performed using 10 µM of SST.

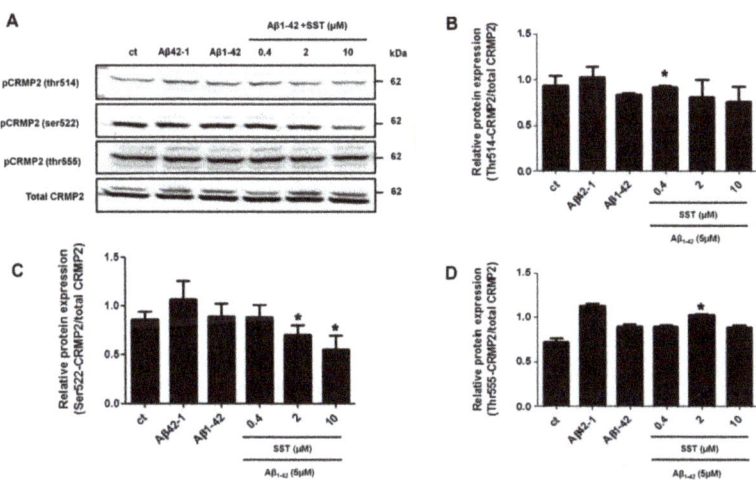

Figure 3. SST-mediated regulation of CRMP2 (Ser522) phosphorylation. (**A**). Representative Western blot showing the decreased phosphorylation level of Ser522-CRMP2 with increasing concentration of SST. Total CRMP2 was used as a loading control. B-D. Graphs represent the densitometry analysis of Western blot data shown in A for Thr514-CRMP2 (**B**), Ser522-CRMP2 (**C**), and Thr555-CRMP2 (**D**). Note that the Ser522-phosphorylation level is inhibited in a dose-dependent manner with increasing concentration of SST in the presence of $A\beta$. The data represent the mean ± SD of three independent experiments. * $p < 0.05$ against $A\beta_{1-42}$ treated alone.

3.3. Somatostatin Inhibits the Activation of CRMP2 in the Presence of Aβ

To determine whether increased CRMP2 phosphorylation at Ser522 is associated with neurite formation, the subcellular distribution and colocalization of phosphorylated CRMP2 at Ser522 and neuronal tubulin marker βIII-tubulin was determined. In differentiated cells treated with scramble A$β_{42-1}$, CRMP2-like immunoreactivity was confined primarily to the cell body, along with some punctuated staining in neurites (Figure 4A). The cells were mostly devoid of any colocalization and displayed no detectable changes in the presence of SST. Conversely, treatment with A$β_{1-42}$ induced CRMP2 phosphorylation in neurites and showed colocalization with βIII-tubulin. However, following treatment with A$β_{1-42}$ in combination with SST, CRMP2-like immunoreactivity was decreased, while the cells exhibited an increase in the expression of βIII-tubulin.

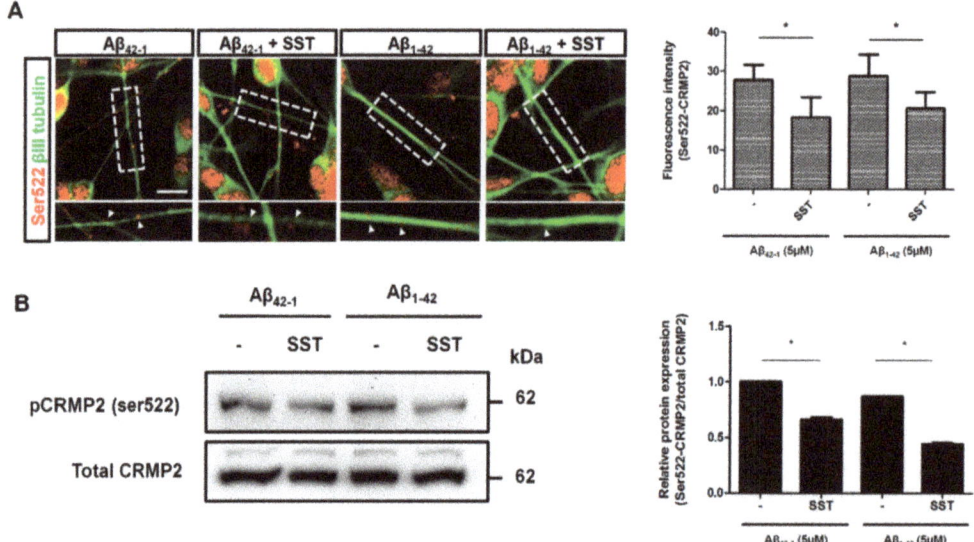

Figure 4. SST inhibits S522-CRMP2 phosphorylation. (**A**). Immunofluorescence staining image of Ser522-CRMP2 (red) co-stained with neuronal tubulin marker βIII-tubulin (green). The colocalization of Ser522-CRMP2 on neurites with βIII-tubulin is indicated (arrowhead; inset), and the average fluorescence intensity of S522-CRMP2 (in red) is shown on the bar graph. (**B**). Representative Western blot showing reduced phosphorylation at Ser522-CRMP2 in the presence of SST (bottom panel). The densitometry analysis of the Western blot is corroborated with a significant reduction in the phosphorylation level in the presence of SST in both A$β_{42-1}$ and A$β_{1-42}$ treated cells (upper panel). The data represent the mean ± SD of three independent experiments. * $p < 0.05$ against respective control; Scale bar = 20 μm.

To further validate whether CRMP2 phosphorylation at Ser522 in the presence of Aβ is abolished by SST, differentiated SH-SY5Y cells were treated with SST alone or in combination with A$β_{42-1}$ or A$β_{1-42}$, and the cell lysate prepared was processed for immunoblot analysis. As shown in Figure 4B, cells treated with SST displayed significant inhibition on A$β_{1-42}$-mediated CRMP2 phosphorylation at Ser522 in comparison to cells treated with A$β_{42-1}$. A quantitative analysis of the changes in CRMP2 phosphorylation (Ser522) was determined by a densitometric analysis (Figure 4B). These results suggest that SST suppresses the subcellular distribution of CRMP2 in SH-SY5Y cells and prompt the dissociation from βIII-tubulin in neurite formation.

3.4. SST Inhibits the Aβ$_{1-42}$-Induced Over-Expression of SSTR4

The biological effects of SST are mediated by binding to five different receptor subtypes (SSTR1-5). We recently reported the role of SSTR2 and 4 in promoting the RA-induced neuronal differentiation of SH-SY5Y cells [40]. Here, accordingly, we monitored the changes in the expression of SSTR2 and 4 following treatment with either $A\beta_{1-42}$ alone or in combination with SST. Scrambled $A\beta_{42-1}$ was used as a control. SH-SY5Y cells were treated with $A\beta_{42-1}$ (5 µM) and $A\beta_{1-42}$ (5 µM) in the presence and absence of SST (10 µM) for 24 h. Post-treatment, cell lysates were collected and processed for immunoblot analyses for the expression of SSTR2 and 4. As shown in Figure 5, the cells treated with $A\beta_{42-1}$ in the presence of SST exhibited an increase in SSTR2 expression without any discernible changes in SSTR4 expression. In contrast, the SH-SY5Y cells treated with $A\beta_{1-42}$ displayed an increased expression of both SSTR2 and 4 when compared to the cells treated with $A\beta_{42-1}$. In the cells treated with SST in combination with $A\beta_{1-42}$, SSTR2 expression remained higher than $A\beta_{42-1}$-treated cells but was comparable to the cells treated with $A\beta_{1-42}$ alone. Interestingly, the cells treated with $A\beta_{1-42}$ in combination with SST showed a significant reduction of SSTR4 expression when compared to cells treated with $A\beta_{1-42}$ alone. These results indicate SST-induced changes in subtype-specific receptor internalization, desensitization, and degradation.

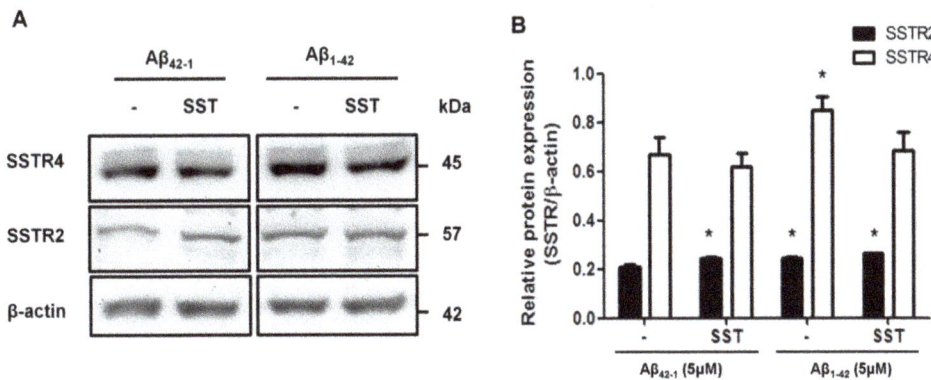

Figure 5. SST-induced changes in SSTR2 and SSTR4 expressions. (**A**). Representative Western blot showing the effect of SST in the expression of SSTR2 and 4. (**B**). The densitometry analysis of the Western blot shows that the treatment of cells with SST resulted in a significant increase in SSTR2 expression in the presence of either $A\beta_{42-1}$ or $A\beta_{1-42}$. SSTR4 expression increased following the treatment with $A\beta_{1-42}$. In contrast, the co-treatment of cells with $A\beta_{1-42}$ and SST resulted in the inhibition of $A\beta_{1-42}$-induced upregulation of SSTR4. The data represent the mean ± SD of three independent experiments. * $p < 0.05$ against respective control.

3.5. SSTR-Subtypes-Mediated Changes in CRMP2 Phosphorylation

To determine which receptor subtype is involved in the SST-mediated inhibition of CRMP2 activation, differentiated SH-SY5Y cells were treated with SSTR2 and 4 specific agonists alone or in the presence of Aβ for 24 hr. Post-treatment, cell lysates collected from controls and treated cells were processed for Western blot analysis to assess CRMP2 phosphorylation. As shown in Figure 6A, in comparison to the control, CRMP2 phosphorylation increased significantly in cells treated with $A\beta_{1-42}$. Receptor agonists induced concentration-dependent changes on CRMP2 phosphorylation in a receptor-specific manner. As shown in Figure 6A, in the absence of $A\beta_{1-42}$, at the lowest concentration (3 nM), SSTR2-specific agonist (L-779976) inhibits CRMP2 phosphorylation at Ser522, whereas at higher concentrations (10, 30 nM), a moderate increase in CRMP2 phosphorylation was observed. The differentiated SH-SY5Y cells treated with SSTR2 agonist (3 nM) in the presence of $A\beta_{1-42}$ displayed inhibition of CRMP2 phosphorylation when compared to the cells treated with $A\beta_{1-42}$ alone. However, in the presence of $A\beta_{1-42}$ and SSTR2 agonist at higher concentrations (10 and 30 nM), no significant change in CRMP2 phosphorylation was observed when compared to $A\beta_{1-42}$ treatment alone. Notably, a higher concentration of SSTR2 agonist displayed no apparent difference in the levels of CRMP2 phosphorylation with or without Aβ$_{1-42}$.

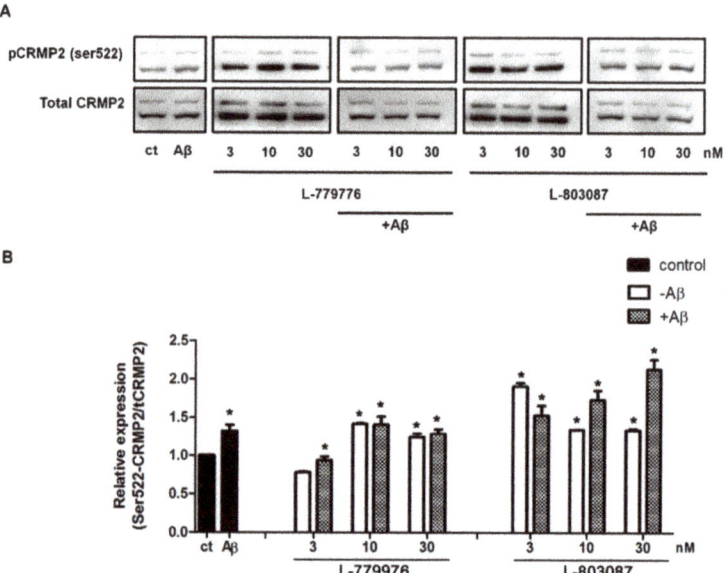

Figure 6. SSTR specific agonist effect on Ser522-CRMP2 phosphorylation. (**A**). Representative Western blot showing changes in the level of S522-CRMP2 phosphorylation in cells, following treatment with increasing concentrations of SSTR2 and SSTR4-specific agonist (3, 10, 30 nM) in the presence or absence of Aβ$_{1-42}$ (5 μM). (**B**). The densitometry analysis of Western blot shows a significant inhibition of Ser522 phosphorylation upon treatment with L-779976 (3 nM) in the absence or presence of Aβ$_{1-42}$. L-779976 (10 and 30 nM) alone, which resulted in the moderate elevation of phosphorylation at the Ser522 site compared to the untreated control. In the presence of Aβ$_{1-42}$, L-779976 (10 and 30 nM) displayed moderate changes when compared to the cells treated with Aβ$_{1-42}$. In the presence of Aβ$_{1-42}$, L-803087 induced a dose-dependent increase of Ser522 phosphorylation, resulting in the highest level of expression at 30 nM treatment of L-803087. The data represent the mean ± SD of three independent experiments. * $p < 0.05$ against respective control.

As shown in Figure 6A, differentiated SH-SY5Y cells treated with SSTR4 agonist (L-803087) displayed significantly higher CRMP2 phosphorylation in comparison to controls. However, such enhanced status of CRMP2 phosphorylation was relatively higher at a lower concentration (3 nM), in contrast to a higher concentration, without any distinguishable difference between 10 and 30 nM. Next, we determined whether Aβ$_{1-42}$ activated CRMP2 phosphorylation is suppressed in the presence of SSTR4 agonist. As shown in Figure 6B, the status of CRMP2 phosphorylation in cells treated with SSTR4 agonist in combination with Aβ$_{1-42}$ exhibited a concentration-dependent increase that was significantly higher than both controls and cells treated with Aβ$_{1-42}$ alone.

3.6. Somatostatin-Mediated Inhibition of Ser522-CRMP2 Is Regulated Through the Calcium Pathway

Increased intracellular Ca^{2+} accumulation is a well-documented mechanism of Aβ-mediated toxicity via inducing calpain activity, over-activation of CDK5, and hyper-phosphorylation of CRMP2 at Ser522, leading to the disassembly of the CRMP2 complex. Previous studies have suggested that SST inhibits Ca^{2+} by binding to SSTR2 [47–49]. To assess whether SST inhibits Aβ induced an increase in the Ca^{2+} influx, and the intracellular Ca^{2+} content was monitored using Fluo-4 in RA differentiated SH-SY5Y cells. In the cells treated with SST alone (10 µM), the intracellular Ca^{2+} level was comparable to the control. The cells treated with $A\beta_{1-42}$ alone (5 µM) had no significant effect on intracellular Ca^{2+} levels at early time points (data not shown), whereas treatment with $A\beta_{1-42}$ alone at a higher concentration of 20 µM induced a time-dependent increase in intracellular Ca^{2+} level within a short treatment duration (Figure 7A). The intracellular Ca^{2+} influx was suppressed and maintained at a lower level in cells treated with $A\beta_{1-42}$ (20 µM) in combination with SST (10 µM) when compared to $A\beta_{1-42}$ alone (Figure 7A). These results indicate that SST potentially inhibits an $A\beta_{1-42}$-induced increase in the Ca^{2+} influx and supports possible mechanisms of SST-mediated neuroprotection in $A\beta$-induced toxicity.

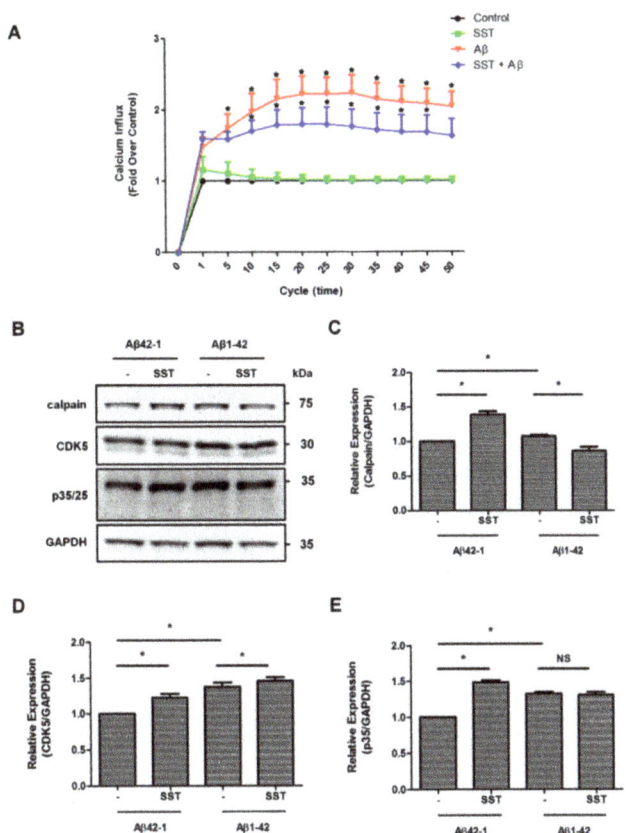

Figure 7. SST-mediated effects on calcium signaling and downstream mediators. (**A**). The intracellular level of Ca^{2+} was assessed using the Fluo-4 calcium indicator. Cells treated with $A\beta_{1-42}$ resulted in an increased Ca^{2+} influx compared to the SST or untreated control. Cells treated with $A\beta_{1-42}$ in the presence of SST resulted in a noticeable inhibition of the Ca^{2+} influx compared to the cells treated with $A\beta_{1-42}$ alone. B. Representative Western blot displaying the changes in the expression of calpain, CDK5, and p35/25 expression in cells treated with $A\beta_{1-42}$ in the presence or absence of SST. (**C–E**). Histograms represent the densitometry analysis of the Western blot shown in (**B**). Data represent the mean ± SD of three independent experiments. * $p < 0.05$ against respective control, Two-way ANOVA with Bonferroni post-hoc tests.

Whether SST-mediated changes in the intracellular Ca^{2+} affected resulted in changes in calpain expression and CDK5 activity and their downstream p35/25 expression is not known. As shown in Figure 7B–E, differentiated SH-SY5Y cells treated with $A\beta_{42-1}$ in combination with SST showed a significant increase in calpain expression in comparison to Aβ_{42-1} alone. The calpain expression in differentiated SH-SY5Y cells upon treatment with Aβ_{1-42} alone was not changed as compared to scramble. However, cells treated with Aβ_{1-42} in combination with SST displayed a significant inhibition of calpain expression in comparison to the cells treated with Aβ_{1-42} alone (Figure 7C). The CDK5 expression was also increased in the presence of SST and Aβ_{42-1} in combination when compared to the cells treated with Aβ_{42-1} (Figure 7D). In particular, the cells treated with Aβ_{1-42} and SST together also resulted in a significant increase in CDK5 expression compared to the cells treated with Aβ_{1-42} alone. Interestingly, such changes in calpain expression did not translate into changes in p35 expression. Instead, p35 expression increased significantly in the presence of SST in combination with Aβ_{42-1} as well as with Aβ_{1-42} alone or in combination with SST (Figure 7E). Taken together, in differentiated SH-SY5Y cells, these events are supposed to be interconnected but function independently.

4. Discussion

We recently described the role of SST in RA-induced neurite growth in SH-SY5Y cells and established a possible interaction with the changes in MAP2/Tau and TUJ1, as well as an ERK1/2 signaling pathway. We also uncovered that the cells displaying colocalization between SST and TUJ1 exhibited a more extended neurite growth than cells devoid of colocalization [40]. The intact neurite formation is essential for a normal neuronal function. In contrast, disrupted neurite organizations are often observed in neurological diseases, including AD, and are associated with impaired cognitive function and memory loss. Whether SST is involved in improving neurite outgrowth and maintaining neuronal integrity in Aβ-induced neurotoxicity is not known. In the present study, using differentiated SH-SY5Y cells, we describe the role of SST in Aβ-induced toxicity and the molecular determinants, including CRMP2, Ca^{2+} influx, CDK5, calpain, and P35/25, that might be associated with neurite outgrowth and cell viability. We demonstrate that SST improves cell viability and inhibits Aβ activated caspase 3/7 activity. We did not observe significant changes in metabolic activity as a proxy for Aβ-induced toxicity, and this might require higher concentrations of Aβ [50,51]. Furthermore, SST downregulates the influx of calcium level, which plays a pivotal role in the CDK5 activity. Our data suggest that SST mediates changes in CRMP2 phosphorylation and Aβ_{1-42}-induced toxicity via the regulation of calcium in differentiated SH-SY5Y cells. This newly discovered mechanism might be involved in improving microtubules' organization and neurite outgrowth in AD pathogenesis.

Amongst the neuropeptides studied to date, SST is one of the most significant peptides that changes during the onset and progression of AD, with a consistent reduction in both the cerebrospinal fluid and brain tissues of AD patients [52–59]. We have previously reported the neuroprotective role of SST against various neurotoxic insults, such as pro-inflammatory lipopolysaccharide and Aβ_{1-42} in a human cerebral micro-vessel cell line (hCMEC/D3), cultured cortical neurons, and cultured striatal neurons, as well as QUIN- and NMDA-induced excitotoxicity and cell death [43,60–63]. An intracerebroventricular (i.c.v) infusion of Aβ in rats led to the significant reduction of SST-positive neurons in various brain regions, including the hippocampus and the temporal and frontoparietal cortex [64–67]. Furthermore, studies have also shown colocalization between the somatostatinergic-neurons and Aβ plaques in brain regions, including the amygdala, cortex, and hippocampus, of AD patients [68,69]. Saito et al. reported that the activity of a potent inhibitor of Aβ accumulation, neprilysin, was elevated following the introduction of SST, resulting in a subsequent reduction of Aβ aggregation [70]. Consistent with these observations, in the present study, the SST-induced amelioration of the toxic effect of Aβ was corroborated via various toxicity assays, including MTT, caspase-3/7 activity assay, and LIVE/DEAD toxicity assay. Collectively, these findings suggest a significant neuroprotective role of SST against Aβ-induced toxicity.

The impaired CRMP2 expression or activity may lead to a significant disruption in the overall neurite structure and a decline in cognitive function. CRMP2 is associated with various characteristics of neurite homeostasis, such as formation, outgrowth, and guidance, as well as maintaining the proper microtubule assembly by binding to the microtubule heterodimers and inducing polymerization while directly regulating tubulin GTPase activity [13,21,71–73]. The hyperphosphorylation of CRMP2 has been observed in NFTs as well as in the soluble fragments of the brain tissues derived from AD patients [2,74]. Furthermore, transgenic mouse models of AD, including (PSEN1 (M146V) KI, Thy1.2-AβPP (swe) and triple (PSEN1 (M146V) KI, Thy1.2- AβPP (swe), and Thy1.2-tau (P301L), exhibit a significant increase in CRMP2 phosphorylation in the hippocampus and cortex [2]. On the other hand, other transgenic mouse models of AD, such as Tg2576, P301L, or P301s tau, fail to show an increase in CRMP2 phosphorylation, suggesting that the combination of AβPP and PSEN1 mutation may be a prerequisite for dysfunctional CRMP2 phosphorylation. Consistent with these studies and in support of SST-mediated neuroprotective and neurite outgrowth promoting effects, we observed here that SST downregulated CRMP2 hyperphosphorylation in the presence of $A\beta_{1-42}$. Reduced CRMP2 phosphorylation, along with the increased expression of βIII-tubulin and its dissociation from CRMP2 in neurites upon treatment with SST, is an indication that tubulin is a prerequisite in the neurite elongation. It was not surprising to note that no significant elevation in CRMP2- Ser522 phosphorylation levels in SH-SY5Y cells was observed following treatment with $A\beta_{1-42}$ in our study. A previous study has reported that the phosphorylation of CRMP2 at the T555 site was significantly elevated in the presence of $A\beta_{1-40}$ in SH-SY5Y cells. The study reported no such changes at Thr514 and Ser522 sites and linked such variations to the Aβ species-dependent mechanism [75]. However, despite the differences in the CRMP2 phosphorylation levels, both $A\beta_{1-40}$ and $A\beta_{1-42}$ potentially impacted neurite length and elicit similar cellular outcomes [75]. Therefore, the role of $A\beta_{1-42}$, $A\beta_{1-40}$, or $A\beta_{25-35}$ on the phosphorylation of various CRMP2 sites could be potentially explored in future studies.

Increased activation of CRMP2 in the presence of SSTR2 and 4 specific agonists is surprising and warrants future research. We have previously shown that both SSTR2 and 4 internalize in response to ligand binding [76,77]. Our past studies have shown that SSTR2 exists predominantly as homodimers on the cell surface, whereas SSTR4 exists as both monomers and homodimers [76,77]. The inhibition of CRMP2 phosphorylation at this lower dose of SSTR2 agonist suggests that SSTR2 internalization is not prompted at this concentration, but triggered at a higher concentration. Moreover, in the presence of SSTR4 agonist, the receptor internalization is expected at all the concentrations used and followed by degradation, which may account for CRMP2 phosphorylation, which may be even higher in the presence of Aβ. We have previously demonstrated that SSTR2 and SSTR4 exist as homo- and heterodimers on the cell surface, whereas agonist treatment leads to changes in the receptor dimerization and enhanced internalization [76,77]. Consistent with these observations, it is highly possible that the dissociation of SSTR2 and 4 homo- and heteromeric complexes at the cell surface in response to receptor activation resulted in enhanced CRMP2 phosphorylation.

Previous studies have shown increased phosphorylation of CRMP2 by CDK5 and GSK3β in AD patients when compared to the age-matched controls [2]. CDK5 is a serine/threonine kinase that is activated upon association with its substrate p35 or p39. The abnormal CDK5 expression or activity has been closely associated with neurotoxicity in various neurodegenerative diseases, including AD, HIV neurotoxicity, and prion-related encephalopathies [37,78,79]. Furthermore, the disruptions in intracellular calcium homeostasis have also been associated with the onset and progression of AD and other amyloidogenic diseases, such as Parkinson's disease [80–82]. Various mechanisms have been suggested for the Aβ-mediated increase in calcium influx, including the disruption of lipid integrity [83], the formation of cation-selective channels by Aβ [81,84], or the activation of selective cell surface receptors to calcium [80,85,86]. These studies further emphasize that the Aβ-induced increase in calcium influx is not solely dependent on one particular pathway, but mediated through a complex network. In particular, the excess Ca^{2+} influx in the presence of Aβ leads to the calpain-mediated truncation of CDK5 substrate p35 into the much more stable form of p25, leading to the prolonged activation of CDK5, followed by the hyper-phosphorylation of downstream mediators such as CRMP2 [35,87,88].

SST through SSTR2 is known to inhibit the Ca^{2+} influx [47–49]. In agreement with previous studies, we found an increased expression of SSTR2 upon treatment with SST in the presence or absence of Aβ, supporting SSTR2 as the essential receptor involved in the SST-mediated inhibition of Ca^{2+} influx. Although the observed inhibitory changes in Ca^{2+} influx were not significantly different between $Aβ_{1-42}$ alone or in combination with SST-14 due to higher deviations, a similar trend was observed in all the experiments performed. We predict that the assay's high sensitivity and changes in the baseline due to experimental variability might be the reason for such observation. Furthermore, we have also observed a significant inhibition of calpain expression in cells co-treated with Aβ and SST compared to the cells treated with Aβ alone. This inhibition of calpain expression by SST did not result in the inhibition of CDK5 expression. Still, it resulted in a significant decrease of CRMP2 phosphorylation at Ser522, suggesting that SST might inhibit the hyperphosphorylation of CRMP2 by interfering with Ca^{2+} homeostasis. Furthermore, as the CDK5-mediated phosphorylation of downstream targets such as CRMP2 depends on the activity rather than the expression level of CDK5, a significant change in CDK5 activity mediated by SST is conceivable, and future studies are warranted in this direction.

The activation of CRMP2 (Ser522) upon treatment with SSTR2 and 4 specific agonists, in contrast to SST-mediated attenuation, is intriguing. However, the molecular mechanism associated with such contradicting results is not known. Whether the SST-mediated suppression of CRMP2 (Ser522) phosphorylation is due to the direct or indirect activation of multiple SSTR subtypes warrants further research. Furthermore, it is possible that unlike SST, which is highly associated with the Ca^{2+} uptake, specific SSTRs may work independently of the calcium pathway and via the modulation of downstream signaling pathways. Importantly, the role of other CRMP phosphorylation sites and isoforms, specifically CRMP5, cannot be avoided from the discussion. Previous studies have shown that CRMP5 inhibits neurite outgrowth and antagonizes CRMP2-mediated axonal and dendrite growth [89]. It is highly possible that SSTR2 and 4 agonists might inhibit CRMP5, resulting in enhanced CRMP2 phosphorylation.

5. Conclusions

In conclusion, the findings from the current study elucidate the mechanistic regulatory role of SST in intracellular calcium homeostasis, CRMP2 phosphorylation, and neurite formation and integrity. These observations corroborate the neuroprotective role of SST in neurotoxicity and neurodegenerative diseases by suggesting a novel mode of action. Furthermore, as disrupted calcium homeostasis is restricted to the neurodegenerative disease, the effective regulation of calcium levels by SST may have significant therapeutic applicability.

Author Contributions: Conceptualization, S.P. and U.K.; Formal analysis, S.P., R.K.S., S.Z., and H.A.O.; Funding acquisition, S.P. and U.K.; Methodology, S.P., R.K.S., S.Z., and H.A.O.; Resources, U.K.; Supervision, U.K.; Writing—original draft, S.P.; Writing—review & editing, S.P., R.K.S., and U.K. All authors have read and agreed to the published version of the manuscript.

Funding: This work was supported by grants from the Canadian Institute of Health Research (MOP 74465) and NSERC (402594-11 and 16-05171) Canada to UK. S.P. is the recipient of a CIHR Doctoral Research Award (GSD 134858) and a UBC 4-Year Fellowship.

Institutional Review Board Statement: Not applicable.

Informed Consent Statement: Not applicable.

Data Availability Statement: The data supporting the findings of this study are available within the article.

Acknowledgments: SH-SY5Y cells were kindly provided by Neil Cashman, UBC.

Conflicts of Interest: The authors declare no conflict of interest. The funders had no role in the design of the study; in the collection, analyses, or interpretation of data; in the writing of the manuscript, or in the decision to publish the results.

References

1. Chung, M.A.; Lee, J.E.; Lee, J.Y.; Ko, M.J.; Lee, S.T.; Kim, H.J. Alteration of collapsin response mediator protein-2 expression in focal ischemic rat brain. *Neuroreport* **2005**, *16*, 1647–1653. [CrossRef] [PubMed]
2. Cole, A.R.; Noble, W.; van Aalten, L.; Plattner, F.; Meimaridou, R.; Hogan, D.; Taylor, M.; LaFrancois, J.; Gunn-Moore, F.; Verkhratsky, A.; et al. Collapsin response mediator protein-2 hyperphosphorylation is an early event in Alzheimer's disease progression. *J. Neurochem.* **2007**, *103*, 1132–1144. [CrossRef] [PubMed]
3. Jorm, A.F.; Jolley, D. The incidence of dementia: A meta-analysis. *Neurology* **1998**, *51*, 728–733. [CrossRef] [PubMed]
4. Cork, L.C.; Sternberger, N.H.; Sternberger, L.A.; Casanova, M.F.; Struble, R.G.; Price, D.L. Phosphorylated neurofilament antigens in neurofibrillary tangles in Alzheimer's disease. *J. Neuropathol. Exp. Neurol.* **1986**, *45*, 56–64. [CrossRef] [PubMed]
5. Sternberger, N.H.; Sternberger, L.A.; Ulrich, J. Aberrant neurofilament phosphorylation in Alzheimer disease. *Proc. Natl. Acad. Sci. USA* **1985**, *82*, 4274–4276. [CrossRef] [PubMed]
6. Haass, C.; Selkoe, D.J. Soluble protein oligomers in neurodegeneration: Lessons from the Alzheimer's amyloid beta-peptide. *Nat. Rev. Mol. Cell Biol.* **2007**, *8*, 101–112. [CrossRef] [PubMed]
7. Palop, J.J.; Mucke, L. Amyloid-beta-induced neuronal dysfunction in Alzheimer's disease: From synapses toward neural networks. *Nat. Neurosci.* **2010**, *13*, 812–818. [CrossRef]
8. Solomon, A.; Mangialasche, F.; Richard, E.; Andrieu, S.; Bennett, D.A.; Breteler, M.; Fratiglioni, L.; Hooshmand, B.; Khachaturian, A.S.; Schneider, L.S.; et al. Advances in the prevention of Alzheimer's disease and dementia. *J. Intern. Med.* **2014**, *275*, 229–250. [CrossRef]
9. Gadhave, K.; Kumar, D.; Uversky, V.N.; Giri, R. A multitude of signaling pathways associated with Alzheimer's disease and their roles in AD pathogenesis and therapy. *Med. Res. Rev.* **2020**. [CrossRef]
10. Arimura, N.; Kaibuchi, K. Neuronal polarity: From extracellular signals to intracellular mechanisms. *Nat. Rev. Neurosci.* **2007**, *8*, 194–205. [CrossRef]
11. Yamashita, N.; Goshima, Y. Collapsin response mediator proteins regulate neuronal development and plasticity by switching their phosphorylation status. *Mol. Neurobiol.* **2012**, *45*, 234–246. [CrossRef] [PubMed]
12. Arimura, N.; Menager, C.; Kawano, Y.; Yoshimura, T.; Kawabata, S.; Hattori, A.; Fukata, Y.; Amano, M.; Goshima, Y.; Inagaki, M.; et al. Phosphorylation by Rho kinase regulates CRMP-2 activity in growth cones. *Mol. Cell. Biol.* **2005**, *25*, 9973–9984. [CrossRef] [PubMed]
13. Fukata, Y.; Itoh, T.J.; Kimura, T.; Menager, C.; Nishimura, T.; Shiromizu, T.; Watanabe, H.; Inagaki, N.; Iwamatsu, A.; Hotani, H.; et al. CRMP-2 binds to tubulin heterodimers to promote microtubule assembly. *Nat. Cell Biol.* **2002**, *4*, 583–591. [CrossRef] [PubMed]
14. Tan, M.; Cha, C.; Ye, Y.; Zhang, J.; Li, S.; Wu, F.; Gong, S.; Guo, G. CRMP4 and CRMP2 Interact to Coordinate Cytoskeleton Dynamics, Regulating Growth Cone Development and Axon Elongation. *Neural Plast.* **2015**, *2015*, 947423. [CrossRef]
15. Varrin-Doyer, M.; Nicolle, A.; Marignier, R.; Cavagna, S.; Benetollo, C.; Wattel, E.; Giraudon, P. Human T lymphotropic virus type 1 increases T lymphocyte migration by recruiting the cytoskeleton organizer CRMP2. *J. Immunol. (Baltim. MD 1950)* **2012**, *188*, 1222–1233. [CrossRef]
16. Kimura, T.; Watanabe, H.; Iwamatsu, A.; Kaibuchi, K. Tubulin and CRMP-2 complex is transported via Kinesin-1. *J. Neurochem.* **2005**, *93*, 1371–1382. [CrossRef]
17. Namba, T.; Nakamuta, S.; Funahashi, Y.; Kaibuchi, K. The role of selective transport in neuronal polarization. *Dev. Neurobiol.* **2011**, *71*, 445–457. [CrossRef]
18. Brown, M.; Jacobs, T.; Eickholt, B.; Ferrari, G.; Teo, M.; Monfries, C.; Qi, R.Z.; Leung, T.; Lim, L.; Hall, C. Alpha2-chimaerin, cyclin-dependent Kinase 5/p35, and its target collapsin response mediator protein-2 are essential components in semaphorin 3A-induced growth-cone collapse. *J. Neurosci. Off. J. Soc. Neurosci.* **2004**, *24*, 8994–9004. [CrossRef]
19. Cole, A.R.; Knebel, A.; Morrice, N.A.; Robertson, L.A.; Irving, A.J.; Connolly, C.N.; Sutherland, C. GSK-3 phosphorylation of the Alzheimer epitope within collapsin response mediator proteins regulates axon elongation in primary neurons. *J. Biol. Chem.* **2004**, *279*, 50176–50180. [CrossRef]
20. Uchida, Y.; Ohshima, T.; Sasaki, Y.; Suzuki, H.; Yanai, S.; Yamashita, N.; Nakamura, F.; Takei, K.; Ihara, Y.; Mikoshiba, K.; et al. Semaphorin3A signalling is mediated via sequential Cdk5 and GSK3beta phosphorylation of CRMP2: Implication of common phosphorylating mechanism underlying axon guidance and Alzheimer's disease. *Genes Cells Devoted Mol. Cell. Mech.* **2005**, *10*, 165–179. [CrossRef]
21. Yoshimura, T.; Kawano, Y.; Arimura, N.; Kawabata, S.; Kikuchi, A.; Kaibuchi, K. GSK-3beta regulates phosphorylation of CRMP-2 and neuronal polarity. *Cell* **2005**, *120*, 137–149. [CrossRef] [PubMed]
22. Cole, A.R.; Soutar, M.P.; Rembutsu, M.; van Aalten, L.; Hastie, C.J.; McLauchlan, H.; Peggie, M.; Balastik, M.; Lu, K.P.; Sutherland, C. Relative resistance of Cdk5-phosphorylated CRMP2 to dephosphorylation. *J. Biol. Chem.* **2008**, *283*, 18227–18237. [CrossRef] [PubMed]

23. Brittain, J.M.; Wang, Y.; Eruvwetere, O.; Khanna, R. Cdk5-mediated phosphorylation of CRMP-2 enhances its interaction with CaV2.2. *FEBS Lett.* **2012**, *586*, 3813–3818. [CrossRef] [PubMed]
24. Fischer, A.; Sananbenesi, F.; Pang, P.T.; Lu, B.; Tsai, L.H. Opposing roles of transient and prolonged expression of p25 in synaptic plasticity and hippocampus-dependent memory. *Neuron* **2005**, *48*, 825–838. [CrossRef]
25. Jessberger, S.; Aigner, S.; Clemenson, G.D., Jr.; Toni, N.; Lie, D.C.; Karalay, O.; Overall, R.; Kempermann, G.; Gage, F.H. Cdk5 regulates accurate maturation of newborn granule cells in the adult hippocampus. *PLoS Biol.* **2008**, *6*, e272. [CrossRef]
26. Johansson, J.U.; Lilja, L.; Chen, X.L.; Higashida, H.; Meister, B.; Noda, M.; Zhong, Z.G.; Yokoyama, S.; Berggren, P.O.; Bark, C. Cyclin-dependent kinase 5 activators p35 and p39 facilitate formation of functional synapses. *Brain Res. Mol. Brain Res.* **2005**, *138*, 215–227. [CrossRef]
27. Lagace, D.C.; Benavides, D.R.; Kansy, J.W.; Mapelli, M.; Greengard, P.; Bibb, J.A.; Eisch, A.J. Cdk5 is essential for adult hippocampal neurogenesis. *Proc. Natl. Acad. Sci. USA* **2008**, *105*, 18567–18571. [CrossRef]
28. Samuels, B.A.; Hsueh, Y.P.; Shu, T.; Liang, H.; Tseng, H.C.; Hong, C.J.; Su, S.C.; Volker, J.; Neve, R.L.; Yue, D.T.; et al. Cdk5 promotes synaptogenesis by regulating the subcellular distribution of the MAGUK family member CASK. *Neuron* **2007**, *56*, 823–837. [CrossRef]
29. Xie, Z.; Sanada, K.; Samuels, B.A.; Shih, H.; Tsai, L.H. Serine 732 phosphorylation of FAK by Cdk5 is important for microtubule organization, nuclear movement, and neuronal migration. *Cell* **2003**, *114*, 469–482. [CrossRef]
30. Hisanaga, S.; Saito, T. The regulation of cyclin-dependent kinase 5 activity through the metabolism of p35 or p39 Cdk5 activator. *Neuro-Signals* **2003**, *12*, 221–229. [CrossRef]
31. Sherr, C.J.; Roberts, J.M. CDK inhibitors: Positive and negative regulators of G1-phase progression. *Genes Dev.* **1999**, *13*, 1501–1512. [CrossRef] [PubMed]
32. Cicero, S.; Herrup, K. Cyclin-dependent kinase 5 is essential for neuronal cell cycle arrest and differentiation. *J. Neurosci. Off. J. Soc. Neurosci.* **2005**, *25*, 9658–9668. [CrossRef] [PubMed]
33. Copani, A.; Uberti, D.; Sortino, M.A.; Bruno, V.; Nicoletti, F.; Memo, M. Activation of cell-cycle-associated proteins in neuronal death: A mandatory or dispensable path? *Trends Neurosci.* **2001**, *24*, 25–31. [CrossRef]
34. Fischer, A.; Sananbenesi, F.; Spiess, J.; Radulovic, J. Cdk5 in the adult non-demented brain. *Curr. Drug Targets CNS Neurol. Disord.* **2003**, *2*, 375–381. [CrossRef]
35. Lee, M.S.; Kwon, Y.T.; Li, M.; Peng, J.; Friedlander, R.M.; Tsai, L.H. Neurotoxicity induces cleavage of p35 to p25 by calpain. *Nature* **2000**, *405*, 360–364. [CrossRef]
36. Neve, R.L.; McPhie, D.L. The cell cycle as a therapeutic target for Alzheimer's disease. *Pharmacol. Ther.* **2006**, *111*, 99–113. [CrossRef]
37. Patrick, G.N.; Zukerberg, L.; Nikolic, M.; de la Monte, S.; Dikkes, P.; Tsai, L.H. Conversion of p35 to p25 deregulates Cdk5 activity and promotes neurodegeneration. *Nature* **1999**, *402*, 615–622. [CrossRef]
38. Saito, K.; Elce, J.S.; Hamos, J.E.; Nixon, R.A. Widespread activation of calcium-activated neutral proteinase (calpain) in the brain in Alzheimer disease: A potential molecular basis for neuronal degeneration. *Proc. Natl. Acad. Sci. USA* **1993**, *90*, 2628–2632. [CrossRef]
39. Stutzmann, G.E. The pathogenesis of Alzheimers disease is it a lifelong "calciumopathy"? *Neurosci. Rev. J. Bringing Neurobiol. Neurol. Psychiatry* **2007**, *13*, 546–559. [CrossRef]
40. Paik, S.; Somvanshi, R.K.; Kumar, U. Somatostatin-Mediated Changes in Microtubule-Associated Proteins and Retinoic Acid-Induced Neurite Outgrowth in SH-SY5Y Cells. *J. Mol. Neurosci. MN* **2019**, *68*, 120–134. [CrossRef]
41. Encinas, M.; Iglesias, M.; Liu, Y.; Wang, H.; Muhaisen, A.; Cena, V.; Gallego, C.; Comella, J.X. Sequential treatment of SH-SY5Y cells with retinoic acid and brain-derived neurotrophic factor gives rise to fully differentiated, neurotrophic factor-dependent, human neuron-like cells. *J. Neurochem.* **2000**, *75*, 991–1003. [CrossRef] [PubMed]
42. War, S.A.; Somvanshi, R.K.; Kumar, U. Somatostatin receptor-3 mediated intracellular signaling and apoptosis is regulated by its cytoplasmic terminal. *Biochimica Biophysica Acta* **2011**, *1813*, 390–402. [CrossRef] [PubMed]
43. Paik, S.; Somvanshi, R.K.; Kumar, U. Somatostatin Maintains Permeability and Integrity of Blood-Brain Barrier in beta-Amyloid Induced Toxicity. *Mol. Neurobiol.* **2018**. [CrossRef]
44. Ferriero, D.M.; Sheldon, R.A.; Messing, R.O. Somatostatin enhances nerve growth factor-induced neurite outgrowth in PC12 cells. *Brain Res. Dev. Brain Res.* **1994**, *80*, 13–18. [CrossRef]
45. Crews, L.; Ruf, R.; Patrick, C.; Dumaop, W.; Trejo-Morales, M.; Achim, C.L.; Rockenstein, E.; Masliah, E. Phosphorylation of collapsin response mediator protein-2 disrupts neuronal maturation in a model of adult neurogenesis: Implications for neurodegenerative disorders. *Mol. Neurodegener.* **2011**, *6*, 67. [CrossRef]
46. Mokhtar, S.H.; Bakhuraysah, M.M.; Cram, D.S.; Petratos, S. The Beta-amyloid protein of Alzheimer's disease: Communication breakdown by modifying the neuronal cytoskeleton. *Int. J. Alzheimer's Dis.* **2013**, *2013*, 910502. [CrossRef]
47. Johnson, J.; Caravelli, M.L.; Brecha, N.C. Somatostatin inhibits calcium influx into rat rod bipolar cell axonal terminals. *Vis. Neurosci.* **2001**, *18*, 101–108. [CrossRef]
48. Petrucci, C.; Resta, V.; Fieni, F.; Bigiani, A.; Bagnoli, P. Modulation of potassium current and calcium influx by somatostatin in rod bipolar cells isolated from the rabbit retina via sst2 receptors. *Naunyn-Schmiedeberg's Arch. Pharmacol.* **2001**, *363*, 680–694. [CrossRef]

49. Reisine, T. Cellular mechanisms of somatostatin inhibition of calcium influx in the anterior pituitary cell line AtT-20. *J. Pharmacol. Exp. Ther.* **1990**, *254*, 646–651.
50. Daniels, W.M.; Hendricks, J.; Salie, R.; Taljaard, J.J. The role of the MAP-kinase superfamily in beta-amyloid toxicity. *Metab. Brain Dis.* **2001**, *16*, 175–185. [CrossRef]
51. Suttisansanee, U.; Charoenkiatkul, S.; Jongruaysup, B.; Tabtimsri, S.; Siriwan, D.; Temviriyanukul, P. Mulberry Fruit Cultivar 'Chiang Mai' Prevents Beta-Amyloid Toxicity in PC12 Neuronal Cells and in a Drosophila Model of Alzheimer's Disease. *Molecules* **2020**, *25*, 1837. [CrossRef] [PubMed]
52. Beal, M.F.; Mazurek, M.F.; Svendsen, C.N.; Bird, E.D.; Martin, J.B. Widespread reduction of somatostatin-like immunoreactivity in the cerebral cortex in Alzheimer's disease. *Ann. Neurol.* **1986**, *20*, 489–495. [CrossRef] [PubMed]
53. Bissette, G.; Cook, L.; Smith, W.; Dole, K.C.; Crain, B.; Nemeroff, C.B. Regional Neuropeptide Pathology in Alzheimer's Disease: Corticotropin-Releasing Factor and Somatostatin. *J. Alzheimer's Dis.* **1998**, *1*, 91–105. [CrossRef] [PubMed]
54. Bissette, G.; Myers, B. Somatostatin in Alzheimer's disease and depression. *Life Sci.* **1992**, *51*, 1389–1410. [CrossRef]
55. Davies, P.; Katzman, R.; Terry, R.D. Reduced somatostatin-like immunoreactivity in cerebral cortex from cases of Alzheimer disease and Alzheimer senile dementa. *Nature* **1980**, *288*, 279–280. [CrossRef]
56. Davis, K.L.; Davidson, M.; Yang, R.K.; Davis, B.M.; Siever, L.J.; Mohs, R.C.; Ryan, T.; Coccaro, E.; Bierer, L.; Targum, S.D. CSF somatostatin in Alzheimer's disease, depressed patients, and control subjects. *Biol. Psychiatry* **1988**, *24*, 710–712. [CrossRef]
57. Molchan, S.E.; Hill, J.L.; Martinez, R.A.; Lawlor, B.A.; Mellow, A.M.; Rubinow, D.R.; Bissette, G.; Nemeroff, C.B.; Sunderland, T. CSF somatostatin in Alzheimer's disease and major depression: Relationship to hypothalamic-pituitary-adrenal axis and clinical measures. *Psychoneuroendocrinology* **1993**, *18*, 509–519. [CrossRef]
58. Nemeroff, C.B.; Knight, D.L.; Bissette, G. Somatostatin: A neuropeptide system pathologically altered in Alzheimer's disease and depression. *Clin. Neuropharmacol.* **1992**, *15* (Suppl. 1), 311a–312a. [CrossRef]
59. Nilsson, C.L.; Brinkmalm, A.; Minthon, L.; Blennow, K.; Ekman, R. Processing of neuropeptide Y, galanin, and somatostatin in the cerebrospinal fluid of patients with Alzheimer's disease and frontotemporal dementia. *Peptides* **2001**, *22*, 2105–2112. [CrossRef]
60. Basivireddy, J.; Somvanshi, R.K.; Romero, I.A.; Weksler, B.B.; Couraud, P.O.; Oger, J.; Kumar, U. Somatostatin preserved blood brain barrier against cytokine induced alterations: Possible role in multiple sclerosis. *Biochem. Pharmacol.* **2013**, *86*, 497–507. [CrossRef]
61. Geci, C.; How, J.; Alturaihi, H.; Kumar, U. Beta-amyloid increases somatostatin expression in cultured cortical neurons. *J. Neurochem.* **2007**, *101*, 664–673. [CrossRef] [PubMed]
62. Kumar, U. Characterization of striatal cultures with the effect of QUIN and NMDA. *Neurosci. Res.* **2004**, *49*, 29–38. [CrossRef] [PubMed]
63. Kumar, U. Expression of somatostatin receptor subtypes (SSTR1-5) in Alzheimer's disease brain: An immunohistochemical analysis. *Neuroscience* **2005**, *134*, 525–538. [CrossRef] [PubMed]
64. Aguado-Llera, D.; Arilla-Ferreiro, E.; Campos-Barros, A.; Puebla-Jimenez, L.; Barrios, V. Protective effects of insulin-like growth factor-I on the somatostatinergic system in the temporal cortex of beta-amyloid-treated rats. *J. Neurochem.* **2005**, *92*, 607–615. [CrossRef]
65. Burgos-Ramos, E.; Hervas-Aguilar, A.; Puebla-Jimenez, L.; Boyano-Adanez, M.C.; Arilla-Ferreiro, E. Chronic but not acute intracerebroventricular administration of amyloid beta-peptide (25–35) decreases somatostatin content, adenylate cyclase activity, somatostatin-induced inhibition of adenylate cyclase activity, and adenylate cyclase I levels in the rat hippocampus. *J. Neurosci. Res.* **2007**, *85*, 433–442. [CrossRef]
66. Hervas-Aguilar, A.; Puebla-Jimenez, L.; Burgos-Ramos, E.; Aguado-Llera, D.; Arilla-Ferreiro, E. Effects of single and continuous administration of amyloid beta-peptide (25–35) on adenylyl cyclase activity and the somatostatinergic system in the rat frontal and parietal cortex. *Neuroscience* **2005**, *135*, 181–190. [CrossRef]
67. Nag, S.; Yee, B.K.; Tang, F. Reduction in somatostatin and substance P levels and choline acetyltransferase activity in the cortex and hippocampus of the rat after chronic intracerebroventricular infusion of beta-amyloid (1–40). *Brain Res. Bull.* **1999**, *50*, 251–262. [CrossRef]
68. Armstrong, D.M.; LeRoy, S.; Shields, D.; Terry, R.D. Somatostatin-like immunoreactivity within neuritic plaques. *Brain Res.* **1985**, *338*, 71–79. [CrossRef]
69. Morrison, J.H.; Rogers, J.; Scherr, S.; Benoit, R.; Bloom, F.E. Somatostatin immunoreactivity in neuritic plaques of Alzheimer's patients. *Nature* **1985**, *314*, 90–92. [CrossRef]
70. Saito, T.; Iwata, N.; Tsubuki, S.; Takaki, Y.; Takano, J.; Huang, S.M.; Suemoto, T.; Higuchi, M.; Saido, T.C. Somatostatin regulates brain amyloid beta peptide Abeta42 through modulation of proteolytic degradation. *Nat. Med.* **2005**, *11*, 434–439. [CrossRef]
71. Inagaki, N.; Chihara, K.; Arimura, N.; Menager, C.; Kawano, Y.; Matsuo, N.; Nishimura, T.; Amano, M.; Kaibuchi, K. CRMP-2 induces axons in cultured hippocampal neurons. *Nat. Neurosci.* **2001**, *4*, 781–782. [CrossRef] [PubMed]
72. Nishimura, T.; Fukata, Y.; Kato, K.; Yamaguchi, T.; Matsuura, Y.; Kamiguchi, H.; Kaibuchi, K. CRMP-2 regulates polarized Numb-mediated endocytosis for axon growth. *Nat. Cell Biol.* **2003**, *5*, 819–826. [CrossRef] [PubMed]
73. Chae, Y.C.; Lee, S.; Heo, K.; Ha, S.H.; Jung, Y.; Kim, J.H.; Ihara, Y.; Suh, P.G.; Ryu, S.H. Collapsin response mediator protein-2 regulates neurite formation by modulating tubulin GTPase activity. *Cell. Signal.* **2009**, *21*, 1818–1826. [CrossRef] [PubMed]
74. Yoshida, H.; Watanabe, A.; Ihara, Y. Collapsin response mediator protein-2 is associated with neurofibrillary tangles in Alzheimer's disease. *J. Biol. Chem.* **1998**, *273*, 9761–9768. [CrossRef] [PubMed]

75. Mokhtar, S.H.; Kim, M.J.; Magee, K.A.; Aui, P.M.; Thomas, S.; Bakhuraysah, M.M.; Alrehaili, A.A.; Lee, J.Y.; Steer, D.L.; Kenny, R.; et al. Amyloid-beta-dependent phosphorylation of collapsin response mediator protein-2 dissociates kinesin in Alzheimer's disease. *Neural Regen. Res.* **2018**, *13*, 1066–1080. [CrossRef] [PubMed]
76. Grant, M.; Collier, B.; Kumar, U. Agonist-dependent dissociation of human somatostatin receptor 2 dimers: A role in receptor trafficking. *J. Biol. Chem.* **2004**, *279*, 36179–36183. [CrossRef] [PubMed]
77. Somvanshi, R.K.; Billova, S.; Kharmate, G.; Rajput, P.S.; Kumar, U. C-tail mediated modulation of somatostatin receptor type-4 homo- and heterodimerizations and signaling. *Cell. Signal.* **2009**, *21*, 1396–1414. [CrossRef] [PubMed]
78. Liu, F.; Su, Y.; Li, B.; Zhou, Y.; Ryder, J.; Gonzalez-DeWhitt, P.; May, P.C.; Ni, B. Regulation of amyloid precursor protein (APP) phosphorylation and processing by p35/Cdk5 and p25/Cdk5. *FEBS Lett.* **2003**, *547*, 193–196. [CrossRef]
79. Wang, G.R.; Shi, S.; Gao, C.; Zhang, B.Y.; Tian, C.; Dong, C.F.; Zhou, R.M.; Li, X.L.; Chen, C.; Han, J.; et al. Changes of tau profiles in brains of the hamsters infected with scrapie strains 263 K or 139 A possibly associated with the alteration of phosphate kinases. *BMC Infect. Dis.* **2010**, *10*, 86. [CrossRef]
80. Blanchard, B.J.; Chen, A.; Rozeboom, L.M.; Stafford, K.A.; Weigele, P.; Ingram, V.M. Efficient reversal of Alzheimer's disease fibril formation and elimination of neurotoxicity by a small molecule. *Proc. Natl. Acad. Sci. USA* **2004**, *101*, 14326–14332. [CrossRef]
81. Kawahara, M.; Kuroda, Y.; Arispe, N.; Rojas, E. Alzheimer's beta-amyloid, human islet amylin, and prion protein fragment evoke intracellular free calcium elevations by a common mechanism in a hypothalamic GnRH neuronal cell line. *J. Biol. Chem.* **2000**, *275*, 14077–14083. [CrossRef]
82. Mattson, M.P. Pathways towards and away from Alzheimer's disease. *Nature* **2004**, *430*, 631–639. [CrossRef] [PubMed]
83. Kayed, R.; Sokolov, Y.; Edmonds, B.; McIntire, T.M.; Milton, S.C.; Hall, J.E.; Glabe, C.G. Permeabilization of lipid bilayers is a common conformation-dependent activity of soluble amyloid oligomers in protein misfolding diseases. *J. Biol. Chem.* **2004**, *279*, 46363–46366. [CrossRef] [PubMed]
84. Kagan, B.L.; Hirakura, Y.; Azimov, R.; Azimova, R.; Lin, M.C. The channel hypothesis of Alzheimer's disease: Current status. *Peptides* **2002**, *23*, 1311–1315. [CrossRef]
85. Guo, Q.; Furukawa, K.; Sopher, B.L.; Pham, D.G.; Xie, J.; Robinson, N.; Martin, G.M.; Mattson, M.P. Alzheimer's PS-1 mutation perturbs calcium homeostasis and sensitizes PC12 cells to death induced by amyloid beta-peptide. *Neuroreport* **1996**, *8*, 379–383. [CrossRef] [PubMed]
86. Mattson, M.P.; Chan, S.L. Calcium orchestrates apoptosis. *Nat. Cell Biol.* **2003**, *5*, 1041–1043. [CrossRef] [PubMed]
87. Amin, N.D.; Albers, W.; Pant, H.C. Cyclin-dependent kinase 5 (cdk5) activation requires interaction with three domains of p35. *J. Neurosci. Res.* **2002**, *67*, 354–362. [CrossRef]
88. Dhavan, R.; Tsai, L.H. A decade of CDK5. *Nat. Rev. Mol. Cell Biol.* **2001**, *2*, 749–759. [CrossRef]
89. Brot, S.; Rogemond, V.; Perrot, V.; Chounlamountri, N.; Auger, C.; Honnorat, J.; Moradi-Ameli, M. CRMP5 interacts with tubulin to inhibit neurite outgrowth, thereby modulating the function of CRMP2. *J. Neurosci. Off. J. Soc. Neurosci.* **2010**, *30*, 10639–10654. [CrossRef]

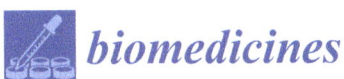

Article

Quinpirole-Mediated Regulation of Dopamine D2 Receptors Inhibits Glial Cell-Induced Neuroinflammation in Cortex and Striatum after Brain Injury

Sayed Ibrar Alam [1,†], Min Gi Jo [1,†], Tae Ju Park [2], Rahat Ullah [1], Sareer Ahmad [1], Shafiq Ur Rehman [1] and Myeong Ok Kim [1,*]

[1] Division of Life Sciences and Applied Life Science (BK21 FOUR), College of Natural Science, Gyeongsang National University, Jinju 52828, Korea; ibrar@gnu.ac.kr (S.I.A.); mingi.cho@gnu.ac.kr (M.G.J.); Rahatullah1414@gnu.ac.kr (R.U.); sareer_50@gnu.ac.kr (S.A.); shafiq.qau.edu@gmail.com (S.U.R.)

[2] Paul O'Gorman Leukaemia Research Centre, Institute of Cancer Sciences, MVLS, University of Glasgow, Glasgow G12 8QQ, UK; 2358860p@student.gla.ac.uk

* Correspondence: mokim@gnu.ac.kr; Tel.: +82-55-772-1345; Fax: +82-55-772-2656

† These authors equally contributed to this paper.

Abstract: Brain injury is a significant risk factor for chronic gliosis and neurodegenerative diseases. Currently, no treatment is available for neuroinflammation caused by the action of glial cells following brain injury. In this study, we investigated the quinpirole-mediated activation of dopamine D2 receptors (D2R) in a mouse model of traumatic brain injury (TBI). We also investigated the neuroprotective effects of quinpirole (a D2R agonist) against glial cell-induced neuroinflammation secondary to TBI in adult mice. After the brain injury, we injected quinpirole into the TBI mice at a dose of 1 mg/kg daily intraperitoneally for 7 days. Our results showed suppression of D2R expression and deregulation of downstream signaling molecules in ipsilateral cortex and striatum after TBI on day 7. Quinpirole administration regulated D2R expression and significantly reduced glial cell-induced neuroinflammation via the D2R/Akt/glycogen synthase kinase 3 beta (GSK3-β) signaling pathway after TBI. Quinpirole treatment concomitantly attenuated increase in glial cells, neuronal apoptosis, synaptic dysfunction, and regulated proteins associated with the blood–brain barrier, together with the recovery of lesion volume in the TBI mouse model. Additionally, our in vitro results confirmed that quinpirole reversed the microglial condition media complex-mediated deleterious effects and regulated D2R levels in HT22 cells. This study showed that quinpirole administration after TBI reduced secondary brain injury-induced glial cell activation and neuroinflammation via regulation of the D2R/Akt/GSK3-β signaling pathways. Our study suggests that quinpirole may be a safe therapeutic agent against TBI-induced neurodegeneration.

Keywords: brain injury; quinpirole; dopamine D2 receptors; glial cell; neuroinflammation; neurodegeneration

1. Introduction

Traumatic brain injury (TBI) is a global risk factor and the leading cause of neurological disability. Recent studies have reported that TBI is associated with several neurodegenerative diseases, such as Alzheimer's and Parkinson's disease [1–3]. TBI leads to a primary injury, which is followed by a secondary brain injury. Primary brain injury refers to the direct mechanical force applied at the time of the initial impact on the brain. Secondary brain injury occurs as a consequence of the initial traumatic events. It refers to the involvement of the brain vasculature as well as the blood–brain barrier (BBB) disruption, which results in significant complications in the brain [4]. Neuroinflammation is the principal hallmark of brain injury, followed by astrocyte and microglia activation and release of pro-inflammatory cytokines and chemokines, which impair the endogenous self-repair ability of the brain and eventually cause neuronal apoptosis and neurodegenerative conditions [5,6]. Several studies have proved that brain injuries precipitate an inflammatory response with activation of neuroinflammatory mediators [7]. Therefore, it is important to develop neuroprotective and neurorestorative agents to treat TBI. Notably, this subject offers much scope for extensive research to treat the TBI-induced neuroinflammatory response and inflammatory cytokine release. Restoration of BBB integrity and treatment of neuroinflammation is the key therapeutic goals in patients with brain injury-induced pathological events.

Dopamine (DA) is a major neurotransmitter that controls abnormal neuronal excitotoxicity and regulates the function of the dopaminergic system in the brain [6,8,9]. Dopamine D2 receptors (D2R) belong to the class of G protein-coupled receptors that are activated by DA and participate in essential functions, including innate immunity and neuroinflammatory responses [10,11]. However, previous studies have reported a significantly increased inflammatory response in D2R-knockout (D2R−/−) mice [12]. D2R is expressed in several regions of the brain, including the cerebral cortex, hippocampus, and striatum [13]. A previous study has shown that DA receptors are expressed on glial and immune cells [14]. Several studies have reported that DA plays a vital role in humans and animals and that cortical dopaminergic dysfunction is associated with attention deficit hyperactivity disorder [15,16]. A recent study has reported that cortical D2R is involved in psychotic and mood disorders and regulates neuronal circuits [17]. Deregulation of the DA system could be a significant contributor to behavioral and cognitive deficits that are observed after TBI. A growing body of evidence suggests that D2R agonists protect against neuroinflammation and immune reactions, perhaps by inhibiting cytokine release [18,19]. An earlier study reported that quinpirole-activated D2R positively affects neuronal activity in the cingulate cortex and striatum [20]. However, limited studies have reported the role of D2R activation in the inhibition of glial cell-induced neuroinflammatory responses following brain injury.

Akt, a serine-threonine kinase, is known to play an essential role in the cell death/survival pathway. Akt phosphorylates and inhibits several substrates, including glycogen synthase kinase 3 beta (GSK3-β) [21]. A previous study investigated the regulation of the Akt pathway by stimulation of DA receptors and reported possible regulation of the Akt/GSK3-β pathway via regulation of D2R [22].

In this study, we investigated the possible regulation of D2R in the cortical region of the brain, which is the primary target of brain injury, and also explored the striatal region in a TBI mouse model. Furthermore, we investigated the therapeutic potential of post-TBI administration of quinpirole hydrochloride [19,23]. We observed that quinpirole administration at a dose of 1 mg/kg could potentially protect against brain injury-induced gliosis, neuroinflammation, neurodegeneration, lesion volume, synaptic dysfunction and and regulated proteins associated with the BBB via stimulation of D2R, particularly in the ipsilateral cortex of TBI mice. We could also confirm microglial involvement in D2R deregulation and that quinpirole at a dose of 20 μM is sufficient to stimulate D2R and regulate Akt levels in neuronal cell lines. This study highlights that quinpirole administration ipsilateral side of TBI mouse brain stimulated D2R and lead to the recovery of brain function via regulation of the Akt/GSK3-β signaling pathway and inhibition of a glial cell-induced neuroinflammatory response.

2. Materials and Methods

2.1. Animals

Male wild-type C57BL/6N mice, 7 weeks of age with 25–30 g weight, were obtained from Samtako Bio Korea. The animals were acclimatized in the animal care center at Gyeongsang National University, South Korea. The animal were maintained in the control environment with 12/12 h light/dark cycle at 23 °C, and 60 ± 10% humidity with free access to food and water. The mice were randomly divided into following different groups; control, TBI, and TBI + quinpirole after a week of acclimatization. The animals were handled carefully according to the guidelines of the Institutional Animal Care and Use committee (IACUC) (5 March 2019. Approval ID: 125), Division of Life Science and Applied Life Science, Gyeongsang National University, Republic of South Korea.

2.2. Quinpirole Treatment for Mice

The treated animals were divided into the following groups:

Saline treated control group, Stab Wound Cortical Injury, Stab Wound Cortical Injury + quinpirole.

Quinpirole was dissolved in distilled water and administered daily intraperitoneally (i.p) at a dose of 1 mg/kg body weight for 7 days. For western blot ($n = 5$) and for confocal experiments ($n = 6$) mice per group were used. The chemical quinpirole was purchased from Tocris-Cookson (Bristol, UK).

2.3. Stab Wound Cortical Injury

The stab wound cortical brain injury mouse model was established as previously described with modification [24]. Briefly, the mice were anesthetized with Rompun (0.05 mL/100 g body weight) and Zoletil (0.1 mL/100 g body weight). The mice were placed on stereotaxic apparatus and the skull was exposed the by making a mid-longitudinal incision. The dental drill was used to make a circular craniotomy 4 mm in diameter (2 mm lateral to the midline and 1 mm posterior to the bregma) in the skull. For stab wound injury, a sharp edge scalpel blade was inserted (3 mm; right hemisphere) in the mouse brain and kept for 1 min in the brain and then removed slowly. The bone wax was applied to cover the rupture skull followed by stitching with a silk suture to close the wound area. Next, the animals were placed carefully by providing continuous heating with a heating lamp until fully recovered from anesthesia and proceeded for further experiments.

2.4. Protein Extraction

After the completion of the mice treatment, all the animals were first anesthetized and then sacrificed carefully. After the surgery brain were immediately collected and froze on dry ice. The ipsilateral cortex of TBI brain tissue was homogenized using PRO-PREP protein extract solution (iNtRON Biotechnology, Burlington, NJ, USA). to extract protein from tissues followed by centrifugation and stored at $-80\ °C$. The samples were centrifuged at speed of $13,000\times g$ rpm at $4\ °C$ for 25 min. The supernatants were collected and stored at $-80\ °C$ for immunoblotting.

2.5. Western Blot Analysis

The western blot analysis was assessed as previously described with minor changes [25–27]. In brief, an equal volume of 20–30 µg of proteins (extracted from the ipsilateral cortex) was mixed with $2\times$ Sample Buffer (Invitrogen). To separate the proteins, an equal volume of the proteins were run on 10% of SDS polyacrylamide gel electrophoresis and transferred to the PVDF membrane followed by blocking in 5% skim milk. The membranes were slightly washed to clear the skim milk. The primary antibody was incubated overnight at $4\ °C$ 1:1000, anti-(D2R), anti-Glycogen synthase kinase 3 (p-GSK3-β) (Ser9), p-Akt (Ser473), anti-Glial fibrillary acidic protein beta (Anti-GFAP), anti-ionized calcium-binding adapter molecule 1 (anti-Iba-1), anti-phospho-c-Jun N-terminal kinase (p-JNK), anti-interleukin-1β (IL-1β), anti-caspase-3, anti-poly (ADP-ribose) polymerase-1 (Anti-PARP-1), anti-Bax, anti-Bcl-2 and anti-β-actin from Santa Cruz Biotechnology. Anti-beta actin was used as a loading control. The next day, the membranes were incubated with horseradish peroxidase-conjugated secondary antibodies diluted in $1\times$ TBST for 1–2 h as appropriate; the immunoblots were developed using an ECL chemiluminescence system, according to the manufacturer's instructions (Amersham Pharmacia Biotech, Uppsala, Sweden).

2.6. Brain Tissue Collection and Sample Preparation

For brain tissue collection, the mice were anesthetized and transcardially perfused with saline followed by (4%) paraformaldehyde and then fixed with (4%) paraformaldehyde for

48 h. Further, the brain tissues were immersed in a 20% sucrose solution for 48 h. Next, the Brain were fixed vertically in the OCT compound medium, Sakura Finetek USA, Inc., Torrance, CA, USA). For the brain cross-section (14 μm in size) using a vibratome (Leica, Nussloch, Germany) and stored at −80 °C.

2.7. Immunofluorescence Staining

The tissue slides were proceeded for immunofluorescence staining as described previously with minor modification [27,28]. Initially, the slides were dried at room temperature and washed twice with PBS 0.01 M solution for 8–10 min. The tissue slides were incubated in proteinase-K (5 min) and then washed twice for 5 min in PBS solution. Next, the protein was blocked for 1 h with 5% normal serum (goat/rabbit) D2R and 0.1% Triton X-100 in 0.01 M PBS solution. The tissue slides were then incubated with primary antibodies (1:100) ratio in 0.01 M PBS solution overnight at 4 °C. The following antibodies were used for the immunofluorescence detection; anti-p-GSK3-β (ser9), anti-p-Akt, anti-D2R, anti-IL1-β, anti-Caspase-3, anti-PSD-95, anti-SNAP-23, anti-ZO-1 anti-CD31. The tissue slides were then incubated for 2 h in the secondary antibody (1:100) fluorescein isothiocyanate (FITC), and tetramethylrhodamine isothiocyanates (TRITC) labeled secondary antibodies (anti-goat, anti-rabbit, and anti-mouse) from Santa Cruz Biotechnology. The 4′,6-diamidino-2-phenylindole (DAPI) was used for nucleus detection (8–10 min). The slides were covered with coverslips using with fluorescent mounting medium. Confocal laser scanning microscopy FluoViewer MPE-1000 (Olympus, Tokyo, Japan) was used to take the images and the maximum fluorescent intensity in the representative field was taken. The images were converted into Tiff format and the fluorescent intensity of the ipsilateral cortex and striatum region was measured and calculated via ImageJ win32 software (version 1.50, NIH, https://imagej.nih.gov/ij/, USA).

2.8. Assessment of Brain Lesion Volume

To measure lesion volume of the cortical area of TBI and TBI + quinpirole groups, the tissue slides were stained with cresyl violet and the images were taken with a simple light microscope and analyzed with ImageJ software. The injured areas of the TBI and TBI plus quinpirole groups were first outlined and then carefully calculated. The lesion volume was attained by multiplying the sum of the ipsilateral hemisphere area by the distance between the sections [24].

2.9. Nissl Staining

To analyze the neuronal cell death and lesion after brain injury, the Nissl staining was performed as described previously [24]. In brief, the slides were washed twice with 0.01 M PBS for 15 min followed by treatment with cresyl violet solution for another 1–15 min. The slides were washed with distilled water and dehydrated with ethanol (70%, 95%, and 100%). The tissue slides were cleared in xylene solution for 3 min and the mounting medium was added to the slides and coverslip was applied. A simple light microscope was used to examine the slides and taken images.

2.10. Cell Culture and Treatment

The Mouse hippocampal cell line HT22 and Microglial cell line BV2 were grown and maintained in Dulbecco's modified Eagle medium (DMEM) medium (Thermo Fisher Scientific, Waltham, MA, USA) supplemented with 10% fetal bovine serum (Gibco, Grand Island, NY, USA). The final formulation comprises an additional 1% penicillin/streptomycin sulfate (Gibco, Grand Island, NY, USA). Cells were cultured in a humidified cell culture incubator equipped with a 5% carbon dioxide supply. Cell media was regularly replaced after every 2 days passaged. The cells were subjected to experimental procedures after confirmation of above 80% confluency.

Cell viability assay of mouse hippocampal neuronal HT22 cells was evaluated as described previously [29]. In brief, to know the effect of quinpirole the cells were cultured in 96 well plates (density of 1×10^4 cells) containing Dulbecco's modified Eagle's medium (DMEM) 100 µL. After 24 h, the attached cells were subjected to microglial conditioned media (MCM). The cells were co-treated with three different concentrations of quinpirole (10 µM, 20 µM, and 40 µM) while the control cells were cultured only in DMEM (0.01%).

2.11. Microglial Conditioned Media

Mouse microglial cell line BV-2 was cultured to above 80% confluency were treated with Lipopolysaccharide (1 µg/mL) (Sigma-Aldrich, St. Louis, MO, USA) dissolved in Cell culturing media. After 24 h, media was aspirated and centrifuged to remove cells and debris. The clear supernatant was collected for further biochemical analysis.

2.12. Statistical Analysis

The western blot band's results were scanned and analyzed by densitometry using sigma gel software (SPSS Inc., Chicago, IL, USA). ImageJ software (National Institutes of Health, Bethesda, MD, USA) was used for immunohistological analysis, and the obtained values were calculated as the mean ± S.E.M. The data analysis was performed by using one-way ANOVA followed by a post-hoc analysis of variance for control, TBI, and treated groups comparison. The data calculation and graphs were determined by using Prism 5 software (Graph Pad Software, Inc., San Diego, CA, USA). The statistical significance values were considered as $p < 0.05$. Note: * significantly different between control and brain injury, # significantly different between brain injury and quinpirole treated group.

3. Results

3.1. Quinpirole Regulated the D2R Expression Level in the Injured Brain and HT22 Cells

Many studies have reported that D2R agonist increases glial and neuronal cell D2R levels and suppresses the release of various inflammatory cytokines [30,31]. Studies have shown that quinpirole (a D2R agonist) activated D2R and suppressed neuroinflammation following brain injury in a mouse model of intracerebral hemorrhage (ICH) with Parkinson's disease [19]. Based on this evidence, we performed Western blot and confocal microscopy analysis to investigate the effects of quinpirole on D2R expression levels especially in the ipsilateral cortex and striatum of brain-injured mice. Our results showed decreased D2R expression levels in the TBI experimental mice group. Notably, quinpirole treatment (1 mg/kg) significantly increased D2R expression in the quinpirole-treated group compared with the non-quinpirole-treated group of TBI mice (Figure 1a).

Deregulation of GSK3β is a critical step in the development and progression of neurodegenerative diseases via activation of neuroinflammatory processes [32]. Accumulating evidence suggests that the regulation of Akt and GSK3-β attenuates neurodegeneration and neuroinflamation [33]. Research has shown that D2R activation regulates the Akt and GSK3β protein levels [22]. Therefore, we performed Western blot analysis to determine the post-TBI expression levels of p-Akt and p-GSK3β and interleukin (IL)-1β. Our results showed increased expression levels of p-GSK3-β at (Ser 9) and IL-1β and decreased expression levels of p-Akt at (Ser 473) in the ipsilateral cortex of injured mouse brains. However, quinpirole treatment significantly regulated Akt/GSK3-β phosphorylation and reduced the IL-1β expression level in ipsilateral cortex of a damaged mouse brain (Figure 1a).

Furthermore, we investigated the protective role of quinpirole in vivo by in vitro studies. We subjected the HT22 cell line to Microglial conditioned media (MCM) treatment, and the cells were collected 24 h after MCM treatment. The HT22 cells were co-treated with three different concentrations of quinpirole (10 µM, 20 µM and 40 µM). Western blot analysis revealed that MCM-induced inflammatory mediators are associated with neuronal D2R deterioration. We observed that the administration of 10 µM or 20 µM reduced the toxic effect of MCM and significantly regulated D2R, which might be associated with the regulatory activity of p-Akt (Figure 1b).

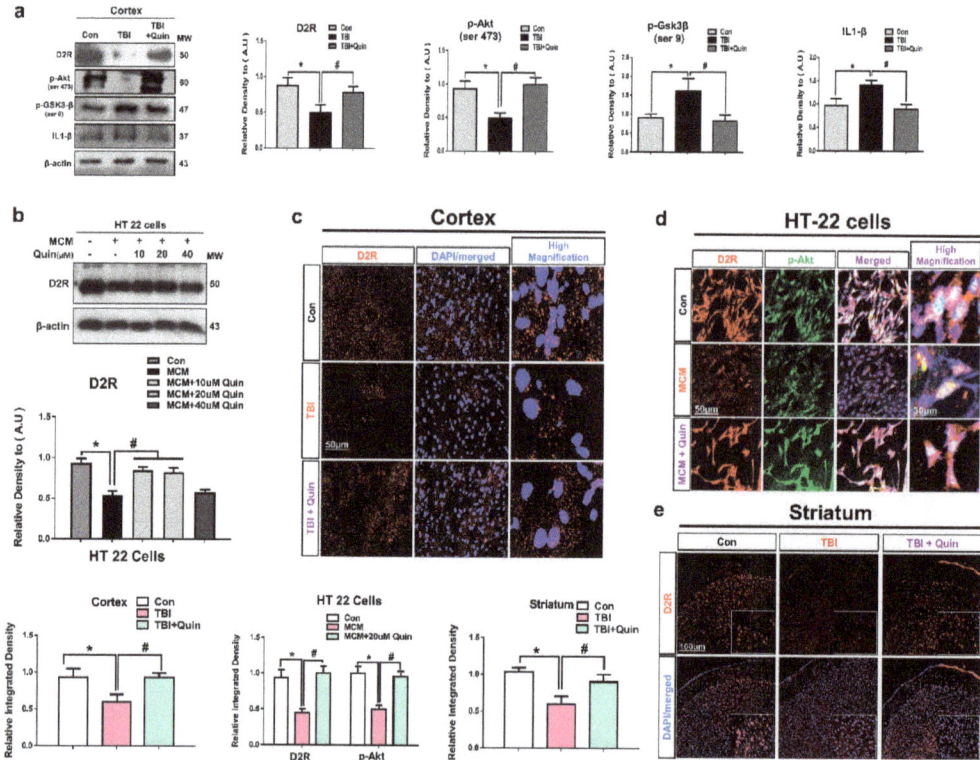

Figure 1. Quinpirole regulates the D2R/Akt/GSK3-β signaling pathway after brain injury. (**a**) Representative Western blot and histogram analysis of D2R, p-Akt, p-GSK3-β, and IL1-β in the ipsilateral cortex of an injured mouse brain. (**b**) Representing the Western blot analysis of D2R in HT22 cells. The β-actin was used as a loading control ($n = 5$). Western blot bands were quantified using the SigmaGel software. (**c**) Image showing results of immunofluorescence testing for D2R expression in the ipsilateral cortex of the control, brain injury, and quinpirole-treated mice groups. (**d**) D2R expression level and p-Akt co-localization in HT22 cells. (**e**) Image showing results of immunofluorescence testing for D2R expression in the ipsilateral striatum of the control, brain injury, and quinpirole-treated mice groups, with respective bar graphs (magnification ×10, $n = 6$). Data were obtained following three independent experiments. The ImageJ software was used for quantitative analysis of the confocal microscopy images and the maximum fluorescent intensity in the representative field was taken(green, FITC; red, TRITC; blue, DAPI). Values are represented as mean ± SEM. We performed the one-way ANOVA test followed by post-hoc analysis. A p value < 0.05 was considered statistically significant. * significantly different between control and brain injury groups, # significantly different between the brain injury and quinpirole-treated groups. ANOVA: analysis of variance, D2R: dopamine D2 receptors, GSK3-β: glycogen synthase kinase 3 beta, IL: interleukin, SEM: standard error of mean.

These results were validated by confocal microscopy. Our results also showed that the immunoreactivity of D2R was lower in the TBI group than in the control group. In contrast, quinpirole treatment improved D2R expression levels in the ipsilateral cortex and striatum after TBI (Figure 1c,e). Co-localization analysis of Akt and D2R revealed that their expression was significantly lesser in the MCM-treated HT22 cells. In contrast, quinpirole at a dose of 20 μM activated D2R and significantly increased Akt expression in HT22 cells (Figure 1d). Next, The p-Akt expression level was analyzed with iba-1, the double Immunofluorescence test result indicated the significantly reduced expression level of p-Akt and significantly increased expression of Iba-1 in the ipsilateral cortex of TBI mouse brain. However, post-TBI quinpirole treatment reversed this effect and significantly regulated the expression level of these markers in the ipsilateral cortex as compared to the TBI group of mice on day 7 (Figure 2a). We also evaluated Akt and IL1-β expression levels, particularly in the ipsilateral cortex, and confocal microscopy analysis revealed that post-TBI quinpirole treatment significantly regulated the expression level of these markers (Figure 2b,c). Moreover, co-localization analysis of p-GSK3β (Ser 9) and IL-1β showed increased expression levels in the ipsilateral striatum of TBI mice and also confirmed that post-TBI quinpirole treatment significantly reduced p-GSK3β and IL-1β expression levels (Figure 2d). Overall, these results confirm that post-TBI quinpirole administration may protects against neurodegenerative conditions via regulation of the D2R/Akt/GSK3β and IL-1β signaling pathways.

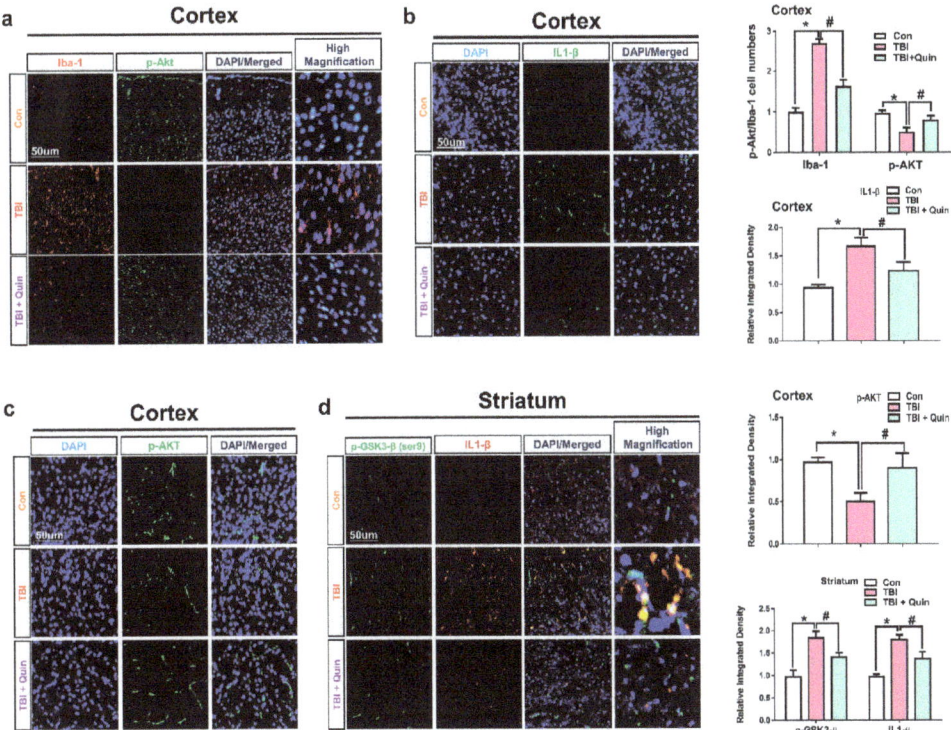

Figure 2. Quinpirole treatment reduces neuroinflammation via activation of the iba-1/p-Akt/p-GSK3-β and IL1-β signaling pathways after brain injury. (**a**) Double IF images of iba-1 and p-Akt in the ipsilateral cortex of brain-injured and quinpirole-treated mice. (**b**,**c**) Images showing results of immunofluorescence testing p-Akt (ser9) and IL1-β in the ipsilateral cortex after brain injury. (**d**) Images showing double immunofluorescence of p-GSK3-β (ser9) (FITC-label, green) and IL1-β (TRITC-label, red) (DAPI-label, blue) in the ipsilateral striatum with respective bar graphs, (magnification ×10, $n = 6$). Data were obtained after following three independent experiments. The ImageJ software was used for quantitative analysis of the confocal microscopy images and the maximum fluorescent intensity in the representative field was taken. Values are expressed as mean ± SEM. We performed the one-way ANOVA test followed by post-hoc analysis. A p value < 0.05 was considered statistically significant. * significantly different between control and brain injury groups, # significantly different between the brain injury and quinpirole-treated groups. ANOVA: analysis of variance, FITC: fluorescein isothiocyanate, GSK3-β: glycogen synthase kinase 3 beta, IL: interleukin, SEM: standard error of mean, TRITC: tetramethylrhodamine-isothiocyanate.

3.2. Quinpirole Reduced Gloisis and Atttenates D2R/Akt Level after Brain Injury

Gliosis plays an important role in the release of pro-inflammatory cytokines, such as IL-1β and tumor necrosis factor (TNF)-α and is a prominent feature of neurodegenerative conditions. Studies have reported that brain injury results in astrocyte and microglial activation, which precipitates further deleterious effects through the release of neuroinflammatory mediators [34–36]. Reportedly, D2R agonists are shown to significantly reduce the activation of astrocytes and the release of TNF-α in the spinal cord of a mouse model of amyotrophic lateral sclerosis and also prevent motor neuron loss (or death). Previously, studies reported the suppression of microglia following D2R activation [37]. While another study was also well suggested that Akt and GSK3β plays an essential role in glial response [38]. Based on these reports, we investigated whether quinpirole treatment could inhibit neuroinflammatory responses in our mouse model of TBI. Therefore, we evaluate glial fibrillary acidic protein (GFAP); a marker of active astrocytes, ionized calcium-binding adaptor molecule 1 (Iba-1); a marker of active microglia together with D2R and p-AKT expression level in ipsilateral or striatum after brain injury. Our double Immunofluorescence test results showed significantly increased immunoreactivity of GFAP and the expression level of D2R and p-AKT was significantly decreased in the ipsilateral cortex of TBI group as compared to saline treated group of mice. However, post-TBI quinpirole treatment reversed this effect, and significantly regulated the expression level of these markers on day 7 (Figure 3a,b). Moreover, we also checked the expression level of iba-1 in the ipsilateral striatum of TBI group of mice. Confocal microscopy result for iba-1 showed the significantly increased expression level of iba-1 in the TBI group of mice. However, the expression level of iba-1 was significantly decreased in quinpirole-treated TBI mice on day 7 (Figure 3c). Interestingly, the results of the Western blot analysis also showed increased Iba-1 and GFAP expression levels, indicating that the number of activated microglia and astrocytes was higher in TBI mice than in mice treated with saline (Figure 3d). Moreover, glial cell activation was significantly lower in the quinpirole-treated group than in the TBI group. Our results show that quinpirole treatment potentially ameliorates TBI-induced glial cell activation on day 7. This condensation of glial cells may be associated with astrocyte and microglial D2R and p-Akt modulation following quinpirole treatment.

3.3. Quinpirole Reduced Neuronal Apoptosis after Brain Injury

Many studies performed in a TBI mouse model have reported neuronal apoptosis after brain injury, particularly in the perilesional areas and striatum [39,40]. Using Western blot analysis, we investigated apoptotic markers, including Bax, Bcl-2, and PARP1 in the ipsilateral cortex (Figure 4a). We observed that compared with saline-treated mice, brain-injured mice showed a marked increase in neuronal apoptosis. Interestingly, we found significantly lower levels of p-JNK and apoptotic markers in the ipsilateral cortex in the quinpirole-treated group than in the non-quinpirole-treated group. These results were further validated by confocal microscopy. Immunofluorescence test results revealed increased expression of caspase-3 ipsilateral cortex and striatum in brain-injured mice.

Additionally, compared with the TBI group, the quinpirole-treated group showed a significant reduction in the high expression of caspase-3 in the ipsilateral cortex and striatum (Figure 4b,c). We performed Nissl staining to further assess neuronal cell death; compared with the control group, the brain-injured mice group showed a reduced number of surviving neurons in the ipsilateral cortex. Notably, quinpirole treatment reversed this effect and significantly increased the number of surviving neurons in the ipsilateral cortex of quinpirole-treated TBI mice (Figure 4d). These results suggest that the impact of brain injury extend to the ipsilateral cortex and striatum, and quinpirole treatment is known to inhibit neuronal apoptosis possibly via D2R activation in ipsilateral side of injured mouse brain.

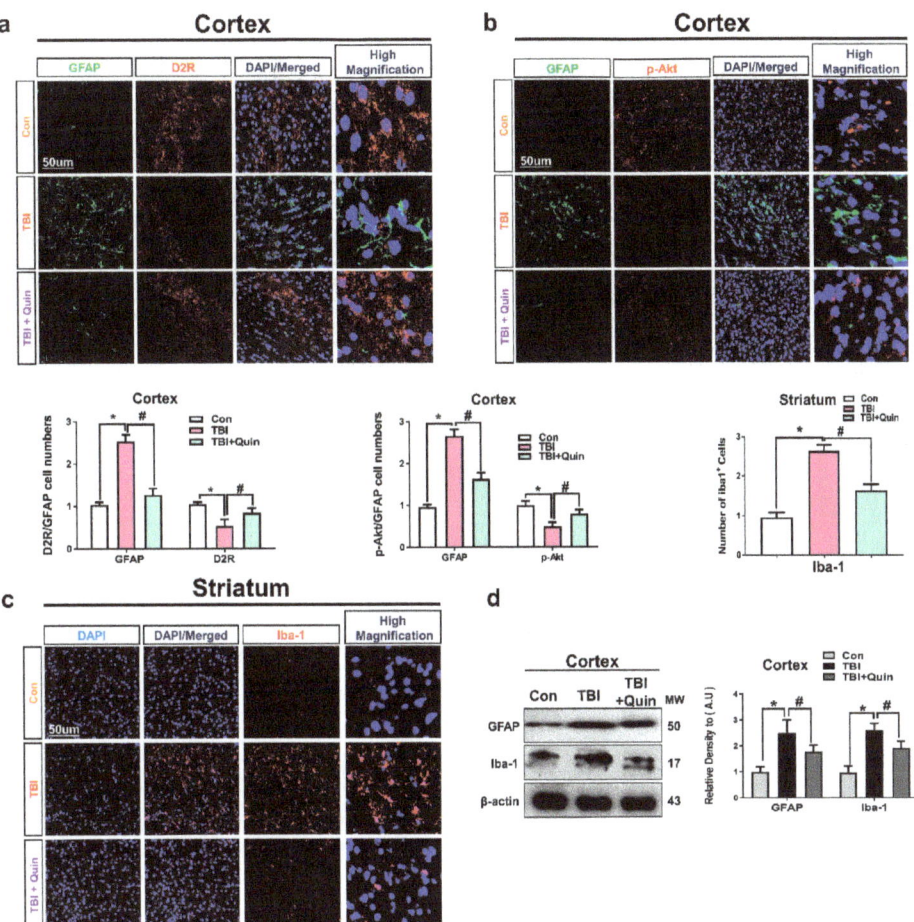

Figure 3. Quinpirole reduces astrocyte and microglia activation after brain injury. (**a**) Representative confocal microscopy images showing double immunoreactivity of GFAP and D2R expression level in ipsilateral cortex of TBI mouse model. (**b**) Images of double immunoreactivity of GFAP and p-Akt expression level in ipsilateral cortex of TBI mouse model (green, FITC; red, TRITC; blue, DAPI). (**c**) Confocal images of Iba-1 in ipsilateral striatum of brain-injured and quinpirole-treated mice, with respective bar graphs, (magnification ×10, $n = 6$). (**d**) Images of Western blot and histogram analysis showing GFAP and Iba-1 expression levels in ipsilateral cortex of brain-injured and quinpirole-treated mice. The β-actin was used as a loading control ($n = 5$). The ImageJ software was used for immunohistological analysis and the number of GFAP and iba-1 cells were quantified that containing D2R and p-Akt in the representative field. Data were obtained following three independent experiments. The ImageJ software was used for quantitative analysis of the confocal microscopy images. Values are expressed as mean ± SEM. We performed the one-way ANOVA test followed by post-hoc analysis. A p value < 0.05 was considered statistically significant. * significantly different between the control and brain injury groups, # significantly different between the brain injury and quinpirole-treated groups. ANOVA: analysis of variance, GFAP: glial fibrillary acidic protein, Iba-1: ionized calcium binding adaptor molecule 1, SEM: standard error of mean.

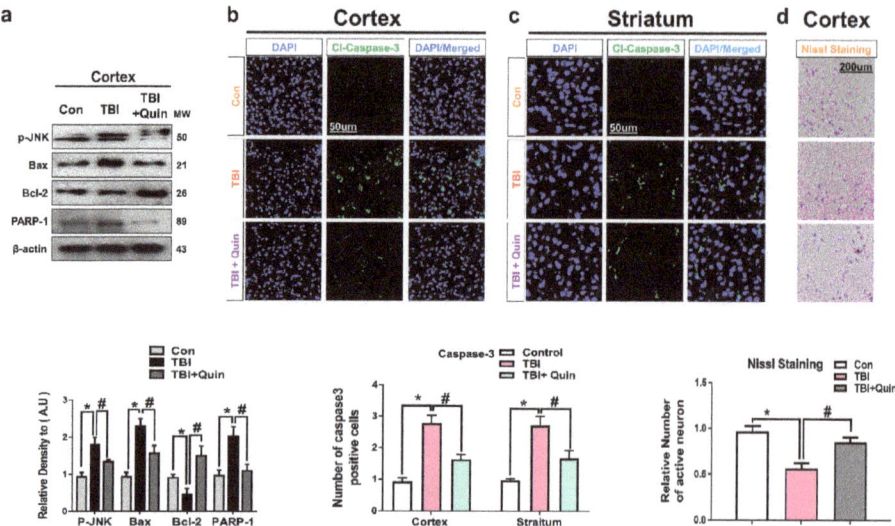

Figure 4. Quinpirole inhibits brain injury-induced neuronal apoptosis in mice brain. (**a**) Representative images showing results of immunoblot and histogram analysis of p-JNK, Bax, Bcl-2, and PARP-1 proteins in the ipsilateral cortex of injured mouse brain. The β-actin was used as a loading control ($n = 5$). (**b,c**) Immunofluorescence test images showing cl-caspase-3 immunoreactivity in the ipsilateral cortex and striatum of injured mouse brain, (green, FITC; blue, DAPI) with respective bar graphs, (magnification ×10, $n = 6$). (**d**) Nissl stain images of the ipsilateral cortex. ImageJ software was used for immunohistological analysis. Data were obtained following three independent experiments. The ImageJ software was used for quantitative analysis of the nissl images and confocal microscopy images. The integrative density of the number of caspase3 positive cells were quantified in the representative field. Values are expressed as mean ± SEM. We performed the one-way ANOVA test followed by post-hoc analysis. A p value < 0.05 was considered statistically significant. * significantly different between the control and brain injury groups, # significantly different between the brain injury and quinpirole-treated groups. ANOVA: analysis of variance, SEM: standard error of mean.

3.4. Quinpirole-Induced Restoration of Blood–Brain Barrier Disruption and Lesion Volume after Brain Injury

Previous research has shown that TBI results in severe BBB disruption, which invariably leads to severe complications in the affected areas [41]. Activation of astrocytic signaling causes BBB injury through the release of cytokines or chemokines and immune cell recruitment. Therefore, we evaluated the BBB breakdown and the possible role of quinpirole in the restoration of the disrupted BBB in our TBI mouse model. On confocal microscopy, co-localization of zonula occludens-1 (ZO-1) and a cluster of differentiation 31 (CD31) proteins showed that compared with the saline-treated control mice, the brain-injured mice showed significantly decreased ZO-1 expression levels in endothelial cells, and compared with brain-injured mice, the quinpirole-treated mice showed elevation of the reduced ZO-1 protein levels and a significant increase in its expression on post-TBI day 7 (Figure 5a). It is well known that brain injury immediately causes gross tissue disruption at the site of injury. Therefore, we also assessed the lesion volume on post-TBI day 7. Histopathological examination of specimens obtained from brain-injured mice showed a marked increase in the contusion and lesion volume in this group, which was significantly reduced following quinpirole treatment (Figure 5b).

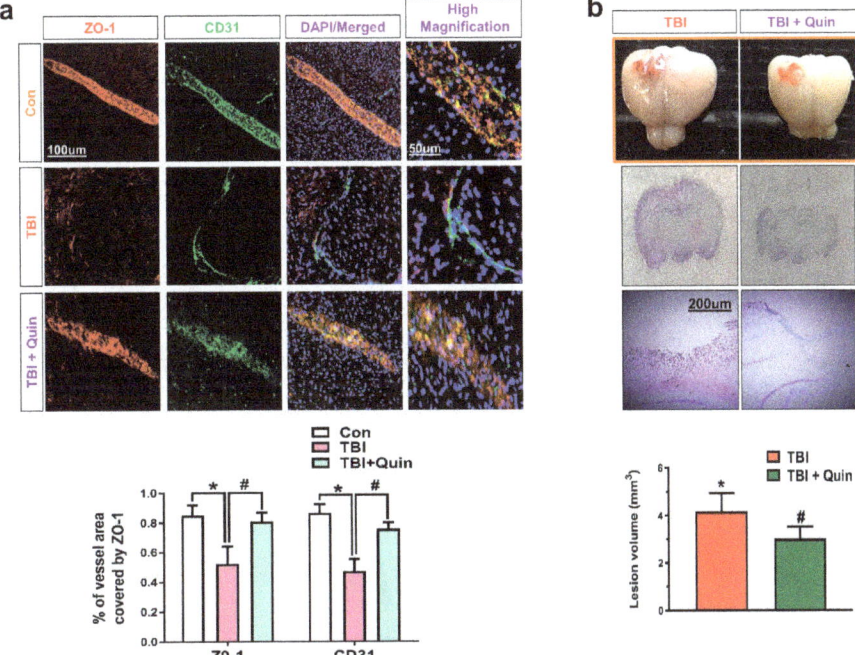

Figure 5. Quinpirole regulates the BBB-associated ZO-1 and CD31 expression levels and lesion volume after brain injury. (**a**) Representative confocal microscopy images for ZO-1 (TRITC-label, red) and CD31 (FITC-label, green) immunofluorescence reactivity in the ipsilateral cortex in injured mouse brain (green, FITC; red, TRITC; blue, DAPI). (**b**) Representative images showing TBI mouse brain after surgery, and Nissl-stained images showing the lesion volume in the brain injury and quinpirole-treated groups, with respective bar graphs, (magnification ×10, $n = 6$). Data were obtained following three independent experiments. The ImageJ software was used for quantitative analysis of the confocal microscopy images and the percentage of vessels were quantified that containing ZO-1 in the representative field. Values are expressed as mean ± SEM. We performed the one-way ANOVA test followed by post-hoc analysis. A p value < 0.05 was considered statistically significant. * significantly different between the control and brain injury groups, # significantly different between the brain injury and quinpirole-treated groups. ANOVA: analysis of variance, BBB: blood–brain barrier, CD31: cluster of differentiation 31, FITC: fluorescein isothiocyanate, SEM: standard error of mean, TRITC: tetramethylrhodamine-isothiocyanate, ZO-1: zonula occludens-1.

3.5. Quinpirole Attenuated Synaptic Dysfunction after Brain Injury

Previous studies have reported that brain injury causes synaptic protein loss, which leads to memory impairment [35,42]. Therefore, we evaluated the expression levels of synaptic proteins, including synaptosomal-associated protein 23 (SNAP-23) and post-synaptic density protein 95 (PSD-95) in our TBI mouse model. We performed confocal microscopy for PSD-95 and SNAP-23 in ipsilateral cortex and striatum respectively. We observed that brain injury significantly decreases synaptic protein expression, whereas quinpirole treatment significantly increased synaptic protein loss in an injured mouse brain (Figure 6a,b). Western blot analysis revealed that compared with saline-treated mice, brain-injured mice showed reduced PSD-95 and SNAP-23 expression in the ipsilateral cortex (Figure 6c). However, quinpirole treatment significantly restored synaptic proteins following brain injury.

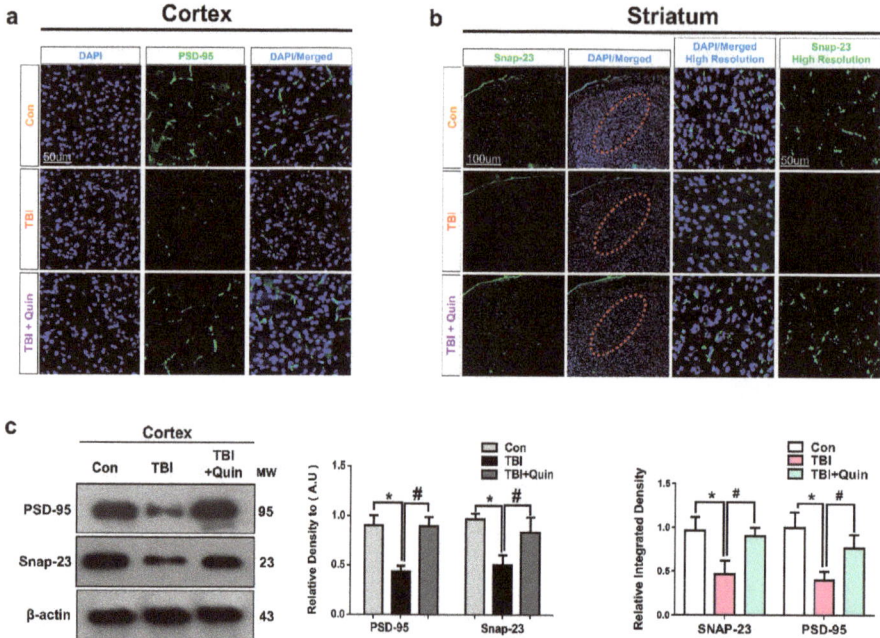

Figure 6. Quinpirole regulates synaptic protein loss after brain injury. (**a,b**) Confocal microscopy images for PSD-95 and SNAP-23 expression in the ipsilateral cortex and striatum of an injured mouse brain (green, FITC; blue, DAPI), with respective bar graphs, the red dotted lines showing the striatum region, (magnification ×10, $n = 6$). The protein band levels were quantified using the SigmaGel software. (**c**) Images showing results of Western blot and histogram analysis for PSD-95 and sanp-23 in ipsilateral cortex of injured mouse brain. The β-actin was used as a loading control ($n = 5$). Data were obtained following three independent experiments. The ImageJ software was used for quantitative analysis of the confocal microscopy images. Values are expressed as mean ± SEM. We performed the one-way ANOVA test followed by post-hoc analysis. A p value < 0.05 was considered statistically significant. * significantly different between the control and brain injury groups, # significantly different between the brain injury and quinpirole-treated groups. ANOVA: analysis of variance, PSD-95: post-synaptic density protein 95, SEM: standard error of mean, SNAP-23: synaptosomal-associated protein 23, TBI: traumatic brain injury.

4. Discussion

An optimal therapeutic approach to brain injuries is unavailable owing to the multifactorial pathogenesis of brain trauma. Brain injuries lead to cognitive dysfunction that can be prevented by DA therapies targeted at the restoration of cognitive impairment [43,44]. The most important neurotransmitters in the central nervous system: glutamate is released from multiple stores after a TBI and the activation of D2Rs could contribute in the modulation of the glutamate release both from neurons than from astrocytes. Hence, activation of D2Rs may play essential role after TBI-induce disturbance in neurotransmitters. In this study, we observed that quinpirole (a D2R agonist) plays a significant role in brain injury-induced neuroinflammation, neurodegeneration, and synaptic dysfunction. We focused on the neuroprotective effect of quinpirole following brain injury in mice. This report shows that post-TBI quinpirole administration attenuates several neuropathological events, such as glial cell activation, neuroinflammation, neuronal apoptosis, and synaptic dysfunction via the D2R/Akt GSK3β/IL-1β signaling pathways. Since the TBI-induced striatal glial activation and expression of pro-inflammatory cytokines and therapeutic potential of D2R activation in the ipsilateral striatum is mostly known previously as compared to the ipsilateral cortex; thus, still it is essential to investigate the therapeutic potential of D2R in the cortex of TBI mouse brain [45]. Therefore, we investigated the neuroprotective effect of D2R activation mainly in the ipsilateral cortex, while we checked slightly the ipsilateral striatum of the injured mouse brain. Our results suggest that quinpirole activates D2R, which plays a crucial role in several neuropathological events particularly in ipsilateral cortex after brain injury.

Brain injury leads to neuroinflammation, which contributes to severe neurodegeneration. Studies have reported chronic neuroinflammatory responses in the cortex and hippocampus of an injured mouse brain [46,47]. In our TBI mouse model, we observed increased neuroinflammation indicated by microglial and astrocyte activation in the ipsilateral cortex and striatum. Interestingly, post-TBI quinpirole treatment significantly reduced the increased gliosis and release of pro-inflammatory markers. Our results are consistent with those reported by previous studies [12]. It is known that the regulation of p-GSK3-β via p-Akt is involved in the cell survival pathway [48]. A previous study showed that injury-induced disruption of Akt and GSK3β expression in glial cells is a major contributor to the mechanistic of glial cell adaptation as well as protection in response to cell damage. Thus Akt and GSK3β play an essential role in glial response and excitotoxic lesion outcome of injury [38]. Another study investigated the role of Akt/GSK3β pathway in acute brain injury after subarachnoid hemorrhage [49,50]. The regulation of GSK3-β and Akt via D2R could be a novel therapeutic approach following brain injury. In the present study, we investigated the protective effect of quinpirole mediated via the D2R/GSK3β/Akt signaling pathway. We found decreased expression of D2R/Akt and increased expression of p-GSK3-β and IL-1β after TBI, based on Western blot and immunofluorescence analysis. However, these levels normalized to the baseline levels in quinpirole-treated mice. A previous study also reported the anti-neuroinflammatory effect of quinpirole via D2R activation in an ICH injury model [19]. The BBB plays a central role in brain homeostasis. However, BBB disruption leads to enhanced cytokine infiltration and neuronal susceptibility.

Several tight junction proteins, including claudin, occludin, and ZO-1, are essential for the maintenance of BBB integrity [51]. BBB breakdown following brain injury is attributable to significant histopathological alterations and tissue loss in the affected areas [52]. Double immunofluorescence staining performed for ZO-1 and CD31 showed significantly low levels of these proteins in the ipsilateral cortex of an injured mouse brain. Notably, quinpirole treatment restored ZO-1 and CD31 levels in the ipsilateral cortex of an injured mouse brain. Quinpirole-regulated restoration of the disrupted BBB is attributable to reduced neuroinflammation and active gliosis. A previous study has reported that brain injury is strongly associated with deregulated tight junction proteins [53]. Brain injury is known to cause marked tissue disruption [34]. We observed increased lesion volume in an injured mouse brain, and that quinpirole treatment significantly reduced the lesion volume, which suggests that quinpirole aids in the repair of the brain after injury and restores tight junction proteins to inhibit infiltration of cytokines and other blood-borne biochemical agents. Moreover, we observed a significant increase in the contusion volume after brain injury, indicating that severe damage is associated with tissue disruption in the ipsilateral cortex of injured mouse brain. Notably, all these effects were ameliorated in brain-injured mice that received quinpirole treatment.

Increasing evidence has shown neuronal apoptosis after brain injury [54]. Our results showed increased expression of neuronal apoptotic markers, including Bax and PARP1, and decreased expression of Bcl-2, an anti-apoptotic protein. Quinpirole treatment significantly reduced the increased levels of pro-apoptotic and increase the reduced level of anti-apoptotic markers in the ipsilateral cortex of brain-injured mice. A previous study supports the protective role of D2/D3 receptor agonist ropinirole protects against apoptosis-induced neurodegeneration via a JNK-dependent pathway [11]. Our results are consistent with those of a previous study in which D2R agonists were shown to reduce neuronal apoptosis [55]. In accordance with the caspase3 result, the nissl staining results also showed the significantly increase number of apoptotic and degenerated neurons in the ipsilateral side of TBI mouse brain as compared to saline- treated control group of mice. However, the number of damage and degenerated neuronal cells were significantly reduced in quinpirole-treated group of mice after TBI on day 7.

Synaptic protein loss is associated with brain injury and leads to cognitive deficits and impaired neurotransmission. A study has reported that DR activation protects against amyloid-β oligomer-mediated synaptic dysfunction. Therefore, we evaluated synaptic protein markers after brain injury. The results of Western blot and immunofluorescence testing showed that quinpirole treatment reversed the deregulated levels of synaptic protein markers, including PSD-95 and SNAP-23 in TBI mice. Moreover, other studies have also reported that D2R is vital for several brain functions, including learning and working memory. We concluded that quinpirole could be a potentially useful therapeutic agent to restore synaptic function after brain injury and to improve the cognitive performance of brain-injured mice.

These results suggest that brain injury may cause D2R suppression, which consequently activates deleterious signaling pathways at a later stage after brain injury, and that quinpirole-mediated D2R activation produces a neuroprotective effect in the ipsilateral cortex and striatum of injured brains.

5. Conclusions

This study highlights the significant role of D2R in neurodegenerative conditions affecting the ipsilateral cortex after brain injury and that D2R regulation might be an effective therapeutic strategy to inhibit glial cell-induced neuroinflammation in a mouse model of brain injury (Figure 7). In this study, we discuss the role of quinpirole (a D2R agonist), that can potentially attenuate several neuropathological processes via D2R/Akt/GSK3-β/IL-1β signaling in the ipsilateral cortex and striatum of an injured mouse brain. Further studies are warranted to gain a deeper understanding of the molecular mechanisms contributing to the neuroprotective effects of quinpirole via D2R activation in neuropathological events associated with brain injury.

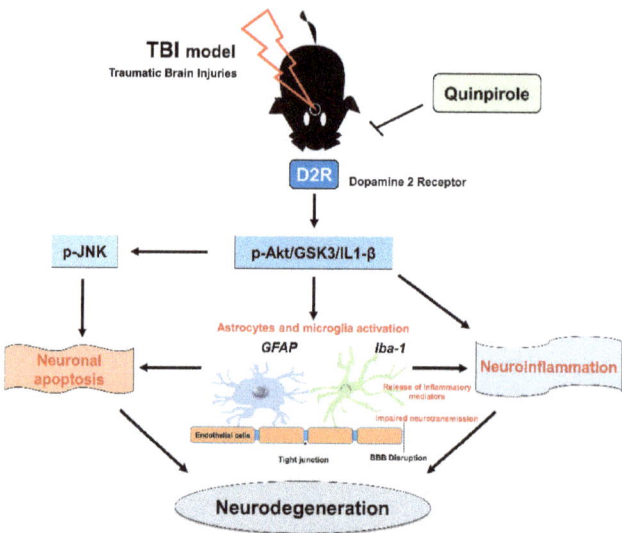

Figure 7. Schematic representation of the proposed mechanism of neuroprotection of quinpirole against brain injury-induced neuroinflammation, BBB disruption and neurodegeneration via D2R and Akt/GSK3-β/IL-1β signaling in the injured mouse brains.

Author Contributions: S.I.A. designed the study, performed the experimental work, and wrote the manuscript. M.G.J. reviewed the manunsript and edited the figures. R.U. and T.J.P. review and edited the manuscript. S.U.R. help in writing the manuscript. S.A. conducted experiment. M.O.K. is a corresponding author, reviewed and approved the manuscript, and holds all the responsibilities related to this manuscript. All authors have read and agreed to the published version of the manuscript.

Funding: This research was supported by the Neurological Disorder Research Program of the National Research Foundation (NRF) funded by the Korean Government (MSIT) (2020M3E5D9080660).

Institutional Review Board Statement: This study was carried out in animals in accordance with approved guidelines (Approval ID: 125) by the animal ethics committee (IACUC) of the Division of Applied Life Science, Gyeongsang National University, South Korea.

Informed Consent Statement: Not applicable.

Data Availability Statement: The authors hereby declares that the data presented in this study will be presented upon request from the corresponding author.

Acknowledgments: Not applicable.

Conflicts of Interest: The authors declare no conflict of interest.

References

1. Delic, V.; Beck, K.D.; Pang, K.C.H.; Citron, B.A. Biological links between traumatic brain injury and Parkinson's disease. *Acta Neuropathol. Commun.* **2020**, *8*, 45. [CrossRef] [PubMed]
2. Graham, N.S.; Sharp, D.J. Understanding neurodegeneration after traumatic brain injury: From mechanisms to clinical trials in dementia. *J. Neurol. Neurosurg. Psychiatry* **2019**, *90*, 1221–1233. [CrossRef] [PubMed]
3. McKee, A.C.; Daneshvar, D.H. The neuropathology of traumatic brain injury. *Handb. Clin. Neurol.* **2015**, *127*, 45–66. [CrossRef] [PubMed]
4. Wallenquist, U.; Holmqvist, K.; Hanell, A.; Marklund, N.; Hillered, L.; Forsberg-Nilsson, K. Ibuprofen attenuates the inflammatory response and allows formation of migratory neuroblasts from grafted stem cells after traumatic brain injury. *Restor. Neurol. Neurosci.* **2012**, *30*, 9–19. [CrossRef] [PubMed]
5. Campos-Pires, R.; Hirnet, T.; Valeo, F.; Ong, B.E.; Radyushkin, K.; Aldhoun, J.; Saville, J.; Edge, C.J.; Franks, N.P.; Thal, S.C.; et al. Xenon improves long-term cognitive function, reduces neuronal loss and chronic neuroinflammation, and improves survival after traumatic brain injury in mice. *Br. J. Anaesth.* **2019**, *123*, 60–73. [CrossRef] [PubMed]
6. Tajiri, N.; Hernandez, D.; Acosta, S.; Shinozuka, K.; Ishikawa, H.; Ehrhart, J.; Diamandis, T.; Gonzales-Portillo, C.; Borlongan, M.C.; Tan, J.; et al. Suppressed cytokine expression immediatey following traumatic brain injury in neonatal rats indicates an expeditious endogenous anti-inflammatory response. *Brain Res.* **2014**, *1559*, 65–71. [CrossRef] [PubMed]
7. Lloyd, E.; Somera-Molina, K.; Van Eldik, L.J.; Watterson, D.M.; Wainwright, M.S. Suppression of acute proinflammatory cytokine and chemokine upregulation by post-injury administration of a novel small molecule improves long-term neurologic outcome in a mouse model of traumatic brain injury. *J. Neuroinflamm.* **2008**, *5*, 28. [CrossRef]
8. Becker, A.; Grecksch, G.; Thiemann, W.; Hollt, V. Pentylenetetrazol-kindling modulates stimulated dopamine release in the nucleus accumbens of rats. *Pharmacol. Biochem. Behav.* **2000**, *66*, 425–428. [CrossRef]
9. Sellnow, R.C.; Newman, J.H.; Chambers, N.; West, A.R.; Steece-Collier, K.; Sandoval, I.M.; Benskey, M.J.; Bishop, C.; Manfredsson, F.P. Regulation of dopamine neurotransmission from serotonergic neurons by ectopic expression of the dopamine D2 autoreceptor blocks levodopa-induced dyskinesia. *Acta Neuropathol. Commun.* **2019**, *7*, 8. [CrossRef]
10. Bibb, J.A. Decoding dopamine signaling. *Cell* **2005**, *122*, 153–155. [CrossRef]
11. Chen, S.; Zhang, X.; Yang, D.; Du, Y.; Li, L.; Li, X.; Ming, M.; Le, W. D2/D3 receptor agonist ropinirole protects dopaminergic cell line against rotenone-induced apoptosis through inhibition of caspase-and JNK-dependent pathways. *FEBS Lett.* **2008**, *582*, 603–610. [CrossRef] [PubMed]
12. Shao, W.; Zhang, S.Z.; Tang, M.; Zhang, X.H.; Zhou, Z.; Yin, Y.Q.; Zhou, Q.B.; Huang, Y.Y.; Liu, Y.J.; Wawrousek, E.; et al. Suppression of neuroinflammation by astrocytic dopamine D2 receptors via alphaB-crystallin. *Nature* **2013**, *494*, 90–94. [CrossRef] [PubMed]
13. Takahashi, H.; Kato, M.; Takano, H.; Arakawa, R.; Okumura, M.; Otsuka, T.; Kodaka, F.; Hayashi, M.; Okubo, Y.; Ito, H. Differential contributions of prefrontal and hippocampal dopamine D1 and D2 receptors in human cognitive functions. *J. Neurosci.* **2008**, *28*, 12032–12038. [CrossRef] [PubMed]
14. Sarkar, C.; Basu, B.; Chakroborty, D.; Dasgupta, P.S.; Basu, S. The immunoregulatory role of dopamine: An update. *Brain Behav. Immun.* **2010**, *24*, 525–528. [CrossRef] [PubMed]
15. Del Campo, N.; Chamberlain, S.R.; Sahakian, B.J.; Robbins, T.W. The roles of dopamine and noradrenaline in the pathophysiology and treatment of attention-deficit/hyperactivity disorder. *Biol. Psychiatry* **2011**, *69*, e145–e157. [CrossRef]

16. Russell, V.A.; Sagvolden, T.; Johansen, E.B. Animal models of attention-deficit hyperactivity disorder. *Behav. Brain Funct.* **2005**, *1*, 9. [CrossRef]
17. Khlghatyan, J.; Quintana, C.; Parent, M.; Beaulieu, J.M. High Sensitivity Mapping of Cortical Dopamine D2 Receptor Expressing Neurons. *Cereb. Cortex* **2018**, *29*, 3813–3827. [CrossRef]
18. Kuric, E.; Wieloch, T.; Ruscher, K. Dopamine receptor activation increases glial cell line-derived neurotrophic factor in experimental stroke. *Exp. Neurol.* **2013**, *247*, 202–208. [CrossRef]
19. Zhang, Y.; Chen, Y.; Wu, J.; Manaenko, A.; Yang, P.; Tang, J.; Fu, W.; Zhang, J.H. Activation of Dopamine D2 Receptor Suppresses Neuroinflammation Through alphaB-Crystalline by Inhibition of NF-kappaB Nuclear Translocation in Experimental ICH Mice Model. *Stroke* **2015**, *46*, 2637–2646. [CrossRef]
20. Huang, J.J.; Yen, C.T.; Liu, T.L.; Tsao, H.W.; Hsu, J.W.; Tsai, M.L. Effects of dopamine D2 agonist quinpirole on neuronal activity of anterior cingulate cortex and striatum in rats. *Psychopharmacology* **2013**, *227*, 459–466. [CrossRef]
21. Datta, S.R.; Dudek, H.; Tao, X.; Masters, S.; Fu, H.; Gotoh, Y.; Greenberg, M.E. Akt phosphorylation of BAD couples survival signals to the cell-intrinsic death machinery. *Cell* **1997**, *91*, 231–241. [CrossRef]
22. Beaulieu, J.M.; Tirotta, E.; Sotnikova, T.D.; Masri, B.; Salahpour, A.; Gainetdinov, R.R.; Borrelli, E.; Caron, M.G. Regulation of Akt signaling by D2 and D3 dopamine receptors in vivo. *J. Neurosci.* **2007**, *27*, 881–885. [CrossRef] [PubMed]
23. Koller, W.; Herbster, G.; Anderson, D.; Wack, R.; Gordon, J. Quinpirole hydrochloride, a potential anti-parkinsonism drug. *Neuropharmacology* **1987**, *26*, 1031–1036. [CrossRef]
24. Alam, S.I.; Rehman, S.U.; Kim, M.O. Nicotinamide Improves Functional Recovery via Regulation of the RAGE/JNK/NF-kappaB Signaling Pathway after Brain Injury. *J. Clin. Med.* **2019**, *8*, 271. [CrossRef]
25. Rehman, S.U.; Ali, T.; Alam, S.I.; Ullah, R.; Zeb, A.; Lee, K.W.; Rutten, B.P.F.; Kim, M.O. Ferulic Acid Rescues LPS-Induced Neurotoxicity via Modulation of the TLR4 Receptor in the Mouse Hippocampus. *Mol. Neurobiol.* **2019**, *56*, 2774–2790. [CrossRef]
26. Ahmad, R.; Khan, A.; Lee, H.J.; Ur Rehman, I.; Khan, I.; Alam, S.I.; Kim, M.O. Lupeol, a Plant-Derived Triterpenoid, Protects Mice Brains against Abeta-Induced Oxidative Stress and Neurodegeneration. *Biomedicines* **2020**, *8*, 380. [CrossRef]
27. Shah, S.A.; Yoon, G.H.; Chung, S.S.; Abid, M.N.; Kim, T.H.; Lee, H.Y.; Kim, M.O. Novel osmotin inhibits SREBP2 via the AdipoR1/AMPK/SIRT1 pathway to improve Alzheimer's disease neuropathological deficits. *Mol. Psychiatry* **2017**, *22*, 407–416. [CrossRef]
28. Khan, M.; Rutten, B.P.F.; Kim, M.O. MST1 Regulates Neuronal Cell Death via JNK/Casp3 Signaling Pathway in HFD Mouse Brain and HT22 Cells. *Int. J. Mol. Sci.* **2019**, *20*, 2504. [CrossRef]
29. Ullah, R.; Jo, M.H.; Riaz, M.; Alam, S.I.; Saeed, K.; Ali, W.; Rehman, I.U.; Ikram, M.; Kim, M.O. Glycine, the smallest amino acid, confers neuroprotection against D-galactose-induced neurodegeneration and memory impairment by regulating c-Jun N-terminal kinase in the mouse brain. *J. Neuroinflamm.* **2020**, *17*, 303. [CrossRef]
30. Han, X.; Li, B.; Ye, X.; Mulatibieke, T.; Wu, J.; Dai, J.; Wu, D.; Ni, J.; Zhang, R.; Xue, J.; et al. Dopamine D2 receptor signalling controls inflammation in acute pancreatitis via a PP2A-dependent Akt/NF-kappaB signalling pathway. *Br. J. Pharmacol.* **2017**, *174*, 4751–4770. [CrossRef]
31. Qiu, J.; Yan, Z.; Tao, K.; Li, Y.; Li, J.; Li, J.; Dong, Y.; Feng, D.; Chen, H. Sinomenine activates astrocytic dopamine D2 receptors and alleviates neuroinflammatory injury via the CRYAB/STAT3 pathway after ischemic stroke in mice. *J. Neuroinflamm.* **2016**, *13*, 263. [CrossRef] [PubMed]
32. Maixner, D.W.; Weng, H.-R. The role of glycogen synthase kinase 3 beta in neuroinflammation and pain. *J. Pharm. Pharmacol.* **2013**, *1*, 001.
33. Amin, F.U.; Shah, S.A.; Kim, M.O. Vanillic acid attenuates Abeta1-42-induced oxidative stress and cognitive impairment in mice. *Sci. Rep.* **2017**, *7*, 40753. [CrossRef] [PubMed]
34. Clement, T.; Lee, J.B.; Ichkova, A.; Rodriguez-Grande, B.; Fournier, M.L.; Aussudre, J.; Ogier, M.; Haddad, E.; Canini, F.; Koehl, M.; et al. Juvenile mild traumatic brain injury elicits distinct spatiotemporal astrocyte responses. *Glia* **2020**, *68*, 528–542. [CrossRef] [PubMed]
35. Villapol, S.; Balarezo, M.G.; Affram, K.; Saavedra, J.M.; Symes, A.J. Neurorestoration after traumatic brain injury through angiotensin II receptor blockage. *Brain* **2015**, *138*, 3299–3315. [CrossRef] [PubMed]
36. Younger, D.; Murugan, M.; Rama Rao, K.V.; Wu, L.J.; Chandra, N. Microglia Receptors in Animal Models of Traumatic Brain Injury. *Mol. Neurobiol.* **2019**, *56*, 5202–5228. [CrossRef] [PubMed]
37. Tanaka, K.; Kanno, T.; Yanagisawa, Y.; Yasutake, K.; Hadano, S.; Yoshii, F.; Ikeda, J.E. Bromocriptine methylate suppresses glial inflammation and moderates disease progression in a mouse model of amyotrophic lateral sclerosis. *Exp. Neurol.* **2011**, *232*, 41–52. [CrossRef] [PubMed]
38. Kim, D.W.; Lee, J.H.; Park, S.K.; Yang, W.M.; Jeon, G.S.; Lee, Y.H.; Chung, C.K.; Cho, S.S. Astrocytic expressions of phosphorylated Akt, GSK3beta and CREB following an excitotoxic lesion in the mouse hippocampus. *Neurochem. Res.* **2007**, *32*, 1460–1468. [CrossRef] [PubMed]
39. Gerbatin, R.D.R.; Cassol, G.; Dobrachinski, F.; Ferreira, A.P.O.; Quines, C.B.; Pace, I.D.D.; Busanello, G.L.; Gutierres, J.M.; Nogueira, C.W.; Oliveira, M.S.; et al. Guanosine Protects Against Traumatic Brain Injury-Induced Functional Impairments and Neuronal Loss by Modulating Excitotoxicity, Mitochondrial Dysfunction, and Inflammation. *Mol. Neurobiol.* **2017**, *54*, 7585–7596. [CrossRef]

40. Villapol, S.; Byrnes, K.R.; Symes, A.J. Temporal dynamics of cerebral blood flow, cortical damage, apoptosis, astrocyte-vasculature interaction and astrogliosis in the pericontusional region after traumatic brain injury. *Front. Neurol.* **2014**, *5*, 82. [CrossRef]
41. Gao, W.; Zhao, Z.; Yu, G.; Zhou, Z.; Zhou, Y.; Hu, T.; Jiang, R.; Zhang, J. VEGI attenuates the inflammatory injury and disruption of blood–brain barrier partly by suppressing the TLR4/NF-kappaB signaling pathway in experimental traumatic brain injury. *Brain Res.* **2015**, *1622*, 230–239. [CrossRef] [PubMed]
42. Neuwelt, E.; Abbott, N.J.; Abrey, L.; Banks, W.A.; Blakley, B.; Davis, T.; Engelhardt, B.; Grammas, P.; Nedergaard, M.; Nutt, J.; et al. Strategies to advance translational research into brain barriers. *Lancet Neurol.* **2008**, *7*, 84–96. [CrossRef]
43. Bales, J.W.; Yan, H.Q.; Ma, X.; Li, Y.; Samarasinghe, R.; Dixon, C.E. The dopamine and cAMP regulated phosphoprotein, 32 kDa (DARPP-32) signaling pathway: A novel therapeutic target in traumatic brain injury. *Exp. Neurol.* **2011**, *229*, 300–307. [CrossRef] [PubMed]
44. Shin, S.S.; Bray, E.R.; Dixon, C.E. Effects of nicotine administration on striatal dopamine signaling after traumatic brain injury in rats. *J. Neurotrauma* **2012**, *29*, 843–850. [CrossRef]
45. Huang, Y.N.; Yang, L.Y.; Greig, N.H.; Wang, Y.C.; Lai, C.C.; Wang, J.Y. Neuroprotective effects of pifithrin-alpha against traumatic brain injury in the striatum through suppression of neuroinflammation, oxidative stress, autophagy, and apoptosis. *Sci. Rep.* **2018**, *8*, 2368. [CrossRef]
46. Bachstetter, A.D.; Webster, S.J.; Goulding, D.S.; Morton, J.E.; Watterson, D.M.; Van Eldik, L.J. Attenuation of traumatic brain injury-induced cognitive impairment in mice by targeting increased cytokine levels with a small molecule experimental therapeutic. *J. Neuroinflamm.* **2015**, *12*, 69. [CrossRef]
47. Webster, S.J.; Van Eldik, L.J.; Watterson, D.M.; Bachstetter, A.D. Closed head injury in an age-related Alzheimer mouse model leads to an altered neuroinflammatory response and persistent cognitive impairment. *J. Neurosci.* **2015**, *35*, 6554–6569. [CrossRef]
48. Martin, M.; Rehani, K.; Jope, R.S.; Michalek, S.M. Toll-like receptor-mediated cytokine production is differentially regulated by glycogen synthase kinase 3. *Nat. Immunol.* **2005**, *6*, 777–784. [CrossRef]
49. Endo, H.; Nito, C.; Kamada, H.; Yu, F.; Chan, P.H. Akt/GSK3beta survival signaling is involved in acute brain injury after subarachnoid hemorrhage in rats. *Stroke* **2006**, *37*, 2140–2146. [CrossRef]
50. Shlosberg, D.; Benifla, M.; Kaufer, D.; Friedman, A. Blood–brain barrier breakdown as a therapeutic target in traumatic brain injury. *Nat. Rev. Neurol.* **2010**, *6*, 393. [CrossRef]
51. Rehman, S.U.; Ahmad, A.; Yoon, G.H.; Khan, M.; Abid, M.N.; Kim, M.O. Inhibition of c-Jun N-Terminal Kinase Protects Against Brain Damage and Improves Learning and Memory After Traumatic Brain Injury in Adult Mice. *Cereb. Cortex* **2018**, *28*, 2854–2872. [CrossRef] [PubMed]
52. De Beaumont, L.; Tremblay, S.; Poirier, J.; Lassonde, M.; Theoret, H. Altered bidirectional plasticity and reduced implicit motor learning in concussed athletes. *Cereb. Cortex* **2012**, *22*, 112–121. [CrossRef] [PubMed]
53. Lutton, E.M.; Razmpour, R.; Andrews, A.M.; Cannella, L.A.; Son, Y.-J.; Shuvaev, V.V.; Muzykantov, V.R.; Ramirez, S.H. Acute administration of catalase targeted to ICAM-1 attenuates neuropathology in experimental traumatic brain injury. *Sci. Rep.* **2017**, *7*, 3846. [CrossRef] [PubMed]
54. Liu, W.; Chen, Y.; Meng, J.; Wu, M.; Bi, F.; Chang, C.; Li, H.; Zhang, L. Ablation of caspase-1 protects against TBI-induced pyroptosis in vitro and in vivo. *J. Neuroinflamm.* **2018**, *15*, 48. [CrossRef] [PubMed]
55. OLANOW, C.W.; Sealfon, S.C. Activation of phosphoinositide 3-kinase by D2 receptor prevents apoptosis in dopaminergic cell lines. *Biochem. J.* **2003**, *373*, 25–32.

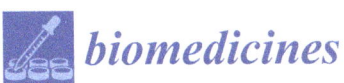

Review

Relevance of Autophagy and Mitophagy Dynamics and Markers in Neurodegenerative Diseases

Carlotta Giorgi [1], Esmaa Bouhamida [1], Alberto Danese [1], Maurizio Previati [2], Paolo Pinton [1] and Simone Patergnani [1,*]

[1] Laboratory for Technologies of Advanced Therapies, Department of Medical Sciences, University of Ferrara, 44121 Ferrara, Italy; carlotta.giorgi@unife.it (C.G.); esmaa.bouhamida@unife.it (E.B.); alberto.danese@unife.it (A.D.); paolo.pinton@unife.it (P.P.)

[2] Surgery and Experimental Medicine, Section of Human Anatomy and Histology, Laboratory for Technologies of Advanced Therapies (LTTA), Department of Morphology, University of Ferrara, 44121 Ferrara, Italy; maurizio.previati@unife.it

* Correspondence: simone.patergnani@unife.it

Abstract: During the past few decades, considerable efforts have been made to discover and validate new molecular mechanisms and biomarkers of neurodegenerative diseases. Recent discoveries have demonstrated how autophagy and its specialized form mitophagy are extensively associated with the development, maintenance, and progression of several neurodegenerative diseases. These mechanisms play a pivotal role in the homeostasis of neural cells and are responsible for the clearance of intracellular aggregates and misfolded proteins and the turnover of organelles, in particular, mitochondria. In this review, we summarize recent advances describing the importance of autophagy and mitophagy in neurodegenerative diseases, with particular attention given to multiple sclerosis, Parkinson's disease, and Alzheimer's disease. We also review how elements involved in autophagy and mitophagy may represent potential biomarkers for these common neurodegenerative diseases. Finally, we examine the possibility that the modulation of autophagic and mitophagic mechanisms may be an innovative strategy for overcoming neurodegenerative conditions. A deeper knowledge of autophagic and mitophagic mechanisms could facilitate diagnosis and prognostication as well as accelerate the development of therapeutic strategies for neurodegenerative diseases.

Keywords: autophagy; mitophagy; neurodegeneration; multiple sclerosis; Alzheimer's disease; Parkinson's disease; biomarker; therapy

Citation: Giorgi, C.; Bouhamida, E.; Danese, A.; Previati, M.; Pinton, P.; Patergnani, S. Relevance of Autophagy and Mitophagy Dynamics and Markers in Neurodegenerative Diseases. *Biomedicines* **2021**, *9*, 149. https://doi.org/10.3390/biomedicines9020149

Academic Editor: Arnab Ghosh
Received: 30 December 2020
Accepted: 1 February 2021
Published: 4 February 2021

Publisher's Note: MDPI stays neutral with regard to jurisdictional claims in published maps and institutional affiliations.

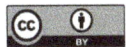

Copyright: © 2021 by the authors. Licensee MDPI, Basel, Switzerland. This article is an open access article distributed under the terms and conditions of the Creative Commons Attribution (CC BY) license (https://creativecommons.org/licenses/by/4.0/).

1. Introduction

Neurodegenerative disorders refer to a large group of pathological conditions in which components of the nervous system lose their structure and function. These diseases are primarily classified according to the clinical features (dementia, tremor, rigidity, and bradykinesia) but especially according to the anatomic distribution of the neurodegenerative lesions [1]. The aggregation of misfolded brain proteins represents the main cause of neuronal damage in hereditary and sporadic neurodegenerative disorders (Figure 1) [2]. Alzheimer's disease (AD) is a late-onset form of dementia and is considered the most frequent type of neurodegeneration worldwide: nearly 50 million people live with AD and related dementia. AD is characterized by a progressive loss of neurons determined by the aberrant accumulation of tau protein and beta-amyloid protein (Aβ protein) [3]. Human brains express six isoforms of tau, whose cellular function is to stabilize the interactions of microtubules with other proteins. To exert this function, tau protein must be phosphorylated. However, in AD, tau is hyperphosphorylated, a condition that induces conformational changes and the aggregation of the tau protein [3]. The second most common neurodegenerative disease is Parkinson's disease (PD). Persons affected by this disease present some common symptoms (such as anxiety, depression, rigidity, and tremor) that worsen over time [4]. PD belongs to a class of neurodegenerative diseases named "synucleinopathies", since the protein aggregations typical of the disease, Lewy bodies (LBs), are formed by different types of proteins, and α-synuclein (α-syn) is the major constituent. Several studies have demonstrated that the aggregation and oligomerization of α-syn are determined by alternative splicing events and by post-translation modifications, such as ubiquitination, oxidative nitration, truncation, and phosphorylation [5]. Furthermore, genetic studies on the familial form of PD have unveiled that specific mutations in the encoding gene, SNCA, accelerate the production of insoluble aggregates and oligomers [4]. Neuronal damage, neuronal loss, and a reduction in brain volume are also important factors inducing long-term disability in patients affected by multiple sclerosis (MS), a complex and multifactorial disorder leading to severe physical or cognitive disabilities and neurological defects [6]. Unlike other types of neurodegenerative disorders, MS is not due to the excessive accumulation of misfolded proteins but is the result of a state of persistent inflammation and adverse immune-mediated processes that activates a cascade of molecular events that provoke demyelination in the white as well as gray matter and subsequent axonal and neuronal damage [7]. Despite the existence of fundamental differences among these neurodegenerative conditions, a growing body of evidence demonstrates that they share important pathogenic mechanisms, of which mitochondrial (dys)function, inflammation, infection, and immune responses are the most frequent [8–10]. In addition, in recent years, the autophagy process has also been found to be particularly associated with neurodegeneration [11]. Autophagy is a cellular catabolic pathway in which cytosolic components, bacteria, viruses, macromolecules, and whole organelles are transported to lysosomes for degradation. To exert these multiple functions, specialized forms of autophagy also exist, the most studied being mitophagy (the selective removal of damaged mitochondria) [12]. Autophagy itself and its specialized forms play important roles in physiological as well as pathological conditions. Under normal conditions, autophagy removes unnecessary material, regulates the physiological turnover of organelles, and meets energetic demand. In pathological conditions, autophagy may have both favorable and deleterious roles. As demonstrated, a loss/gain of function in the autophagic process and increase/decrease in the expression of crucial autophagic mediators have been associated with diverse human disorders, particularly cancer [13,14] and neurodegeneration [15]. Most importantly, different studies have not only confirmed the importance of autophagic dynamics during neurodegeneration but also suggested that several proteins involved in this catabolic process may be considered potential markers for predicting neurodegenerative conditions [16,17]. Analysis of the distribution of autophagy partners and regulators along the different pathologic steps of neurodegenerative disorders may improve the knowledge of the contribution of autophagic processes to neurodegenerative conditions. In addition, we may develop innovative neuroprotective therapies and unveil new potential biomarkers for the early diagnosis and clinical management of these diseases. In this review, we discuss the roles of autophagy and its specialized form mitophagy in different neurological disorders. We explore the possibility of using molecular partners of autophagy and mitophagy as biomarkers for neurodegenerative disease status. Finally, the pharmacological modulation of these processes is discussed as a potential strategy for building new therapeutic approaches against neurodegeneration.

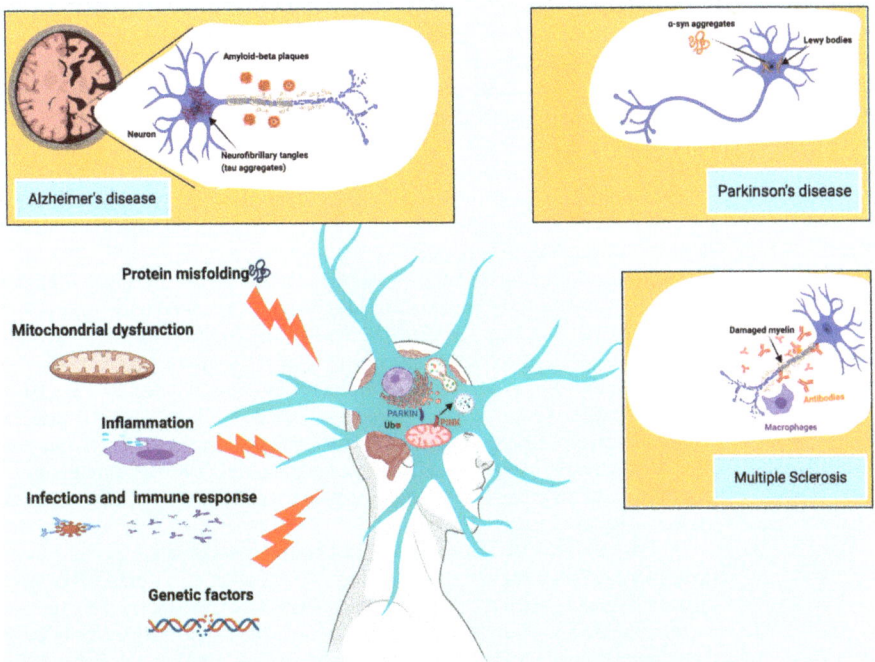

Figure 1. Causes and risk factors of Alzheimer's disease (AD), Parkinson's disease (PD), and multiple sclerosis (MS). AD and PD are the most common neurodegenerative diseases, characterized by an abnormal aggregation of protein inclusions in the brain. While in AD, the progressive loss of neurons is caused by an aberrant accumulation of beta-amyloid and tau protein, PD displays inclusions named Lewy bodies, where α-synuclein (α-syn) is the major constituent. MS is the most frequent cause of disability among young adults after traumatic brain injury. The neurodegenerative condition of MS is not due to an excessive accumulation of misfolded protein but to adverse immune-mediated processes and chronic inflammation that provoke demyelinating and neurodegenerative processes during the entire life of the patient. Among the different molecular mechanisms and risk factors involved in these neurodegenerative conditions, it has been demonstrated that autophagy and mitophagy play an important role.

2. A General Overview of Autophagy

The word autophagy was introduced in late 1963 by the biochemist Christian de Duve [18] and defines a self-degradative cellular pathway whose intent is to degrade and recycle cellular contents. Autophagy exists in three forms that are classified according to their mechanisms and cellular functions: macroautophagy, microautophagy, and chaperone-mediated autophagy (CMA). During microautophagy, the cytosolic material is wrapped and transported directly into the lumen of lysosomes. The main function of microautophagy (mA) is to control cell survival and organellar turnover upon nitrogen restriction. Unfortunately, due to the lack of specific methods for measuring mA (apart from electron microscopy), the effective contributions of mA in mammalian cells remain little studied, and most studies about mA molecular processes are carried out in yeast [19]. Despite this, different investigations suggest that the molecular dynamics of mA existing in yeast may be conserved in mammalian mA. Consistently with this, it has been demonstrated that the endosomal sorting complex required for transport (ESCRT) system is involved in mammalian [20] and yeast mA [21]. Furthermore, a prolonged starvation condition [22,23] as well as cellular treatments with the macrolide compound rapamycin activates mA in both mammalian and yeast cells [21,24,25].

CMA has an important role in protein quality control (QC) and is responsible for degrading a specific subset of oxidized and damaged proteins. The selectivity of CMA is conferred by the existence of a specific pentapeptide motif (KFERQ), which is present in the amino acid sequences of all CMA substrates. This motif is identified by the cytosolic chaperone heat shock-cognate protein of 70 kDa (hSC70), which brings the protein target directly to the lysosome surface [26]. In the last decade, several advances have been made in understanding the molecular mechanisms of CMA. These findings suggest an important contribution of CMA to diverse human diseases, including neurodegeneration [26]. Undoubtedly, the best-characterized and most prevalent form of autophagy in mammalian cells is macroautophagy (hereafter referred to as autophagy), whose multistep process and contribution to the pathophysiology of diverse neurodegenerative conditions will be discussed throughout this review.

Autophagy, a complex intracellular process that is very ancient and has been strongly conserved during evolution, exists to identify and capture a wide group of intracellular components, ranging from low-dimensional biological macromolecules to whole organelles, and bring them to the lysosomal compartment. Its physiological value rests on two main activities. On the one hand, autophagy acts as a QC mechanism that reshapes the cell, ensuring the removal of damaged proteins and organelles [27]. Selective forms of autophagy can specifically target mitochondria (mitophagy), the endoplasmic reticulum (ER; reticulophagy), peroxisomes (pexophagy), and lipid droplets (lipophagy). In addition, autophagy participates in the struggle against invading pathogens (xenophagy), inducing cell defense [12].

On the other hand, lysosomal degradation represents an important source of amino acids and lipids for the de novo synthesis of proteins and lipids. This is of particular importance during starvation, which limits amino acid availability. The limited availability of amino acids affects protein synthesis, which can be performed only in the presence of all the necessary building blocks, in particular, essential amino acids. Under shortage conditions, amino acid pool completeness can be fulfilled only through the degradation of cellular proteins. In such a way, autophagy represents a fundamental survival mechanism, particularly during stress conditions originating from hypoxia or pathogen invasion [27].

Thus, it is not surprising that energy availability can regulate or trigger autophagy and, in particular, that a large number of stimuli converge on metabolic energy sensors, such as mammalian target of rapamycin (mTOR) and 5' adenosine monophosphate-activated protein kinase (AMPK), which, in turn, regulate autophagy [28].

In cells, mTOR exists in two complexes, mTORC1 and mTORC2, which not only are composed of different protein-binding partners but also regulate different pathways. The primary role of mTORC2 is to regulate cell survival and cytoskeletal organization, while its role in autophagy remains poorly understood. Recent work has shed light on this obscure point. Indeed, the transforming growth factor beta (TGFB)/INHB/activin signaling pathway has been recently identified as an upstream regulator of mTORC2. TGFB-INHB/activin mediates mTORC2 inhibition and regulates the autophagic flux and the cardiac functions in a *Drosophila* cardiac-specific knockdown of TGFB-INHB/activin model [29]. Another investigation recently confirmed the importance of mTORC2 for autophagy. In this case, it has been demonstrated that mTORC2 exists on a molecular axis with the serum- and glucocorticoid-inducible kinase 1 (SGK-1) and, in this state, controls autophagy and mitophagy induction. Consistently, mTORC2- or SGK-1 deficient *C. elegans* models present a perturbed mitochondrial homeostasis and aberrant ROS production, which trigger autophagy and mitophagy. Excessive autophagic and mitophagic fluxes, in turn, result in developmental and reproductive deficits in mTORC2- or SGK-1-deficient animals [30]. Oppositely, the primary role of mTORC1 is to play a pivotal role in cellular catabolic pathways, particularly autophagy [31]. To exert its function, mTORC1 integrates different stimuli, including hormonal stimulation, nutrient availability, and the oxygen level. In the presence of normal levels of energy and amino acids, mTOR inhibits autophagy through specific unc-51-like autophagy-activating kinase 1 (ULK1) serine phosphorylation at the phosphorylation site Ser 757. By contrast, in response to nutritional deprivation, oxygen unavailability, and mitochondrial dysfunction, AMPK activates autophagy through the phosphorylation of ULK1 at Ser 317 and Ser 777 [32]. Interestingly, another research group demonstrated that AMPK may phosphorylate ULK in additional sites. Indeed, by employing a bioinformatic approach, it has been found that ULK1 contains a further four potential AMPK sites [33]. Three of them (Ser 555, Ser 637, and Thr 574) were also identified by mass spectrometry in cells pretreated with an AMPK activator, while the site Ser 467 was confirmed by immunoblotting with phosphospecific antibodies [33]. Unfortunately, this work lacks an analysis of the effect of the different phosphorylations on autophagy. By using SILAC (stable isotope labeling with amino acids) technology, other work mapped 13 new phosphorylation sites of ULK1 [34]. All of them were dependent on nutrient availability, but only Ser 638 and Ser 758 displayed the most significant changes. In addition, time course experiments investigating the response to nutrient availability demonstrated that these phosphorylations were differentially regulated and that mTOR mediated both phosphorylations. Intriguingly, the authors also demonstrated that the phosphorylation at Ser 638 was also mediated by AMPK [34]. Altogether, these findings demonstrate that ULK1 is the key regulator of autophagy, and the occurrence of different protein phosphorylation events is crucial for regulating its activity. Furthermore, the concurrent existence of at least two opposite regulatory pathways that converge on ULK1 signaling (mediated by MTOR and AMPK) allows the cell to better adapt to extracellular and intracellular variations but also affects several pathological conditions.

In the cells, ULK1 forms a complex with autophagy-related (ATG) 13/200-kDa focal adhesion kinase family-interacting protein (FIP200) and ATG101. As reported above, ULK1 activity is mainly regulated by phosphorylation/desphosphorylation events mediated by AMPK and mTOR. In addition, it has been demonstrated that ULK1 is able to phosphorylate itself at Thr 180 [35] and FIP200, ATG13, and ATG101 [36,37] and that the phosphorylation events are regulated by protein phosphatase. Protein phosphatase 2A (PP2A) and protein phosphatase 1D magnesium-dependent delta isoform (PPM1D) regulate the ULK1 phosphorylation [38,39]. PP2C phosphatases (Ptc2 and Ptc3) mediate the dephosphorylation of ATG13 30655342. The ULK1/ATG13/FIP200/ATG101 molecular axis represents the most upstream regulatory complex related to double-membrane vacuole (autophagosome) formation [28]. Autophagosomes symbolize the starting moment of the whole autophagic process, which begins with the formation of double-membrane lined vesicles that fuse together to engulf portions of the cytoplasm. The resulting double-membrane vacuoles are autophagosomes, which can fuse with vesicles of the endocytic pathway at different stages of maturation or directly with lysosomes, becoming autolysosomes. In autolysosomes, acidic hydrolases break down macromolecules into smaller constituents that are released back to the cytosol by lysosomal transporters and permeases. Once activated, the ULK1/ATG13/FIP200/ATG101 molecular axis also phosphorylates and activates coiled-coil, moesin-like BCL2 interacting protein (BECN1) [40,41]. BECN1 can be part of a complex including class III phosphatidylinositol 3-kinase (PI3K) and its regulatory proteins vacuolar protein sorting 34 (Vsp34), p150, and ATG14L. Upon activation, this complex is involved in the nucleation and elongation of autophagosomes. The first step occurs on the surface of the membranes of the ER, mitochondria, Golgi complex, endosomes, or plasma membrane [42] and consists of the phosphorylation of phosphatidylinositol to form phosphatidylinositol-3-phosphate (PI3P). This phosphoinositide behaves as a positive regulator of autophagy. In fact, the presence of PI3P at the source membrane triggers the docking of several adaptor proteins, which, in turn, induce and sustain the elongation of the sack-like, omega-shaped structure, which grows, binds, and surrounds the material intended to be digested.

Another interaction of BECN1 can exert an inhibitory effect on autophagy [43]. BECN1 has been reported to bind B-cell lymphoma (BCL)-2, BCL-XL, and other members of the BCL-2 family through the BCL-2-homology-3 (BH3) domain. The consequence of this interaction is a diminution of the interaction between BECN1 and the class III PI3K complex, which prevents the formation of phagophores [43]. Accordingly, BCL-2 phosphorylation can reverse BECN1 sequestration and restore autophagy stimulation [43].

The other two systems, ATG12–ATG5–ATG16L1 and microtubule-associated protein 1A/1B-light chain 3 (LC3)–phosphatidylethanolamine (PE) complexes, seem to play an important role in the elongation and closure of autophagosomes, although the underlying mechanism has not yet been clarified. A key process during autophagosome elongation and closure is the lipidation of the LC3 protein, which is joined to the membrane PE. Once inserted into the autophagosomal membrane, the lipidated complex can further recruit other adaptor proteins. This allows autophagosomes to recognize cargo material, and elongate and close the vesicle. The fusion of the autophagosomes with the lysosome is the subsequent step, which, in a normally operating lysosome, is followed by lysosomal compartment acidification, the degradation of macromolecules by hydrolases and lipases, and the recycling of the base constituents (Figure 2).

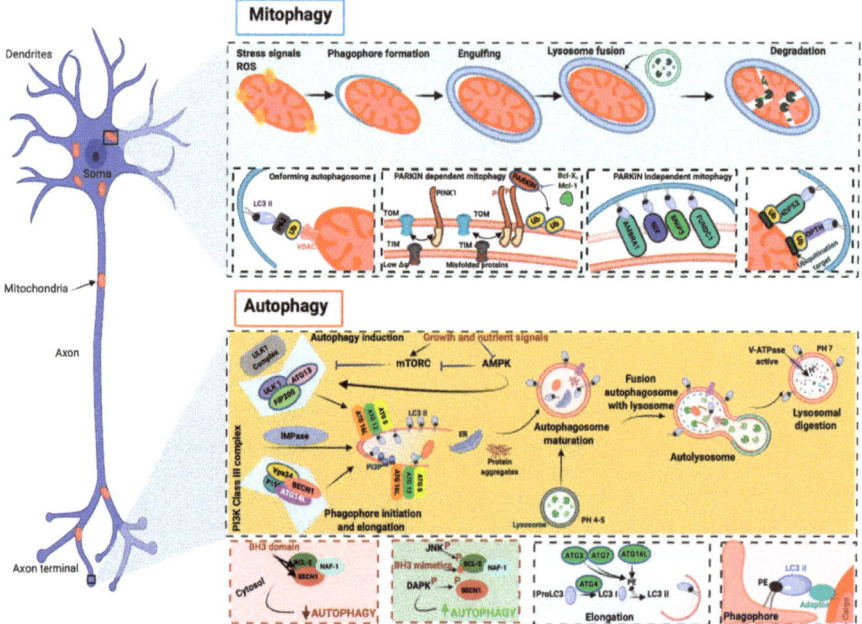

Figure 2. Molecular mechanisms of autophagy and mitophagy. The mammalian target of rapamycin (mTOR) and the 5′ adenosine monophosphate-activated protein kinase (AMPK) are the main negative and positive regulators of autophagy, respectively. One of the primary targets of the action of mTOR and AMPK is the unc-51-like autophagy-activating kinase 1 (ULK1)/autophagy-related (ATG) 13/FIP200 (200-kDa focal adhesion kinase family-interacting protein) complex, which is the main regulator of autophagosomal formation. Other important proteins that participate in this molecular process are the coiled-coil, moesin-like BCL-2 interacting protein (BECN1), class III phosphatidylinositol 3-kinase (PI3K), vacuolar protein sorting 34 (Vsp34), ATG14L, p150, and IMPase. The activity of BECN1 in regulating the autophagy process is also mediated by the interaction with BCL-2. During the elongation of the autophagosome, a series of autophagy-related (ATG) proteins are involved. In particular, two specific complexes were found to be essential for completing autophagosomal formation: (ATG)12–ATG5–ATG16L1 and microtubule-associated protein 1A/1B-light chain 3 (LC3)–phosphatidylethanolamine (PE) complexes. Mitochondria are particularly vulnerable to stress signals, such as ROS, which, in turn, can cause severe mitochondrial dysfunction and activate the mitophagic process. PINK1 senses this mitochondrial damage and phosphorylates and recruits Parkin to the outer mitochondrial membrane of the mitochondria. Phosphorylation converts Parkin to an active ubiquitin (Ub)-dependent enzyme and mediates the phosphorylation of different mitochondrial proteins. During this process intervene different Ub-binding autophagy receptors such as p6, NBR1, NDP52, and optineurin (OPTN), which connect the damaged mitochondria to the forming autophagosomes. Mitophagy may also be executed in a Parkin-independent manner. In this case, different proteins (FUNDC1, AMBRA1, NIX, and BNIP3) intervene to signal the mitochondria that should be degraded.

3. Mitophagy: The Master Regulator of the Mitochondrial Population

Mitochondria are essential intracellular organelles that supply substrates and energy to execute numerous cell functions, such as metabolism, differentiation, apoptosis, cell movement, and differentiation. In contrast to other intracellular components, mitochondria are constituted by two membranes, the outer mitochondrial membrane (OMM) and the inner mitochondrial membrane (IMM), which fully surround the mitochondrial matrix. Between the OMM and IMM, another mitochondrial subcompartment exists, the intermembrane space (IMS) [44]. Another unique feature of mitochondria is that they have their own genome (mitochondrial DNA, mtDNA), which encodes 13 proteins that are essential components of the oxidative phosphorylation (OXPHOS) system, the process by which ATP is formed [45]. A series of members (complexes I-V, C-I-V) of the mitochondrial electron chain (mETC) found in the IMM permit the transfer of electrons from NADH or $FADH_2$ to O_2 [46]. The energy produced during this movement creates a proton gradient that is used by the last component of the mETC (C-V, ATP synthase) to synthesize ATP [46]. The impairment of electron transfer or stress conditions affect the production of reactive oxygen species (ROS), of which C-I and C-III are the main producers [47]. Mitochondria are also central hubs for calcium (Ca^{2+}) signaling [48]. At rest, mitochondria have low Ca^{2+} concentrations [Ca^{2+}] (~100 nM range or lower). However, upon stimulation, mitochondrial [Ca^{2+}] can increase to the range of hundreds in micromolar concentration [49]. This happens due to the highly specialized contact sites (mitochondria-associated membranes, MAMs) that exist between mitochondria and the main intracellular Ca^{2+} store of cells, the ER [50]. These interaction sites represent critical hubs for the regulation of diverse cellular processes (such as energy metabolism, inflammation, redox regulation, and lipid and protein transfer), and recently, MAMs have been described to play an important role in the onset and progression of several human diseases by regulating Ca^{2+} transmission between the ER and mitochondria [51]. Once released from the ER, Ca^{2+} can enter mitochondria owing to the close proximity of the ER to mitochondria, the electrochemical driving force (mitochondrial membrane potential) that is created by electron transfer, and the activity of the components of the mitochondrial Ca^{2+} uniporter (MCU) [52,53]. Mitochondria are normally present in cells in the form of a dynamic network, where the mitochondrial mass increases as a consequence of mitochondrial biogenesis. The control and reshaping of the mitochondrial population can occur through different mechanisms [54]. These mechanisms include (i) the control of protein quality through mitochondrial proteases, the mitochondrial unfolded protein response, or proteasome-dependent degradation; (ii) the budding of mitochondrion-derived vesicles; and (iii) the targeting of some or all mitochondria to lysosomes through mitophagy.

Mitophagy regulation is not yet a completely understood process. During short-term starvation, the mitochondrial pool is not depleted, so as to not further reduce the cellular production of energy, while oxidative metabolism is mainly sustained by general autophagy [28]. This fact necessarily implies a difference in regulation between autophagy and mitophagy that allows the cautious sparing of mitochondria, which are among the principal end-users of the material provided by autophagy. A role in this sense seems to be played by fission restriction. In fact, fragmented mitochondria appear to be a preferred target for mitophagy: when their number is reduced, mitophagy itself is restricted.

When the ultimate goal is to eliminate mitochondria, there are different physiological mechanisms that can be activated. The first example is programmed mitophagy. There are several situations in the cell that can require the activation of programmed mitophagy, independent of the wellness of mitochondria. An example is the mitochondrial depletion that occurs in reticulocytes during differentiation through the activity of NIP3-like protein X (NIX/BNIP3L). Other examples include the elimination of male-derived mitochondria after egg fertilization [55] and the reshaping of the mitochondrial population during cardiomyocyte [56] or muscle cell differentiation, which induces a change from carbohydrate- to fatty acid-driven OXPHOS [57]. Stimulations that can normally trigger mitophagy can be affected by mitochondrial defects, such as a decline in transmembrane potential and excessive ROS production.

Mitophagy involves some fundamental steps. First, as stated above, mitochondria must assume the dimensions necessary to easily enter autophagosome vesicles. Therefore, they are normally resized through fission processes. In addition, they need to be properly displayed on the surface to trigger the formation of vesicles, which will engulf them. Typically, "eat-me signals" can be ubiquitin-dependent or not. The best-known example of a ubiquitin-dependent mechanism is the PTEN-induced kinase 1 (PINK1)/Parkin axis. PINK1 and Parkin belong to a series of genes referred to as PARK genes, which include α-syn (PARK1/4), Parkin (PARK2), PINK1 (PARK6), protein deglycase-1 (DJ-1, PARK7), leucine-rich repeat kinase 2 (LRRK2, PARK8), and ATP13A2 (PARK9). The name of this group of genes (Parkin genes) comes from the finding that mutations in these genes have been linked to familiar forms of PD. In particular, approximately 100 mutations in the Parkin gene have been identified as causing autosomal recessive Parkinsonism [58].

PINK1 is a mitochondrial serine/threonine-protein kinase, and Parkin is an E3 ubiquitin ligase; these proteins induce different functions at the cellular level but act in a common pathway to regulate mitophagy.

PINK1 is a ubiquitous protein characterized by a mitochondrial targeting sequence (MTS), a transmembrane domain, and a highly conserved serine/threonine kinase domain. At present, approximately 30 pathogenic PINK1 mutations that impair its kinase activity and provoke loss of function have been identified [59–62].

Normally, PINK1 is imported into mitochondria via the activity of the translocase of the inner membrane (TIM)–translocase of the outer membrane (TOM) complex. Once PINK1 arrives in the IMM, it is subjected to a series of proteolytic cleavages that reduce the full-length form of PINK1 into fragments, which are then degraded by the proteasome [63–65]. In the presence of alterations in mitochondrial membrane potential, the activity of the TIM/TOM complex is reduced, and PINK1 begins to accumulate on the OMM. Here, after being stabilized by a molecular complex including TOM proteins [66,67], PINK1 phosphorylates Parkin. The phosphorylation converts Parkin from an autoinhibited enzyme to an active ubiquitin (Ub)-dependent enzyme [68,69]. In this state, Parkin actively ubiquitinates several mitochondrial proteins at the OMM. The ubiquitination events promote the recruitment of the Ub-binding autophagy receptors p62/Sequestome, NBR1, NDP52, optineurin (OPTN), and TAX1BP1 (TBK1), which connect damaged mitochondria to phagosomes for clearance in lysosomes [70–72]. In recent years, different studies have identified pathways regulating mitophagy that are PINK1–Parkin-independent. These mechanisms may act in parallel or in addition to PINK1–Parkin-dependent mitophagy and involve a series of OMM mitophagy receptors that bind LC3 and recruit mitochondria to autophagic vesicles. Among them, the most studied are the proapoptotic members of the BCL2 family, NIX and BNIP3 [73,74] and FUNDC1 [75], which regulate the mitophagy process during ischemic/hypoxic conditions, and the BECN1 regulator AMBRA1. Interestingly, it has been proven that AMBRA1 regulates both Parkin-dependent and Parkin-independent mitophagy [76] (Figure 2).

4. Relationship between Autophagy and Mitophagy in MS

Multiple sclerosis (MS) is a progressive and chronic disease that affects approximately 3 million persons worldwide. MS is an inflammatory condition in which activated immune cells enter the central nervous system (CNS) and cause progressive demyelination, gliosis, and neuronal loss. The symptoms vary from individual to individual [77]. The most common symptoms are walking difficulties, sensory disturbances, vision problems, and cognitive and emotional impairments. Typically, MS starts with an unexpected onset of neurological impairments, and the majority of individuals display a relapsing–remitting (RR) course of the disease in which recurrent periods alternate with relapse phases. This course may be followed by a secondary progressive phase in which inflammatory attacks are more frequent and cause irreversible neurological impairments. A small percentage of individuals may present with the primary progressive form of the disease, which is characterized by the absence of remission periods and a progressive worsening of symptoms [78]. Currently, the pathogenesis and etiology of MS are unclear. MS is considered a multifactorial disease, and genetic predisposition and environmental factors may play important roles in disease progression. Furthermore, mitochondrial dysfunction as well as the impairment of the QC systems of mitochondria have been identified in different MS samples and represent evidence that the mitochondrial compartment has a major role in MS [9]. In addition, recent investigations have described an important contribution of autophagic processes. The first evidence that autophagy could be involved in MS was reported in 2009, when a strong correlation was found between the expression of the autophagic marker ATG5 and the clinical disability observed in the experimental autoimmune encephalomyelitis (EAE) MS animal model. Moreover, in this work, the authors found increased expression of ATG5 in T cells obtained from RR-MS patients and in postmortem brain tissue from individuals with secondary progressive MS [79]. Unfortunately, the authors did not address the role of autophagy in T cells and MS. They only speculated that autophagy may help to increase the survival of T cells and help to propagate the immune response. Similarly, other work detected ATG5 increases in terms of both mRNA levels and protein amounts in T cells obtained from MS patients who were treatment naïve [80]. Increases in ATG5 also correlated with the presence of proinflammatory cytokines, thus displaying a possible relationship between the inflammatory status and ATG5 expression in MS. However, they did not perform a detailed analysis of the clinical activity state [80]. T cells present different subpopulations. Among them, T regulatory cells (Treg) are particularly relevant in autoimmune disease because they prevent inflammation and preserve the tolerance to self-antigens. Recently, it has been demonstrated that the autophagic mediator AMBRA1 associates with the protein phosphatase PP2A to sustain Treg differentiation by increasing the expression of Forkhead box P 3 (FOXP3), an essential transcription factor for the differentiation of Treg cells [81]. In addition, the AMBRA1–PP2A–FOXP3 molecular axis was found to be essential for regulating the optimal autophagic levels necessary for T-cell stimulation and differentiation. Consistently, AMBRA1 conditional KO mice display reductions in FOXP3 levels with consequent impairments in Treg differentiation and activity. Most importantly, AMBRA1 deficiency worsens the disease pathogenesis in an EAE MS animal model [81]. Finally, work of Akatsuka et al. not only demonstrates the important role of AMBRA1 in the regulation of T cells, but also highlights decreased mitochondrial functioning and metabolism in these cells [82]. All these findings demonstrate that AMBRA1 is an essential factor that regulates both autophagic and mitochondrial behaviors and, probably, also the mitophagic process in T cells.

In MS, T-cell activities may be modulated by the complement-regulating molecule CD46 [83]. This factor is also described as an autophagic inducer [84], and its levels are documented to be increased in the serum and cerebrospinal fluid (CSF) of MS patients [85]. The increased T-cell autoreactivity in MS may also be promoted by IRGM1, a GTPase that regulates the survival of immune cells through autophagy. Consistent with this finding, IRGM1 deletion increases the apoptosis of T cells, reduces their proliferative capacity, and ameliorates the clinical score of the EAE mouse model [86]. Considering that subsequent studies have demonstrated that IRGM1 is localized to the mitochondrial compartment and regulates the mitochondrial metabolism and mitochondrial fission induced by mitophagy [87,88], the increased T-cell autoreactivity observed in MS may be due to an impairment in the mitophagic process. In addition to its effects on T cells, autophagy plays a role in dendritic cells (DCs), the most potent antigen-presenting cells (APCs) in the immune system. In particular, autophagy starts in response to bacterial and viral infection. By generating transgenic mice with silencing of ATG7 in DCs, Bhattacharya and colleagues demonstrated the importance of DCs and autophagy in MS. Indeed, they showed that the specific loss of autophagy in DCs significantly delayed disease progression and reduced disease severity in EAE mice [89]. As reported above, AMPK is the main positive regulator of autophagy. This kinase works by sensing the AMP/ATP ratio and activates autophagy to combat energetic imbalance. It has been demonstrated that following exposure to proinflammatory cytokines, AMPK activates and triggers autophagy in oligodendrocyte precursor cells (OPCs) [90]. This change is due to a metabolic switch from OXPHOS to glycolysis and impairment of mitochondrial dynamics, leading to increased oxidative stress and reduced mitochondrial Ca^{2+} uptake and ATP production. As a consequence, OPCs fail to differentiate into mature and myelinating oligodendrocytes [90]. In support of these in vitro findings, recent work demonstrated that metabolic stress-induced autophagy is a key element in an in vivo MS model. Indeed, MCU-deficient (MCU-def) mice subjected to EAE displayed elevated clinical scores, excessive inflammation, and demyelination [91]. Morphological and functional analyses performed with the spinal cords of MCU-def mice revealed important mitochondrial damage, accompanied by an elevated presence of autophagosomal markers and a decrease in ATP synthesis and mitochondrial gene expression. Overall, these data confirm that the presence of mitochondrial dysfunction provokes the inhibition of Ca^{2+} buffering, ATP synthesis, and mitochondrial gene expression, causing a metabolic collapse that prompts autophagy and worsens MS-like conditions. Furthermore, since autophagic activation accompanied by the downregulation of PGC1α (a master regulator of mitochondrial biogenesis) has been observed, it is possible to speculate that the mitochondrial QC system is also affected. However, studies have not verified whether autophagy activities lead to autophagic mitochondrial removal.

Markers of autophagic processes may represent reliable potential biomarkers for monitoring the progression of disease. Increased amounts of Parkin, ATG5, and inflammatory cytokines are present in both the serum and CSF obtained from MS patients. Analyses comparing MS patients to healthy individuals and patients affected by other neurodegenerative conditions have been conducted [16]. Moreover, subsequent work demonstrated that increases in both autophagic and mitophagic markers correlated with the active phases of the disease and with circulating lactate levels, demonstrating the presence of an impaired metabolic status in MS patients [92]. Notably, several studies have associated lactate levels with MS progression [93]. Other independent research groups have confirmed that circulating autophagy and mitophagy markers are increased in MS biofluids [94,95]. In addition, the circulating levels of mitochondrial adenine nucleotide translocase 1 (ANT1) and oxidative stress markers have also been investigated. Interestingly, MS patients display increased oxidative stress, accompanied by reduced levels of the mitochondrial marker ANT1, suggesting that the mitochondrial QC systems are activated to promote the removal of nonfunctioning mitochondria. Consistent with this, reduced circulating levels of the OMM protein translocator protein 18 kDa (TSPO) and increased amounts of the mitochondrial disease marker growth/differentiation factor 15 (GDF-15) have been found in MS individuals and correlate with the severity of the disease [96,97] (Table 1).

It is clear that autophagy and mitophagy as well as the mitochondrial quality control system are important contributors in MS. In the last few years, an increasing number of studies have correlated the activities of such molecular mechanisms with the progression of the disease. Furthermore, circulating elements of autophagy and mitophagy may be detected in human samples from MS individuals, thus suggesting the possibility of using them as novel biomarkers. However, MS shows a great heterogeneity with regard to the clinical symptoms as well as therapy response. In addition, MS manifests in different forms (clinically isolated syndrome, RR MS, secondary progressive MS, and primary progressive MS), where the relapse rate and disability progression differentiate one from the other. Only when the dynamics and response of autophagy and mitophagy are well characterized in regard to all these conditions will we be able to claim to have identified the real contributions of them in MS, and we could use autophagic and mitophagic elements as innovative markers for MS disease progression.

Table 1. Summary of autophagy- and mitophagy-related markers in biofluids of MS-, AD-, and PD-affected persons.

Neurodegenerative Condition	Marker	Role	Type of Human Biofluid
MS	Parkin	Mitophagy regulator	Serum, CSF
	ATG5	Autophagy regulator	Serum, CSF
	Mitochondrial adenine nucleotide translocase 1 (ANT1)	Mitochondrial ADP/ATP translocase	Serum, CSF
	Translocator protein 18 kDa (TSPO)	Regulator of mPTP opening	Blood PBMCs
	Growth/differentiation factor 15 (GDF-15)	Mitochondrial disease marker	Serum
	TNFα	Proinflammatory cytokine	Serum, CSF
	Lactate	Mitochondrial dysfunction marker	Serum, CSF
AD	BECN1	Autophagy regulator	Blood PBMCs, serum
	p62	Autophagy regulator	Blood PBMCs
	LC3	Autophagy regulator	Blood PBMCs
	ATG5	Autophagy regulator	Plasma, serum
	Parkin	Mitophagy regulator	Serum
	EEA1, LAMP1, LAMP2, RAB3, and RAB7	Lysosomal regulators	CSF
PD	LC3B	Autophagy regulator	CSF
	BECN1	Autophagy regulator	CSF, blood PBMCs
	ATG5	Autophagy regulator	CSF
	LAMP2	Lysosomal regulator	CSF
	ULK1	Autophagy regulator	Blood PBMCs
	ATG5	Autophagy regulator	Blood PBMCs
	ATG4B	Autophagy regulator	Blood PBMCs
	ATG16L1	Autophagy regulator	Blood PBMCs

5. Involvement of Autophagy Mechanisms in AD Progression

AD was first described in the early 20th century and is characterized by a progressive deterioration of cognitive function. Memory loss and dementia represent the most common symptoms. The cardinal pathological hallmarks of AD are extracellular (amyloid) plaques and intracellular and extracellular neurofibrillary tangles (NFTs). Amyloid plaques are composed of deposits of Aβ, α-syn, Ub, and apolipoprotein E. NFTs are characterized by hyperphosphorylated tau protein and apolipoprotein E. These aggregates induce neuronal toxicity by impeding neural communication and provoking cell death either directly or by preventing the delivery of an optimal nutrient supply to brain cells [3].

At present, the origin of AD and the mechanisms occurring in the pathogenesis of AD are not well defined. Inflammation seems to play an important role: mediators of inflammation, such as cytokines, adhesion molecules, and prostaglandins, drive degeneration in different neural AD models [98]. Consistent with this finding, aggregated peptides increase proinflammatory agent production, and inflammatory molecules are detected in the CSF, serum, and plaques obtained from AD patients. Oxidative and nitrosylative damage provoked by ROS and reactive nitrogen species (RNS) are determinants of the initiation and progression of AD [99]. Oxidatively damaged membrane phospholipids and increased oxidative stress in neurons are frequently present in neurons exposed to Aβ [100]. Furthermore, AD brains extracted at autopsy have decreased amounts of vitamins A and E and β-carotene [101] and display a higher production of free radicals and increased expression of neuronal nitric oxide synthase (nNOS) [102]. This increased nNOS correlates with an increased apoptosis of hippocampal neurons. In the last 10 years, an increasing number of studies have demonstrated the critical contributions of autophagy and mitophagy to AD pathogenesis [103]. Several studies have reported an increased presence of Aβ in autophagosomes [104]. Interestingly, autophagosomes also contain amyloid precursor protein (APP) and its processing enzymes, in particular, a component of the γ-secretase complex, suggesting an additional source of Aβ. Consistent with this finding, the induction of autophagy correlates with Aβ production, and autophagy-deficient animals (with ATG7 knockdown) display reduced Aβ secretion [105]. Additionally, the hyperphosphorylation of tau correlates with increased autophagic levels. Indeed, postmortem AD brain samples are characterized by LC3- and p62-positive autophagosomes, and the hyperphosphorylation of tau has been recognized in autophagy-deficient mice [106,107]. Although these observations highlight a dangerous correlation between autophagy and AD, other studies suggest that autophagy and mitophagy may exert beneficial effects against AD [103]. The abnormal accumulation of autophagosome vesicles is present in AD neurons [104]. This accumulation is related to compromised lysosomal function, which results in lysosomes that are no longer able to degrade autophagosomes. The overexpression of Parkin and PINK activates mitophagy, restores mitochondrial function, and reduces Aβ production [108,109]. Similar results have been obtained from another independent experiments that demonstrated that mitophagy is essential for reducing Aβ levels, abolishing tau hyperphosphorylation, preventing cognitive impairments in an AD mouse model, and suppressing neuroinflammation [110].

To confirm the crucial role of autophagic and mitophagic dynamics in AD, different studies have evaluated the presence of elements belonging to these processes in biofluids from persons with AD. The first investigation was performed in 1995, in which ventricular CSF from postmortem AD patients was analyzed. In this study, the authors detected increased levels of the lysosomal protein cathepsin D [111]. However, a subsequent report performed with lumbar CSF samples from living AD patients found no change in the levels of cathepsin B [112]. This finding was confirmed in other work that investigated a broad range of lysosomal proteins in CSF samples from living AD patients and found no variations in diverse cathepsin forms (A, B, D, and L); however, the study did find altered expression for five other lysosomal proteins in the AD samples: early endosomal antigen 1 (EEA1), LAMP1, LAMP2, RAB3, and RAB7 [113]. By contrast, a recent study analyzed the levels of proteins associated with lysosomal function in the CSF of AD persons by conducting solid-phase extraction and parallel reaction monitoring mass spectrometry and found only minor or absent changes in their levels [114]. Unfortunately, the levels of proteins directly related to autophagy and mitophagy processes were not investigated in that study. A follow-up study at 12 and 24 months identified autophagic elements (BECN1, p62, and LC3) in peripheral blood mononuclear cells (PBMCs) obtained from the blood of AD patients and demonstrated that their levels varied during the course of the disease and correlated with the inflammatory environment [115]. Recently, autophagic elements have also been assessed directly in AD blood samples. Indeed, increased levels of the autophagic marker ATG5 are present in the plasma of patients with dementia who meet the criteria for probable AD. Unfortunately, the authors did not identify the subtype of dementia or confirm the AD status. These limitations were overcome in a recent investigation assessing the circulation of autophagic and mitophagic markers in the serum of patients affected by mild–moderate late-onset AD, mild cognitive impairment (MCI), vascular dementia (VAD), and mixed dementia (MD). In this work, the authors found decreased levels of ATG5 and Parkin in patients affected by AD, MCI, and MD. By contrast, they detected increased levels of these markers in VAD patients [17]. This investigation suggests that autophagy and mitophagy markers are possible biomarkers for AD and that they are differentially affected in different dementia types, which may help to discriminate AD-type dementias from VAD. Additionally, the fact that AD samples have decreased levels of autophagy and mitophagy markers confirms the presence of an impaired degradative system in AD persons (Table 1).

Summing up, autophagy and mitophagy represent well-established mechanisms in AD and may exert a protective role. Accordingly, most research highlights the reduced recruitment of both autophagy and mitophagic factors in cell cultures, in vivo AD models, and human samples obtained from AD-affected patients, including in the body fluids of the CSF and blood. Here, autophagic and mitophagic partners also correlate with the inflammatory status and change during the course of the disease, thus opening up the possibility of using autophagic and mitophagic elements as markers for the progression of AD. However, before ascribing merit to these molecules as potential screening, prognostic, diagnostic, or disease-monitoring markers for AD, it is important to consider different aspects. The diagnosis of AD cannot be achieved until the patient displays dementia symptoms. In addition, different dementia types exist and vary between individuals. Very few studies have monitored the variation of circulating markers of autophagy and mitophagy during the different dementia types. Furthermore, these studies lack validation of the investigated markers with accepted methods for diagnosing AD, such as amyloid PET imaging. Again, all the investigations performed did not provide follow-up studies and did not analyze the effects of the disease-modifying drugs commonly used for AD therapy on autophagy and mitophagy circulating markers. Undoubtedly, more detailed analyses and larger cohort studies are necessary to verify whether autophagic and mitophagic circulating elements may represent promising biomarkers for AD.

6. Current Knowledge of the Relationship between PD and Autophagy Dynamics

Resting tremor, bradykinesia, rigidity, and postural instability represent the four cardinal signs of PD, the most common neurological movement disease, and PD is characterized by a progressive loss of dopaminergic neurons in the substantia nigra pars compacta. PD is considered a multifactorial disease since both genetic and environmental factors play important roles. Approximately 90% of the cases are sporadic, while the remaining 10% are caused by monogenic mutations in at least 23 genes. Similarly, a number of cellular mechanisms are involved in PD pathogenesis. Among them, the uncontrolled intracellular aggregation of α-syn, in the form of LBs and Lewy neurites, represents the main hallmark of the disease. It is not surprising that the first evidence of the genetic mechanisms of PD was a mutation in the α-syn gene, and different forms of the α-syn protein (oligomers, protofibrils, and unfolded monomers) have been found in human PD brain samples. α-syn is a presynaptic neuron protein abundantly expressed in the nervous system; it is present in proximity to synaptic vesicles and folds into α-helical structures. The primary role of this protein is to attenuate neurotransmitter release and synaptic vesicle recycling. In PD, α-syn generates β-sheet structures that are prone to aggregation, which leads to pathologic conditions with toxic gain-of-function effects. Mitochondrial dysfunction is another crucial element during PD pathogenesis in both sporadic PD and familial Parkinsonism. Different postmortem studies have highlighted the existence of deficiencies in components of the mETC, and compounds (toxins and pesticides) were found to promote the Parkinsonian phenotype and neuron loss by impairing complex I of the mETC. Furthermore, α-syn alone induces effects by interacting with the mitochondrial membrane, accumulating inside the organelle, and leading to mitochondrial dysfunction and oxidative stress by damaging C-I [116]; alternatively, α-syn can interact with the mitochondrial transporter TOM20 [117]. Another gene causing autosomal dominant PD is LRRK2, a protein involved in diverse signaling pathways, including vesicular trafficking, protein translation, and the control of mitochondrial dynamics. Mutations in this member of the leucine-rich kinase family have been found in approximately 1–2% of sporadic and 5% of familial PD cases. The most frequent mutation of LRRK2 (G2019S) induces an increase in LRRK2 activity. G2019S-LRRK2 PD postmortem human tissues, animal models, and cellular models are characterized by important mitochondrial dysfunction, with impaired ATP production, mitochondrial fragmentation, mtDNA damage, and oxidative stress representing the main features. Recently, it has been demonstrated that this mutation induces impairment in mitophagic clearance [118]. In addition, the loss of function, mutation, and overexpression of the mitophagic regulatory members PINK1 and Parkin provoke impaired mitochondrial turnover and cause autosomal recessive PD. To mediate mitophagy, PINK1 and Parkin cooperate to recognize and label damaged mitochondria with polyubiquitin (p-Ub) chains [119]. Postmortem brains from LB disease patients are characterized by p-Ub chain structures that colocalize with markers of mitochondria and autophagy [120]. Mutant forms of PINK1 are unable to move to mitochondria upon stress signaling, thereby avoiding mitophagic induction. Similarly, Parkin mutations (such as S65N, G12R, and R33Q) decrease the capacity of PINK1 to phosphorylate and activate Parkin itself. Correct mitochondrial turnover is not guaranteed by only the mitophagic process; it is also regulated by fission and fusion events. Among the mitochondrial fusion proteins, the best characterized are mitofusins (MFNs). It has been demonstrated that MFN-1 and MFN-2 are substrates for PINK1 and Parkin and that they can be ubiquitinated by both PINK1 and Parkin [121,122]. Consistent with this, mutations in and the loss of PINK1 and Parkin impair MFN-1/2 ubiquitination in PD patient cells [123]. MFNs also work as bridges between mitochondria and the ER to preserve the appropriate functioning of MAMs. These contact sites between the ER and mitochondria act as primary signaling hubs for cells and regulate lipid homeostasis, calcium dynamics, apoptosis, the stress response, and autophagosome vesicle formation. Diverse recent studies have highlighted a contribution of these contact subdomains in the progression of PD [124]. Several proteins encoded by genes involved in PD (α-syn, Parkin, and PINK1) are located in MAMs and have been found to regulate correct ER–mitochondrion tethering. For example, Parkin deletion increases MFN2 amounts and increases Ca^{2+} transfer from the ER to mitochondria [125]. Notably, this event is a crucial mediator of the regulation of autophagy [126]. In addition, DJ-1, which provokes a rare form of autosomal recessive PD [127], increases ER–mitochondrion communication and preserves the optimal Ca^{2+} transfer between the ER and mitochondria, thereby having a cytoprotective role that is essential for maintaining mitochondrial functioning [128] and, probably, autophagy levels. As reported above, alterations in tau protein are highly related to AD disease. In truth, pathogenic mutations in tau protein are present in different neurodegenerative disorders, defined as tauopathies. Interestingly, different studies suggest that tau mutations are also present in PD. By comparing characterized tau mutations related to tau toxicity and aggregation in PD (P301L and A152T) [129–131], a recent investigation explored, for the first time, the concomitant activity of the three different forms of autophagy (autophagy, CMA, and mA) [132]. Here, the authors found different activity levels for the three autophagic forms and demonstrated that the pathogenic tau mutation A152T resulted in a blockage of both CMA and mA, but caused a compensatory activation of autophagy. Oppositely, the P301L mutation provoked an inhibition of the degradation of tau aggregates by any of the three catabolic pathways [132]. A deeper understanding of the different recruitment of the diverse autophagic forms may help to increase our knowledge of the molecular mechanisms existing in PD as well as in the other tauopathies.

Detecting autophagy- and mitophagy-related proteins in peripheral human biospecimens may represent a promising method for identifying PD statuses and controlling the progression of the disease. Significant decreases in LC3B, BECN1, ATG5, and lysosomal associated membrane protein (LAMP) 2 are present in CSF samples obtained from early-stage PD patients. Interestingly, among these autophagic partners, only LC3B shows a significant correlation with α-syn, total tau levels, and the clinical severity of patients [133]. Notably, recent studies have demonstrated that tau protein also participates in the pathology of PD [134]. A reduction in LAMP2 levels in the CSF of PD patients was found in another study. In this study, the authors found a decrease in LAMP1 levels, but they did not identify variations in LC3 levels [135]. An important difference exists between these two studies. In the first, circulating proteins were detected by using ELISA technology, while the second employed an immunoblotting technique. LAMP2 levels were also analyzed in a study comparing PD patients, PD patients harboring LRRK2 mutations, and healthy control subjects with or without LRRK2 mutations. The main finding of that investigation was that LAMP2 protein levels were reduced in the PD patients harboring LRRK2 mutations. Similar to the study mentioned above, LAMP2 levels were not related to the clinical states of the patients. However, a positive correlation between LAMP2 and oxidative stress has been shown [136]. Autophagic markers and related proteins were analyzed in circulating PBMCs obtained from PD patients. The results demonstrated that the steady-state autophagy in PD patients was profoundly different from that observed in healthy individuals and correlated with augmented expression of α-syn [137]. Unfortunately, investigations aimed at detecting mitophagic elements in human biofluids are lacking. The existing literature can inform us about the "mitochondrial signature" that exists in PD patients. Significant decreases in mtDNA copy number have been observed in patient blood cells and in CSF samples from early-stage PD [138,139]. Increased mtDNA levels were present in the CSF of PD patients carrying LRRK2 mutations [140] and in the sera of PD persons with mutations in Parkin or PINK1. This study demonstrated an association between mitophagy impairment (represented by a Parkin- or PINK1-mutant genotype) and mtDNA in circulating biofluids from PD patients for the first time. Finally, an interesting study found reduced methylated mtDNA in PD patients, suggesting that affected patients may have disrupted mtDNA gene expression and replication [141] (Table 1).

Undoubtedly, the discovery that many genes involved in both autophagy and (in particular) mitophagy are mutated in familial Parkinsonism and in sporadic PD makes these molecular processes fundamental for this neurodegenerative disease. The fact that markers of these catabolic systems may be detected in human samples also opens up the possibility of creating new real-time monitoring approaches for the progression of the disease. However, today, these studies' results are still incomplete, and some of them report controversial results, probably due to the limited sizes of the cohorts analyzed, the different types of samples analyzed, and, most importantly, not always accounting for the clinical history of each single patient. It is thus clear that more detailed and larger longitudinal, stratified, and standardized analyses are needed.

7. Principles and Current Strategies for Targeting Autophagy in Neurodegeneration

Several therapeutic approaches ameliorate the consequences and symptoms of neurodegenerative disorders. Unfortunately, current treatments become less effective as the neurodegenerative status advances, and most importantly, none of them prevents the onset or progression of the disease. The evidence reported in the previous sections demonstrates that autophagy processes have an important role during the development of the most common neurodegenerative diseases. Hence, these findings suggest that the modulation of autophagic and mitophagic processes may be a possible innovative therapeutic approach for combating neurodegeneration (Figure 3).

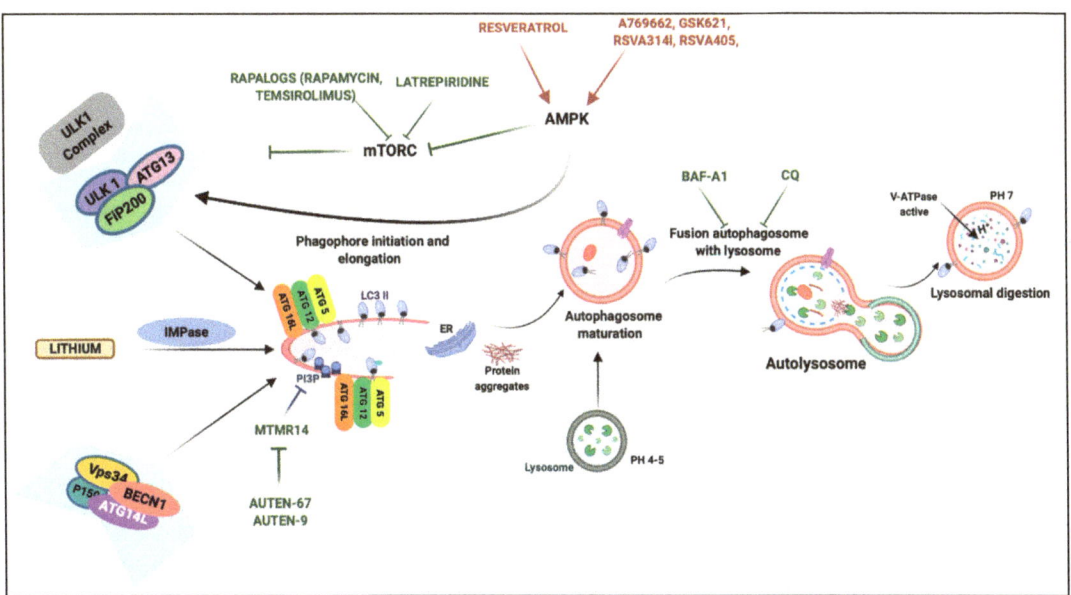

Figure 3. Strategies for targeting autophagy in neurodegeneration.

Autophagy upregulation has been demonstrated to be an effective strategy for increasing the clearance of neurodegenerative disease-causing proteins in different cellular and mouse models, thereby reducing toxicity. Autophagic activation may be induced by blocking mTOR activities. Rapamycin is the best known mTOR inhibitor, and it has been demonstrated that this compound increases the clearance of tau protein and decreases tau toxicity [142,143]. In addition, rapamycin activates autophagy to remove other protein aggregates, such as long polyglutamines and polyalanine-expanded proteins [143]. Unfortunately, one limit of rapamycin is its limited absorption. Different analogs of rapamycin (rapalogs) have been developed in recent years. Among them, temsirolimus has been found to increase the autophagy clearance of hyperphosphorylated tau and ameliorate learning and memory impairments [144]. Another compound mediating mTOR inhibition is the proneurogenic and antihistaminic compound latrepirdine. It has been demonstrated that latrepirdine also improves learning behaviors and reduces Aβ and α-syn aggregates in an AD mouse model [145]. Autophagy can also be activated by mTOR-independent pharmacological agents. For example, resveratrol exerts neuroprotective effects in PD models by increasing autophagy through an AMPK-dependent mechanism [146]. The same effects on AMPK activity are induced by the recently identified small molecules A769662, GSK621, RSVA314, and RSVA405. A769662 and GSK621 promote the autophagic clearance of α-syn aggregates by inducing the phosphorylation of AMPK and ULK1 [147]. RSVA314 and RSVA405 activate AMPK by a CaMKKβ-dependent mechanism to activate autophagy and promote the degradation of Aβ 20852062. The molecule AUTEN-67, which antagonizes the autophagic inhibitor phosphatase MTMR14, increases autophagic flux, promotes neuron longevity, and prevents neurodegenerative symptoms in AD models [148]. Interestingly, the same research group also demonstrated that another molecule, AUTEN-99, is capable of improving autophagy and exerting neuroprotective effects in PD models [149]. Lithium is widely used to treat bipolar disorders and depression. In addition, recent investigations have demonstrated that lithium administration activates autophagy by inhibiting inositol monophosphatase in an mTOR-independent manner [150] and exerts neuroprotection in AD [151]. Consistent with this, a clinical trial evaluating long-term treatment with lithium in AD patients revealed the amelioration of multiple cognitive parameters in the lithium group. Furthermore, analyses conducted with CSF samples revealed a significant reduction in phosphorylated tau [152]. It is clear that an improvement in autophagic machinery should permit an increase in the clearance of protein aggregates. Despite this understanding, studies have also demonstrated that pharmacological interventions aimed at blocking the autophagic process may be useful for counteracting a neurodegenerative status. In an α-syn transgenic mouse model, the overexpression of α-syn reduced dendritic and synaptic markers, which were reduced after exposure to the anti-autophagic compounds bafilomycin-A1 (Baf-A1) and chloroquine (CQ). Interestingly, the authors also found a reduction in α-syn inclusions after treatment with rapamycin. This finding suggests that the aggregation of α-syn is not exclusively mediated by the mTOR-dependent regulation of autophagy. Considering that mTOR is involved in multiple cellular processes, it is possible that other mechanisms are involved in α-syn metabolism [153]. Of note, it is important to specify that both CQ and Baf-A1 have a broad spectrum of biological activities. Similar to what was observed for α-syn aggregates, the inhibition of autophagy promoted by CQ induced a reduction in total tau levels in rat hippocampal extracts. Increase and decreases in tau levels have been observed after rapamycin administration [154]. The inhibition of autophagy also seems to exert beneficial effects in MS. Indeed, by suppressing the inflammatory process in EAE, CQ administration ameliorates the clinical signs of the disease [155]. A subsequent study unveiled that the effect of CQ in reducing the severity of the clinical course of EAE is mediated by a direct effect on DCs. In this work, the authors demonstrated that CQ-treated cells displayed reduced expression of molecules involved in antigen presentation, which resulted in reduced T-cell activation and proliferation [156]. The deleterious role of autophagy in MS has also been demonstrated in the cuprizone (CPZ) demyelination model, which permits us to determine the contribution of other elements independent of the immune system during demyelination/remyelination. The administration of CPZ with rapamycin resulted in increased demyelination compared with treatment with CPZ alone [157]. Furthermore, rapamycin increases axonal damage and leukocyte infiltration when administered together with CPZ [158], suggesting that by administrating agents blocking the autophagic process, it may be possible to reduce demyelination. Despite this finding, other studies have demonstrated that rapamycin ameliorates histological and clinical signs in MS models, particularly EAE models [159]. In addition, a clinical trial in which RR-MS patients received rapamycin for 6 months highlighted some degree of reduction in the volumes of sclerotic plaques, accompanied by a significant decrease in T-responder cells [160]. To the best of our knowledge, there is no specific agent that can modulate the selective autophagic removal of mitochondria during neurodegeneration. Several efforts are ongoing to try to overcome this shortcoming. For example, mitophagy may be improved by small molecules activating the PINK1–Parkin pathway. The ATP analog kinetin triphosphate has been identified as a potent PINK1 activator. Indeed, this neosubstrate accelerates PINK1-dependent Parkin recruitment to damaged mitochondria and prevents the apoptosis induced by oxidative stress in neuronal cells [161]. Unfortunately, long-term oral kinetin administration does not prevent the neurodegeneration induced by α-syn in a PD model [162]. A recent high-throughput screening identified two other small molecules (T0466 and T0467) that affect the PINK1–Parkin axis. These compounds successfully promote Parkin translocation to mitochondria, suppress mitochondrial aggregation in dopaminergic neurons, and improve locomotor defects in the *Drosophila* PINK1 model [163]. Finally, it has been suggested that Rho-associated protein kinase (ROCK) inhibitors may exert a neuroprotective effect by increasing the activity of the Parkin-mediated mitophagy pathway. In one investigation, the authors performed a screen of ~3000 compounds with the aim of identifying compounds that promote Parkin translocation to mitochondria. As a result, they found that several ROCK inhibitors increased the recruitment of Parkin to damaged mitochondria and found compound SR3677 to be the most efficacious. In addition, SR3677 also exerted neuroprotective effects and restored locomotor abilities in a *Drosophila* PD model [164].

The activation of autophagy seems to be efficacious in increasing the clearance of protein aggregates. Autophagic activation may be obtained by using rapamycinRAPAMYCIN and its analogs, such as TEMSIROLIMUS. These compounds permit inhibiting the mammalian target of rapamycin (mTOR). A similar effect was obtained by using the pro-neurogenic and antihistaminic compound LATREPIRIDINE. Autophagy may also be activated by potentiating the activity of 5' adenosine monophosphate-activated protein kinase (AMPK) with RESVERATROL and a series of small molecules (A769662, GSK621, RSVA314, and RSVA405) recently identified. Autophagy activation may also be obtained in an mTOR/AMPK-independent manner. LITHIUM was found to block the pro-autophagic function of inositol monophosphatase (IMPase), and two molecules (AUTEN-69 and -99) antagonize the autophagic inhibitor phosphatase MTMR14. Oppositely, autophagy inhibition represents a possible therapeutic approach against multiple sclerosis (MS). In particular, diverse studies suggest that the anti-autophagic compound chloroquine (CQ) suppresses inflammation and reduces the clinical score of an MS mouse model.

8. Conclusions and Future Perspectives

In this review, we summarize studies showing how autophagy and mitophagy have crucial roles in neurodegenerative disorders. It is clear that compromised autophagy and mitophagy dynamics mediate the pathogenesis and progression of diseases characterized by the uncontrolled accumulation of protein aggregates, such as AD and PD. These mechanisms are in contrast with those in MS, in which the neurodegenerative condition is not due to aberrant protein inclusions and autophagy and mitophagy appear to be excessively activated and to provoke deleterious conditions causing cell death or the impairment of normal cellular functions.

Interestingly, these scenarios are present when autophagy markers or any biochemical or molecular markers are analyzed in body fluids from persons affected by specific neurodegenerative conditions. Indeed, most of the investigations performed highlight a reduced activity of the autophagy processes in AD and PD; however, these processes are increased in human MS samples. Furthermore, autophagy levels correlate with clinical outcomes. Overall, these findings clearly show that changes in autophagy and mitophagy elements may be reliable markers for predicting/controlling disease progression and helping to monitor clinical status. It is, thus, necessary to point out that most of the investigations performed have utilized serum. This biofluid is more accessible and safer and has fewer contraindications than CSF, and it would certainly facilitate the continuous tracking of disease progression. Another point should be highlighted: the findings presented herein also suggest that the modulation of autophagy dynamics with pharmacological strategies may be an effective method for slowing down the progression of some neurodegenerative diseases. Different studies performed in cellular and animal models support this possibility. For instance, the inhibition of autophagy appears to reduce inflammation and clinical signs in MS models, while its activation reduces protein aggregation and consequent motor and learning behavior defects in AD and PD models. Consistent with these findings, long-term treatment with the autophagy inducer lithium in a clinical trial restored multiple cognitive parameters in AD patients.

However, it should be noted that several caveats exist in the studies mentioned above. Currently, there are no good methods for accurately quantifying autophagy and mitophagy levels in samples obtained from human patients. For this reason, it is difficult to understand whether increases or decreases in autophagy levels are not due to the impairment of the correct autophagic flux. Experiments with inhibitors of the autophagosomal fusion with the lysosomal membrane may help to overcome this limitation and may be performed in human tissues, such as skin and muscle biopsies and postmortem brain tissues. However, their application in more accessible human samples, such as sera and CSF, seems very hard to achieve. Similarly, today, it remains difficult to perform real-time monitoring of all the autophagic dynamics, from autophagosomal vesicle formation to degradation, in a patient.

Additionally, it is difficult to ensure that pharmacological agents modulating autophagy in cultured cells and animal models also do so in vivo in patients affected by a neurodegenerative condition. Furthermore, drugs activating/inhibiting autophagy may exert several other effects and modulate gene expression and protein, lipid, and nucleotide synthesis. In addition, to date, no effective treatment aimed at selectively modulating only the mitophagic pathway has been tested. Finally, at first glance, serum may represent a valid alternative to CSF for monitoring clinical status. However, outside of the CSF, the concentrations of markers related to the CNS are often low, and circulating antibodies and proteases may alter the effective concentrations of proteins in peripheral tissues [165].

In summary, more work is required to fully clarify all the connections that exist between autophagy processes and neurodegenerative status. Despite this limitation, the current literature demonstrates that the recent decades have been characterized by a great improvement in the understanding of the connection between autophagic dynamics and neurodegeneration. Currently, autophagy is accepted worldwide to be a fundamental aspect of the onset and progression of almost all neurodegenerative diseases. A better understanding of the molecular partners participating in this cellular process may help to identify susceptible patients, control disease progression, and perform active monitoring of treatment responses. Finally, the pharmacological modulation of autophagy may represent an attractive tool for identifying new disease-modifying therapies to combat different types of neurodegenerative diseases.

Author Contributions: S.P., C.G. and P.P. conceived the article; S.P., A.D., M.P. and E.B. wrote the first version of the manuscript with constructive input from C.G. and P.P.; E.B. prepared the display items ("Created with BioRender.com") under the supervision of S.P. The figures are original and have not been published before. S.P., P.P. and C.G. reviewed and edited the manuscript before submission. All authors have read and agreed to the published version of the manuscript.

Funding: P.P. is grateful to Camilla degli Scrovegni for continuous support. The Signal Transduction Laboratory is supported by the Italian Association for Cancer Research: Grant IG-23670 (to P.P.) and Grant IG-19803 (to C.G.); A-ROSE; the Telethon Grant GGP11139B (to P.P.); Progetti di Rilevante Interesse Nazionale Grants: PRIN2017E5L5P3 (to P.P.) and PRIN20177E9EPY (to C.G.); an Italian Ministry of Health Grant GR-2013-02356747 (to C.G.); a European Research Council Grant 853057-InflaPML (to C.G.); local funds from the University of Ferrara (to P.P. and C.G.); and Fondazione Umberto Veronesi (to S.P.).

Institutional Review Board Statement: Not applicable.

Informed Consent Statement: Not applicable.

Data Availability Statement: Not applicable.

Conflicts of Interest: The authors declare no conflict of interest.

References

1. Dugger, B.N.; Dickson, D.W. Pathology of Neurodegenerative Diseases. *Cold Spring Harbor Perspect. Biol.* **2017**, *9*. [CrossRef]
2. Davis, A.A.; Leyns, C.E.G.; Holtzman, D.M. Intercellular Spread of Protein Aggregates in Neurodegenerative Disease. *Annu. Rev. Cell Dev. Biol.* **2018**, *34*, 545–568. [CrossRef]
3. DeTure, M.A.; Dickson, D.W. The neuropathological diagnosis of Alzheimer's disease. *Mol. Neurodegener.* **2019**, *14*, 32. [CrossRef] [PubMed]
4. Armstrong, M.J.; Okun, M.S. Diagnosis and Treatment of Parkinson Disease: A Review. *JAMA* **2020**, *323*, 548–560. [CrossRef] [PubMed]
5. Beyer, K.; Ariza, A. Alpha-Synuclein posttranslational modification and alternative splicing as a trigger for neurodegeneration. *Mol. Neurobiol.* **2013**, *47*, 509–524. [CrossRef] [PubMed]
6. Patergnani, S.; Fossati, V.; Bonora, M.; Giorgi, C.; Marchi, S.; Missiroli, S.; Rusielewicz, T.; Wieckowski, M.R.; Pinton, P. Mitochondria in Multiple Sclerosis: Molecular Mechanisms of Pathogenesis. *Int. Rev. Cell Mol. Biol.* **2017**, *328*, 49–103. [CrossRef]
7. Lassmann, H. Pathogenic Mechanisms Associated With Different Clinical Courses of Multiple Sclerosis. *Front. Immunol.* **2018**, *9*, 3116. [CrossRef]
8. Burte, F.; Carelli, V.; Chinnery, P.F.; Yu-Wai-Man, P. Disturbed mitochondrial dynamics and neurodegenerative disorders. *Nat. Rev. Neurol.* **2015**, *11*, 11–24. [CrossRef]
9. Missiroli, S.; Genovese, I.; Perrone, M.; Vezzani, B.; Vitto, V.A.M.; Giorgi, C. The Role of Mitochondria in Inflammation: From Cancer to Neurodegenerative Disorders. *J. Clin. Med.* **2020**, *9*, 740. [CrossRef]
10. Chitnis, T.; Weiner, H.L. CNS inflammation and neurodegeneration. *J. Clin. Investig.* **2017**, *127*, 3577–3587. [CrossRef]
11. Menzies, F.M.; Fleming, A.; Caricasole, A.; Bento, C.F.; Andrews, S.P.; Ashkenazi, A.; Fullgrabe, J.; Jackson, A.; Jimenez Sanchez, M.; Karabiyik, C.; et al. Autophagy and Neurodegeneration: Pathogenic Mechanisms and Therapeutic Opportunities. *Neuron* **2017**, *93*, 1015–1034. [CrossRef]
12. Patergnani, S.; Pinton, P. Mitophagy and mitochondrial balance. *Methods Mol. Biol.* **2015**, *1241*, 181–194. [CrossRef]
13. Patergnani, S.; Guzzo, S.; Mangolini, A.; dell'Atti, L.; Pinton, P.; Aguiari, G. The induction of AMPK-dependent autophagy leads to P53 degradation and affects cell growth and migration in kidney cancer cells. *Exp. Cell Res.* **2020**, *395*, 112190. [CrossRef] [PubMed]
14. Xue, J.; Patergnani, S.; Giorgi, C.; Suarez, J.; Goto, K.; Bononi, A.; Tanji, M.; Novelli, F.; Pastorino, S.; Xu, R.; et al. Asbestos induces mesothelial cell transformation via HMGB1-driven autophagy. *Proc. Natl. Acad. Sci. USA* **2020**, *117*, 25543–25552. [CrossRef] [PubMed]
15. Chu, C.T. Mechanisms of selective autophagy and mitophagy: Implications for neurodegenerative diseases. *Neurobiol. Dis.* **2019**, *122*, 23–34. [CrossRef] [PubMed]
16. Patergnani, S.; Castellazzi, M.; Bonora, M.; Marchi, S.; Casetta, I.; Pugliatti, M.; Giorgi, C.; Granieri, E.; Pinton, P. Autophagy and mitophagy elements are increased in body fluids of multiple sclerosis-affected individuals. *J. Neurol. Neurosurg. Psychiatry* **2018**, *89*, 439–441. [CrossRef]
17. Castellazzi, M.; Patergnani, S.; Donadio, M.; Giorgi, C.; Bonora, M.; Bosi, C.; Brombo, G.; Pugliatti, M.; Seripa, D.; Zuliani, G.; et al. Autophagy and mitophagy biomarkers are reduced in sera of patients with Alzheimer's disease and mild cognitive impairment. *Sci. Rep.* **2019**, *9*, 20009. [CrossRef]
18. De Duve, C.; Wattiaux, R. Functions of lysosomes. *Annu. Rev. Physiol.* **1966**, *28*, 435–492. [CrossRef]
19. Mijaljica, D.; Prescott, M.; Devenish, R.J. Microautophagy in mammalian cells: Revisiting a 40-year-old conundrum. *Autophagy* **2011**, *7*, 673–682. [CrossRef]
20. Sahu, R.; Kaushik, S.; Clement, C.C.; Cannizzo, E.S.; Scharf, B.; Follenzi, A.; Potolicchio, I.; Nieves, E.; Cuervo, A.M.; Santambrogio, L. Microautophagy of cytosolic proteins by late endosomes. *Dev. Cell* **2011**, *20*, 131–139. [CrossRef]
21. Morshed, S.; Tasnin, M.N.; Ushimaru, T. ESCRT machinery plays a role in microautophagy in yeast. *BMC Mol. Cell Biol.* **2020**, *21*, 70. [CrossRef]

22. Sato, M.; Seki, T.; Konno, A.; Hirai, H.; Kurauchi, Y.; Hisatsune, A.; Katsuki, H. Fluorescent-based evaluation of chaperone-mediated autophagy and microautophagy activities in cultured cells. *Genes Cells Devoted Mol. Cell. Mech.* **2016**, *21*, 861–873. [CrossRef] [PubMed]
23. Olsvik, H.L.; Svenning, S.; Abudu, Y.P.; Brech, A.; Stenmark, H.; Johansen, T.; Mejlvang, J. Endosomal microautophagy is an integrated part of the autophagic response to amino acid starvation. *Autophagy* **2019**, *15*, 182–183. [CrossRef] [PubMed]
24. Sato, M.; Seki, T.; Konno, A.; Hirai, H.; Kurauchi, Y.; Hisatsune, A.; Katsuki, H. Rapamycin activates mammalian microautophagy. *J. Pharmacol. Sci.* **2019**, *140*, 201–204. [CrossRef] [PubMed]
25. Rahman, M.A.; Terasawa, M.; Mostofa, M.G.; Ushimaru, T. The TORC1-Nem1/Spo7-Pah1/lipin axis regulates microautophagy induction in budding yeast. *Biochem. Biophys. Res. Commun.* **2018**, *504*, 505–512. [CrossRef]
26. Kaushik, S.; Cuervo, A.M. The coming of age of chaperone-mediated autophagy. *Nat. Rev. Mol. Cell Biol.* **2018**, *19*, 365–381. [CrossRef]
27. Dikic, I.; Elazar, Z. Mechanism and medical implications of mammalian autophagy. *Nat. Rev. Mol. Cell Biol.* **2018**, *19*, 349–364. [CrossRef]
28. Hosokawa, N.; Hara, T.; Kaizuka, T.; Kishi, C.; Takamura, A.; Miura, Y.; Iemura, S.; Natsume, T.; Takehana, K.; Yamada, N.; et al. Nutrient-dependent mTORC1 association with the ULK1-Atg13-FIP200 complex required for autophagy. *Mol. Biol. Cell* **2009**, *20*, 1981–1991. [CrossRef]
29. Chang, K.; Kang, P.; Liu, Y.; Huang, K.; Miao, T.; Sagona, A.P.; Nezis, I.P.; Bodmer, R.; Ocorr, K.; Bai, H. TGFB-INHB/activin signaling regulates age-dependent autophagy and cardiac health through inhibition of MTORC2. *Autophagy* **2020**, *16*, 1807–1822. [CrossRef]
30. Aspernig, H.; Heimbucher, T.; Qi, W.; Gangurde, D.; Curic, S.; Yan, Y.; Donner von Gromoff, E.; Baumeister, R.; Thien, A. Mitochondrial Perturbations Couple mTORC2 to Autophagy in C. elegans. *Cell Rep.* **2019**, *29*, 1399–1409.e5. [CrossRef]
31. Jhanwar-Uniyal, M.; Wainwright, J.V.; Mohan, A.L.; Tobias, M.E.; Murali, R.; Gandhi, C.D.; Schmidt, M.H. Diverse signaling mechanisms of mTOR complexes: mTORC1 and mTORC2 in forming a formidable relationship. *Adv. Biol. Regul.* **2019**, *72*, 51–62. [CrossRef]
32. Kim, J.; Kundu, M.; Viollet, B.; Guan, K.L. AMPK and mTOR regulate autophagy through direct phosphorylation of Ulk1. *Nat. Cell Biol.* **2011**, *13*, 132–141. [CrossRef] [PubMed]
33. Egan, D.F.; Shackelford, D.B.; Mihaylova, M.M.; Gelino, S.; Kohnz, R.A.; Mair, W.; Vasquez, D.S.; Joshi, A.; Gwinn, D.M.; Taylor, R.; et al. Phosphorylation of ULK1 (hATG1) by AMP-activated protein kinase connects energy sensing to mitophagy. *Science* **2011**, *331*, 456–461. [CrossRef] [PubMed]
34. Shang, L.; Chen, S.; Du, F.; Li, S.; Zhao, L.; Wang, X. Nutrient starvation elicits an acute autophagic response mediated by Ulk1 dephosphorylation and its subsequent dissociation from AMPK. *Proc. Natl. Acad. Sci. USA* **2011**, *108*, 4788–4793. [CrossRef] [PubMed]
35. Bach, M.; Larance, M.; James, D.E.; Ramm, G. The serine/threonine kinase ULK1 is a target of multiple phosphorylation events. *Biochem. J.* **2011**, *440*, 283–291. [CrossRef]
36. Egan, D.F.; Chun, M.G.; Vamos, M.; Zou, H.; Rong, J.; Miller, C.J.; Lou, H.J.; Raveendra-Panickar, D.; Yang, C.C.; Sheffler, D.J.; et al. Small Molecule Inhibition of the Autophagy Kinase ULK1 and Identification of ULK1 Substrates. *Mol. Cell* **2015**, *59*, 285–297. [CrossRef]
37. Jung, C.H.; Jun, C.B.; Ro, S.H.; Kim, Y.M.; Otto, N.M.; Cao, J.; Kundu, M.; Kim, D.H. ULK-Atg13-FIP200 complexes mediate mTOR signaling to the autophagy machinery. *Mol. Biol. Cell* **2009**, *20*, 1992–2003. [CrossRef]
38. Wong, P.M.; Feng, Y.; Wang, J.; Shi, R.; Jiang, X. Regulation of autophagy by coordinated action of mTORC1 and protein phosphatase 2A. *Nat. Commun.* **2015**, *6*, 8048. [CrossRef]
39. Torii, S.; Yoshida, T.; Arakawa, S.; Honda, S.; Nakanishi, A.; Shimizu, S. Identification of PPM1D as an essential Ulk1 phosphatase for genotoxic stress-induced autophagy. *EMBO Rep.* **2016**, *17*, 1552–1564. [CrossRef]
40. Park, J.M.; Seo, M.; Jung, C.H.; Grunwald, D.; Stone, M.; Otto, N.M.; Toso, E.; Ahn, Y.; Kyba, M.; Griffin, T.J.; et al. ULK1 phosphorylates Ser30 of BECN1 in association with ATG14 to stimulate autophagy induction. *Autophagy* **2018**, *14*, 584–597. [CrossRef]
41. Russell, R.C.; Tian, Y.; Yuan, H.; Park, H.W.; Chang, Y.Y.; Kim, J.; Kim, H.; Neufeld, T.P.; Dillin, A.; Guan, K.L. ULK1 induces autophagy by phosphorylating Beclin-1 and activating VPS34 lipid kinase. *Nat. Cell Biol.* **2013**, *15*, 741–750. [CrossRef]
42. Tooze, S.A.; Yoshimori, T. The origin of the autophagosomal membrane. *Nat. Cell Biol.* **2010**, *12*, 831–835. [CrossRef]
43. Xu, H.D.; Qin, Z.H. Beclin 1, Bcl-2 and Autophagy. *Adv. Exp. Med. Biol.* **2019**, *1206*, 109–126. [CrossRef] [PubMed]
44. Kuhlbrandt, W. Structure and function of mitochondrial membrane protein complexes. *BMC Biol.* **2015**, *13*, 89. [CrossRef] [PubMed]
45. Gammage, P.A.; Frezza, C. Mitochondrial DNA: The overlooked oncogenome? *BMC Biol.* **2019**, *17*, 53. [CrossRef] [PubMed]
46. Chaban, Y.; Boekema, E.J.; Dudkina, N.V. Structures of mitochondrial oxidative phosphorylation supercomplexes and mechanisms for their stabilisation. *Biochim. Biophys. Acta* **2014**, *1837*, 418–426. [CrossRef]
47. Rimessi, A.; Previati, M.; Nigro, F.; Wieckowski, M.R.; Pinton, P. Mitochondrial reactive oxygen species and inflammation: Molecular mechanisms, diseases and promising therapies. *Int. J. Biochem. Cell Biol.* **2016**, *81*, 281–293. [CrossRef]
48. Patergnani, S.; Danese, A.; Bouhamida, E.; Aguiari, G.; Previati, M.; Pinton, P.; Giorgi, C. Various Aspects of Calcium Signaling in the Regulation of Apoptosis, Autophagy, Cell Proliferation, and Cancer. *Int. J. Mol. Sci.* **2020**, *21*, 8323. [CrossRef]

49. Giorgi, C.; Danese, A.; Missiroli, S.; Patergnani, S.; Pinton, P. Calcium Dynamics as a Machine for Decoding Signals. *Trends Cell Biol.* **2018**, *28*, 258–273. [CrossRef]
50. Perrone, M.; Caroccia, N.; Genovese, I.; Missiroli, S.; Modesti, L.; Pedriali, G.; Vezzani, B.; Vitto, V.A.M.; Antenori, M.; Lebiedzinska-Arciszewska, M.; et al. The role of mitochondria-associated membranes in cellular homeostasis and diseases. *Int. Rev. Cell Mol. Biol.* **2020**, *350*, 119–196. [CrossRef]
51. Patergnani, S.; Missiroli, S.; Marchi, S.; Giorgi, C. Mitochondria-Associated Endoplasmic Reticulum Membranes Microenvironment: Targeting Autophagic and Apoptotic Pathways in Cancer Therapy. *Front. Oncol.* **2015**, *5*, 173. [CrossRef]
52. Marchi, S.; Giorgi, C.; Galluzzi, L.; Pinton, P. Ca^{2+} Fluxes and Cancer. *Mol. Cell* **2020**, *78*, 1055–1069. [CrossRef]
53. Giorgi, C.; Marchi, S.; Pinton, P. The machineries, regulation and cellular functions of mitochondrial calcium. *Nat. Rev. Mol. Cell Biol.* **2018**, *19*, 713–730. [CrossRef] [PubMed]
54. Picca, A.; Mankowski, R.T.; Burman, J.L.; Donisi, L.; Kim, J.S.; Marzetti, E.; Leeuwenburgh, C. Mitochondrial quality control mechanisms as molecular targets in cardiac ageing. *Nat. Rev. Cardiol.* **2018**, *15*, 543–554. [CrossRef] [PubMed]
55. Sato, K.; Sato, M. Multiple ways to prevent transmission of paternal mitochondrial DNA for maternal inheritance in animals. *J. Biochem.* **2017**, *162*, 247–253. [CrossRef]
56. Porter, G.A., Jr.; Hom, J.; Hoffman, D.; Quintanilla, R.; de Mesy Bentley, K.; Sheu, S.S. Bioenergetics, mitochondria, and cardiac myocyte differentiation. *Prog. Pediatric Cardiol.* **2011**, *31*, 75–81. [CrossRef] [PubMed]
57. Sin, J.; Andres, A.M.; Taylor, D.J.; Weston, T.; Hiraumi, Y.; Stotland, A.; Kim, B.J.; Huang, C.; Doran, K.S.; Gottlieb, R.A. Mitophagy is required for mitochondrial biogenesis and myogenic differentiation of C_2C_{12} myoblasts. *Autophagy* **2016**, *12*, 369–380. [CrossRef] [PubMed]
58. Kitada, T.; Asakawa, S.; Hattori, N.; Matsumine, H.; Yamamura, Y.; Minoshima, S.; Yokochi, M.; Mizuno, Y.; Shimizu, N. Mutations in the parkin gene cause autosomal recessive juvenile parkinsonism. *Nature* **1998**, *392*, 605–608. [CrossRef]
59. Ishihara-Paul, L.; Hulihan, M.M.; Kachergus, J.; Upmanyu, R.; Warren, L.; Amouri, R.; Elango, R.; Prinjha, R.K.; Soto, A.; Kefi, M.; et al. PINK1 mutations and parkinsonism. *Neurology* **2008**, *71*, 896–902. [CrossRef] [PubMed]
60. Klein, C.; Djarmati, A.; Hedrich, K.; Schafer, N.; Scaglione, C.; Marchese, R.; Kock, N.; Schule, B.; Hiller, A.; Lohnau, T.; et al. PINK1, Parkin, and DJ-1 mutations in Italian patients with early-onset parkinsonism. *Eur. J. Hum. Genet.* **2005**, *13*, 1086–1093. [CrossRef]
61. Hatano, Y.; Li, Y.; Sato, K.; Asakawa, S.; Yamamura, Y.; Tomiyama, H.; Yoshino, H.; Asahina, M.; Kobayashi, S.; Hassin-Baer, S.; et al. Novel PINK1 mutations in early-onset parkinsonism. *Ann. Neurol.* **2004**, *56*, 424–427. [CrossRef]
62. Ibanez, P.; Lesage, S.; Lohmann, E.; Thobois, S.; De Michele, G.; Borg, M.; Agid, Y.; Durr, A.; Brice, A.; French Parkinson's Disease Genetics Study Group. Mutational analysis of the PINK1 gene in early-onset parkinsonism in Europe and North Africa. *Brain J. Neurol.* **2006**, *129*, 686–694. [CrossRef]
63. Jin, S.M.; Lazarou, M.; Wang, C.; Kane, L.A.; Narendra, D.P.; Youle, R.J. Mitochondrial membrane potential regulates PINK1 import and proteolytic destabilization by PARL. *J. Cell Biol.* **2010**, *191*, 933–942. [CrossRef]
64. Deas, E.; Plun-Favreau, H.; Gandhi, S.; Desmond, H.; Kjaer, S.; Loh, S.H.; Renton, A.E.; Harvey, R.J.; Whitworth, A.J.; Martins, L.M.; et al. PINK1 cleavage at position A103 by the mitochondrial protease PARL. *Hum. Mol. Genet.* **2011**, *20*, 867–879. [CrossRef]
65. Yamano, K.; Youle, R.J. PINK1 is degraded through the N-end rule pathway. *Autophagy* **2013**, *9*, 1758–1769. [CrossRef]
66. Hasson, S.A.; Kane, L.A.; Yamano, K.; Huang, C.H.; Sliter, D.A.; Buehler, E.; Wang, C.; Heman-Ackah, S.M.; Hessa, T.; Guha, R.; et al. High-content genome-wide RNAi screens identify regulators of parkin upstream of mitophagy. *Nature* **2013**, *504*, 291–295. [CrossRef] [PubMed]
67. Lazarou, M.; Jin, S.M.; Kane, L.A.; Youle, R.J. Role of PINK1 binding to the TOM complex and alternate intracellular membranes in recruitment and activation of the E3 ligase Parkin. *Dev. Cell* **2012**, *22*, 320–333. [CrossRef]
68. Okatsu, K.; Oka, T.; Iguchi, M.; Imamura, K.; Kosako, H.; Tani, N.; Kimura, M.; Go, E.; Koyano, F.; Funayama, M.; et al. PINK1 autophosphorylation upon membrane potential dissipation is essential for Parkin recruitment to damaged mitochondria. *Nat. Commun.* **2012**, *3*, 1016. [CrossRef] [PubMed]
69. Kondapalli, C.; Kazlauskaite, A.; Zhang, N.; Woodroof, H.I.; Campbell, D.G.; Gourlay, R.; Burchell, L.; Walden, H.; Macartney, T.J.; Deak, M.; et al. PINK1 is activated by mitochondrial membrane potential depolarization and stimulates Parkin E3 ligase activity by phosphorylating Serine 65. *Open Biol.* **2012**, *2*, 120080. [CrossRef] [PubMed]
70. Geisler, S.; Holmstrom, K.M.; Skujat, D.; Fiesel, F.C.; Rothfuss, O.C.; Kahle, P.J.; Springer, W. PINK1/Parkin-mediated mitophagy is dependent on VDAC1 and p62/SQSTM1. *Nat. Cell Biol.* **2010**, *12*, 119–131. [CrossRef] [PubMed]
71. Pickles, S.; Vigie, P.; Youle, R.J. Mitophagy and Quality Control Mechanisms in Mitochondrial Maintenance. *Curr. Biol.* **2018**, *28*, R170–R185. [CrossRef]
72. Lazarou, M.; Sliter, D.A.; Kane, L.A.; Sarraf, S.A.; Wang, C.; Burman, J.L.; Sideris, D.P.; Fogel, A.I.; Youle, R.J. The ubiquitin kinase PINK1 recruits autophagy receptors to induce mitophagy. *Nature* **2015**, *524*, 309–314. [CrossRef]
73. Yuan, Y.; Zheng, Y.; Zhang, X.; Chen, Y.; Wu, X.; Wu, J.; Shen, Z.; Jiang, L.; Wang, L.; Yang, W.; et al. BNIP3L/NIX-mediated mitophagy protects against ischemic brain injury independent of PARK2. *Autophagy* **2017**, *13*, 1754–1766. [CrossRef]
74. Shi, R.Y.; Zhu, S.H.; Li, V.; Gibson, S.B.; Xu, X.S.; Kong, J.M. BNIP3 interacting with LC3 triggers excessive mitophagy in delayed neuronal death in stroke. *CNS Neurosci. Ther.* **2014**, *20*, 1045–1055. [CrossRef]
75. Liu, L.; Feng, D.; Chen, G.; Chen, M.; Zheng, Q.; Song, P.; Ma, Q.; Zhu, C.; Wang, R.; Qi, W.; et al. Mitochondrial outer-membrane protein FUNDC1 mediates hypoxia-induced mitophagy in mammalian cells. *Nat. Cell Biol.* **2012**, *14*, 177–185. [CrossRef]

76. Strappazzon, F.; Nazio, F.; Corrado, M.; Cianfanelli, V.; Romagnoli, A.; Fimia, G.M.; Campello, S.; Nardacci, R.; Piacentini, M.; Campanella, M.; et al. AMBRA1 is able to induce mitophagy via LC3 binding, regardless of PARKIN and p62/SQSTM1. *Cell Death Differ.* **2015**, *22*, 419–432. [CrossRef]
77. Lublin, F.D.; Reingold, S.C.; Cohen, J.A.; Cutter, G.R.; Sorensen, P.S.; Thompson, A.J.; Wolinsky, J.S.; Balcer, L.J.; Banwell, B.; Barkhof, F.; et al. Defining the clinical course of multiple sclerosis: The 2013 revisions. *Neurology* **2014**, *83*, 278–286. [CrossRef]
78. Lublin, F.D. New multiple sclerosis phenotypic classification. *Eur. Neurol.* **2014**, *72* (Suppl. S1), 1–5. [CrossRef] [PubMed]
79. Alirezaei, M.; Fox, H.S.; Flynn, C.T.; Moore, C.S.; Hebb, A.L.; Frausto, R.F.; Bhan, V.; Kiosses, W.B.; Whitton, J.L.; Robertson, G.S.; et al. Elevated ATG5 expression in autoimmune demyelination and multiple sclerosis. *Autophagy* **2009**, *5*, 152–158. [CrossRef] [PubMed]
80. Paunovic, V.; Petrovic, I.V.; Milenkovic, M.; Janjetovic, K.; Pravica, V.; Dujmovic, I.; Milosevic, E.; Martinovic, V.; Mesaros, S.; Drulovic, J.; et al. Autophagy-independent increase of ATG5 expression in T cells of multiple sclerosis patients. *J. Neuroimmunol.* **2018**, *319*, 100–105. [CrossRef] [PubMed]
81. Becher, J.; Simula, L.; Volpe, E.; Procaccini, C.; La Rocca, C.; D'Acunzo, P.; Cianfanelli, V.; Strappazzon, F.; Caruana, I.; Nazio, F.; et al. AMBRA1 Controls Regulatory T-Cell Differentiation and Homeostasis Upstream of the FOXO3-FOXP3 Axis. *Dev. Cell* **2018**, *47*, 592–607.e6. [CrossRef] [PubMed]
82. Akatsuka, H.; Kuga, S.; Masuhara, K.; Davaadorj, O.; Okada, C.; Iida, Y.; Okada, Y.; Fukunishi, N.; Suzuki, T.; Hosomichi, K.; et al. AMBRA1 is involved in T cell receptor-mediated metabolic reprogramming through an ATG7-independent pathway. *Biochem. Biophys. Res. Commun.* **2017**, *491*, 1098–1104. [CrossRef]
83. Astier, A.L. T-cell regulation by CD46 and its relevance in multiple sclerosis. *Immunology* **2008**, *124*, 149–154. [CrossRef] [PubMed]
84. Joubert, P.E.; Meiffren, G.; Gregoire, I.P.; Pontini, G.; Richetta, C.; Flacher, M.; Azocar, O.; Vidalain, P.O.; Vidal, M.; Lotteau, V.; et al. Autophagy induction by the pathogen receptor CD46. *Cell Host Microbe* **2009**, *6*, 354–366. [CrossRef] [PubMed]
85. Soldan, S.S.; Fogdell-Hahn, A.; Brennan, M.B.; Mittleman, B.B.; Ballerini, C.; Massacesi, L.; Seya, T.; McFarland, H.F.; Jacobson, S. Elevated serum and cerebrospinal fluid levels of soluble human herpesvirus type 6 cellular receptor, membrane cofactor protein, in patients with multiple sclerosis. *Ann. Neurol.* **2001**, *50*, 486–493. [CrossRef] [PubMed]
86. Xu, H.; Wu, Z.Y.; Fang, F.; Guo, L.; Chen, D.; Chen, J.X.; Stern, D.; Taylor, G.A.; Jiang, H.; Yan, S.S. Genetic deficiency of Irgm1 (LRG-47) suppresses induction of experimental autoimmune encephalomyelitis by promoting apoptosis of activated CD4+ T cells. *FASEB J.* **2010**, *24*, 1583–1592. [CrossRef]
87. Singh, S.B.; Ornatowski, W.; Vergne, I.; Naylor, J.; Delgado, M.; Roberts, E.; Ponpuak, M.; Master, S.; Pilli, M.; White, E.; et al. Human IRGM regulates autophagy and cell-autonomous immunity functions through mitochondria. *Nat. Cell Biol.* **2010**, *12*, 1154–1165. [CrossRef]
88. Guo, X.; Zhang, W.; Wang, C.; Zhang, B.; Li, R.; Zhang, L.; Zhao, K.; Li, Y.; Tian, L.; Li, B.; et al. IRGM promotes the PINK1-mediated mitophagy through the degradation of Mitofilin in SH-SY5Y cells. *FASEB J.* **2020**, *34*, 14768–14779. [CrossRef]
89. Bhattacharya, A.; Parillon, X.; Zeng, S.; Han, M.; Eissa, N.T. Deficiency of autophagy in dendritic cells protects against experimental autoimmune encephalomyelitis. *J. Biol. Chem.* **2014**, *289*, 26525–26532. [CrossRef]
90. Bonora, M.; De Marchi, E.; Patergnani, S.; Suski, J.M.; Celsi, F.; Bononi, A.; Giorgi, C.; Marchi, S.; Rimessi, A.; Duszynski, J.; et al. Tumor necrosis factor-alpha impairs oligodendroglial differentiation through a mitochondria-dependent process. *Cell Death Differ.* **2014**, *21*, 1198–1208. [CrossRef]
91. Holman, S.P.; Lobo, A.S.; Novorolsky, R.J.; Nichols, M.; Fiander, M.D.J.; Konda, P.; Kennedy, B.E.; Gujar, S.; Robertson, G.S. Neuronal mitochondrial calcium uniporter deficiency exacerbates axonal injury and suppresses remyelination in mice subjected to experimental autoimmune encephalomyelitis. *Exp. Neurol.* **2020**, *333*, 113430. [CrossRef]
92. Castellazzi, M.; Patergnani, S.; Donadio, M.; Giorgi, C.; Bonora, M.; Fainardi, E.; Casetta, I.; Granieri, E.; Pugliatti, M.; Pinton, P. Correlation between auto/mitophagic processes and magnetic resonance imaging activity in multiple sclerosis patients. *J. Neuroinflamm.* **2019**, *16*, 131. [CrossRef]
93. Albanese, M.; Zagaglia, S.; Landi, D.; Boffa, L.; Nicoletti, C.G.; Marciani, M.G.; Mandolesi, G.; Marfia, G.A.; Buttari, F.; Mori, F.; et al. Cerebrospinal fluid lactate is associated with multiple sclerosis disease progression. *J. Neuroinflamm.* **2016**, *13*, 36. [CrossRef]
94. Joodi Khanghah, O.; Nourazarian, A.; Khaki-Khatibi, F.; Nikanfar, M.; Laghousi, D.; Vatankhah, A.M.; Moharami, S. Evaluation of the Diagnostic and Predictive Value of Serum Levels of ANT1, ATG5, and Parkin in Multiple Sclerosis. *Clin. Neurol. Neurosurg.* **2020**, *197*, 106197. [CrossRef]
95. Hassanpour, M.; Cheraghi, O.; Laghusi, D.; Nouri, M.; Panahi, Y. The relationship between ANT1 and NFL with autophagy and mitophagy markers in patients with multiple sclerosis. *J. Clin. Neurosci.* **2020**, *78*, 307–312. [CrossRef]
96. Harberts, E.; Datta, D.; Chen, S.; Wohler, J.E.; Oh, U.; Jacobson, S. Translocator protein 18 kDa (TSPO) expression in multiple sclerosis patients. *J. Neuroimmune Pharmacol.* **2013**, *8*, 51–57. [CrossRef]
97. Nohara, S.; Ishii, A.; Yamamoto, F.; Yanagiha, K.; Moriyama, T.; Tozaka, N.; Miyake, Z.; Yatsuga, S.; Koga, Y.; Hosaka, T.; et al. GDF-15, a mitochondrial disease biomarker, is associated with the severity of multiple sclerosis. *J. Neurol. Sci.* **2019**, *405*, 116429. [CrossRef] [PubMed]
98. Vezzani, B.; Carinci, M.; Patergnani, S.; Pasquin, M.P.; Guarino, A.; Aziz, N.; Pinton, P.; Simonato, M.; Giorgi, C. The Dichotomous Role of Inflammation in the CNS: A Mitochondrial Point of View. *Biomolecules* **2020**, *10*, 1437. [CrossRef] [PubMed]
99. Huang, W.J.; Zhang, X.; Chen, W.W. Role of oxidative stress in Alzheimer's disease. *Biomed. Rep.* **2016**, *4*, 519–522. [CrossRef] [PubMed]

100. Mark, R.J.; Pang, Z.; Geddes, J.W.; Uchida, K.; Mattson, M.P. Amyloid beta-peptide impairs glucose transport in hippocampal and cortical neurons: Involvement of membrane lipid peroxidation. *J. Neurosci.* **1997**, *17*, 1046–1054. [CrossRef]
101. De Wilde, M.C.; Vellas, B.; Girault, E.; Yavuz, A.C.; Sijben, J.W. Lower brain and blood nutrient status in Alzheimer's disease: Results from meta-analyses. *Alzheimer's Dement.* **2017**, *3*, 416–431. [CrossRef]
102. Luth, H.J.; Munch, G.; Arendt, T. Aberrant expression of NOS isoforms in Alzheimer's disease is structurally related to nitrotyrosine formation. *Brain Res.* **2002**, *953*, 135–143. [CrossRef]
103. Kerr, J.S.; Adriaanse, B.A.; Greig, N.H.; Mattson, M.P.; Cader, M.Z.; Bohr, V.A.; Fang, E.F. Mitophagy and Alzheimer's Disease: Cellular and Molecular Mechanisms. *Trends Neurosci.* **2017**, *40*, 151–166. [CrossRef]
104. Nixon, R.A.; Wegiel, J.; Kumar, A.; Yu, W.H.; Peterhoff, C.; Cataldo, A.; Cuervo, A.M. Extensive involvement of autophagy in Alzheimer disease: An immuno-electron microscopy study. *J. Neuropathol. Exp. Neurol.* **2005**, *64*, 113–122. [CrossRef]
105. Nilsson, P.; Loganathan, K.; Sekiguchi, M.; Matsuba, Y.; Hui, K.; Tsubuki, S.; Tanaka, M.; Iwata, N.; Saito, T.; Saido, T.C. Abeta secretion and plaque formation depend on autophagy. *Cell Rep.* **2013**, *5*, 61–69. [CrossRef]
106. Piras, A.; Collin, L.; Gruninger, F.; Graff, C.; Ronnback, A. Autophagic and lysosomal defects in human tauopathies: Analysis of post-mortem brain from patients with familial Alzheimer disease, corticobasal degeneration and progressive supranuclear palsy. *Acta Neuropathol. Commun.* **2016**, *4*, 22. [CrossRef] [PubMed]
107. Inoue, K.; Rispoli, J.; Kaphzan, H.; Klann, E.; Chen, E.I.; Kim, J.; Komatsu, M.; Abeliovich, A. Macroautophagy deficiency mediates age-dependent neurodegeneration through a phospho-tau pathway. *Mol. Neurodegener.* **2012**, *7*, 48. [CrossRef]
108. Kesharwani, R.; Sarmah, D.; Kaur, H.; Mounika, L.; Verma, G.; Pabbala, V.; Kotian, V.; Kalia, K.; Borah, A.; Dave, K.R.; et al. Interplay between Mitophagy and Inflammasomes in Neurological Disorders. *ACS Chem. Neurosci.* **2019**, *10*, 2195–2208. [CrossRef] [PubMed]
109. Martin-Maestro, P.; Gargini, R.; Perry, G.; Avila, J.; Garcia-Escudero, V. PARK2 enhancement is able to compensate mitophagy alterations found in sporadic Alzheimer's disease. *Hum. Mol. Genet.* **2016**, *25*, 792–806. [CrossRef]
110. Fang, E.F.; Hou, Y.; Palikaras, K.; Adriaanse, B.A.; Kerr, J.S.; Yang, B.; Lautrup, S.; Hasan-Olive, M.M.; Caponio, D.; Dan, X.; et al. Mitophagy inhibits amyloid-beta and tau pathology and reverses cognitive deficits in models of Alzheimer's disease. *Nat. Neurosci.* **2019**, *22*, 401–412. [CrossRef] [PubMed]
111. Schwagerl, A.L.; Mohan, P.S.; Cataldo, A.M.; Vonsattel, J.P.; Kowall, N.W.; Nixon, R.A. Elevated levels of the endosomal-lysosomal proteinase cathepsin D in cerebrospinal fluid in Alzheimer disease. *J. Neurochem.* **1995**, *64*, 443–446. [CrossRef]
112. Sundelof, J.; Sundstrom, J.; Hansson, O.; Eriksdotter-Jonhagen, M.; Giedraitis, V.; Larsson, A.; Degerman-Gunnarsson, M.; Ingelsson, M.; Minthon, L.; Blennow, K.; et al. Higher cathepsin B levels in plasma in Alzheimer's disease compared to healthy controls. *J. Alzheimer's Dis.* **2010**, *22*, 1223–1230. [CrossRef]
113. Armstrong, A.; Mattsson, N.; Appelqvist, H.; Janefjord, C.; Sandin, L.; Agholme, L.; Olsson, B.; Svensson, S.; Blennow, K.; Zetterberg, H.; et al. Lysosomal network proteins as potential novel CSF biomarkers for Alzheimer's disease. *Neuromol. Med.* **2014**, *16*, 150–160. [CrossRef]
114. Sjodin, S.; Brinkmalm, G.; Ohrfelt, A.; Parnetti, L.; Paciotti, S.; Hansson, O.; Hardy, J.; Blennow, K.; Zetterberg, H.; Brinkmalm, A. Endo-lysosomal proteins and ubiquitin CSF concentrations in Alzheimer's and Parkinson's disease. *Alzheimer's Res. Ther.* **2019**, *11*, 82. [CrossRef]
115. Francois, A.; Julian, A.; Ragot, S.; Dugast, E.; Blanchard, L.; Brishoual, S.; Terro, F.; Chassaing, D.; Page, G.; Paccalin, M. Inflammatory Stress on Autophagy in Peripheral Blood Mononuclear Cells from Patients with Alzheimer's Disease during 24 Months of Follow-Up. *PLoS ONE* **2015**, *10*, e0138326. [CrossRef]
116. Devi, L.; Raghavendran, V.; Prabhu, B.M.; Avadhani, N.G.; Anandatheerthavarada, H.K. Mitochondrial import and accumulation of alpha-synuclein impair complex I in human dopaminergic neuronal cultures and Parkinson disease brain. *J. Biol. Chem.* **2008**, *283*, 9089–9100. [CrossRef]
117. Di Maio, R.; Barrett, P.J.; Hoffman, E.K.; Barrett, C.W.; Zharikov, A.; Borah, A.; Hu, X.; McCoy, J.; Chu, C.T.; Burton, E.A.; et al. alpha-Synuclein binds to TOM20 and inhibits mitochondrial protein import in Parkinson's disease. *Sci. Transl. Med.* **2016**, *8*, 342ra378. [CrossRef]
118. Walter, J.; Bolognin, S.; Antony, P.M.A.; Nickels, S.L.; Poovathingal, S.K.; Salamanca, L.; Magni, S.; Perfeito, R.; Hoel, F.; Qing, X.; et al. Neural Stem Cells of Parkinson's Disease Patients Exhibit Aberrant Mitochondrial Morphology and Functionality. *Stem Cell Rep.* **2019**, *12*, 878–889. [CrossRef] [PubMed]
119. Ordureau, A.; Sarraf, S.A.; Duda, D.M.; Heo, J.M.; Jedrychowski, M.P.; Sviderskiy, V.O.; Olszewski, J.L.; Koerber, J.T.; Xie, T.; Beausoleil, S.A.; et al. Quantitative proteomics reveal a feedforward mechanism for mitochondrial PARKIN translocation and ubiquitin chain synthesis. *Mol. Cell* **2014**, *56*, 360–375. [CrossRef] [PubMed]
120. Hou, X.; Fiesel, F.C.; Truban, D.; Castanedes Casey, M.; Lin, W.L.; Soto, A.I.; Tacik, P.; Rousseau, L.G.; Diehl, N.N.; Heckman, M.G.; et al. Age- and disease-dependent increase of the mitophagy marker phospho-ubiquitin in normal aging and Lewy body disease. *Autophagy* **2018**, *14*, 1404–1418. [CrossRef] [PubMed]
121. McLelland, G.L.; Goiran, T.; Yi, W.; Dorval, G.; Chen, C.X.; Lauinger, N.D.; Krahn, A.I.; Valimehr, S.; Rakovic, A.; Rouiller, I.; et al. Mfn2 ubiquitination by PINK1/parkin gates the p97-dependent release of ER from mitochondria to drive mitophagy. *Elife* **2018**, *7*. [CrossRef] [PubMed]
122. Chen, Y.; Dorn, G.W., 2nd. PINK1-phosphorylated mitofusin 2 is a Parkin receptor for culling damaged mitochondria. *Science* **2013**, *340*, 471–475. [CrossRef]

123. Rakovic, A.; Grunewald, A.; Kottwitz, J.; Bruggemann, N.; Pramstaller, P.P.; Lohmann, K.; Klein, C. Mutations in PINK1 and Parkin impair ubiquitination of Mitofusins in human fibroblasts. *PLoS ONE* **2011**, *6*, e16746. [CrossRef]
124. Rodriguez-Arribas, M.; Yakhine-Diop, S.M.S.; Pedro, J.M.B.; Gomez-Suaga, P.; Gomez-Sanchez, R.; Martinez-Chacon, G.; Fuentes, J.M.; Gonzalez-Polo, R.A.; Niso-Santano, M. Mitochondria-Associated Membranes (MAMs): Overview and Its Role in Parkinson's Disease. *Mol. Neurobiol.* **2017**, *54*, 6287–6303. [CrossRef] [PubMed]
125. Gautier, C.A.; Erpapazoglou, Z.; Mouton-Liger, F.; Muriel, M.P.; Cormier, F.; Bigou, S.; Duffaure, S.; Girard, M.; Foret, B.; Iannielli, A.; et al. The endoplasmic reticulum-mitochondria interface is perturbed in PARK2 knockout mice and patients with PARK2 mutations. *Hum. Mol. Genet.* **2016**, *25*, 2972–2984. [CrossRef]
126. Missiroli, S.; Bonora, M.; Patergnani, S.; Poletti, F.; Perrone, M.; Gafa, R.; Magri, E.; Raimondi, A.; Lanza, G.; Tacchetti, C.; et al. PML at Mitochondria-Associated Membranes Is Critical for the Repression of Autophagy and Cancer Development. *Cell Rep.* **2016**, *16*, 2415–2427. [CrossRef]
127. Bonifati, V.; Rizzu, P.; van Baren, M.J.; Schaap, O.; Breedveld, G.J.; Krieger, E.; Dekker, M.C.; Squitieri, F.; Ibanez, P.; Joosse, M.; et al. Mutations in the DJ-1 gene associated with autosomal recessive early-onset parkinsonism. *Science* **2003**, *299*, 256–259. [CrossRef] [PubMed]
128. Ottolini, D.; Cali, T.; Negro, A.; Brini, M. The Parkinson disease-related protein DJ-1 counteracts mitochondrial impairment induced by the tumour suppressor protein p53 by enhancing endoplasmic reticulum-mitochondria tethering. *Hum. Mol. Genet.* **2013**, *22*, 2152–2168. [CrossRef]
129. Kara, E.; Ling, H.; Pittman, A.M.; Shaw, K.; de Silva, R.; Simone, R.; Holton, J.L.; Warren, J.D.; Rohrer, J.D.; Xiromerisiou, G.; et al. The MAPT p.A152T variant is a risk factor associated with tauopathies with atypical clinical and neuropathological features. *Neurobiol. Aging* **2012**, *33*, 2231.e7–2231.e14. [CrossRef]
130. Lewis, J.; McGowan, E.; Rockwood, J.; Melrose, H.; Nacharaju, P.; Van Slegtenhorst, M.; Gwinn-Hardy, K.; Paul Murphy, M.; Baker, M.; Yu, X.; et al. Neurofibrillary tangles, amyotrophy and progressive motor disturbance in mice expressing mutant (P301L) tau protein. *Nat. Genet.* **2000**, *25*, 402–405. [CrossRef]
131. Walker, R.H.; Friedman, J.; Wiener, J.; Hobler, R.; Gwinn-Hardy, K.; Adam, A.; DeWolfe, J.; Gibbs, R.; Baker, M.; Farrer, M.; et al. A family with a tau P301L mutation presenting with parkinsonism. *Parkinsonism Relat. Disord.* **2002**, *9*, 121–123. [CrossRef]
132. Caballero, B.; Wang, Y.; Diaz, A.; Tasset, I.; Juste, Y.R.; Stiller, B.; Mandelkow, E.M.; Mandelkow, E.; Cuervo, A.M. Interplay of pathogenic forms of human tau with different autophagic pathways. *Aging Cell* **2018**, *17*. [CrossRef] [PubMed]
133. Youn, J.; Lee, S.B.; Lee, H.S.; Yang, H.O.; Park, J.; Kim, J.S.; Oh, E.; Park, S.; Jang, W. Cerebrospinal Fluid Levels of Autophagy-related Proteins Represent Potentially Novel Biomarkers of Early-Stage Parkinson's Disease. *Sci. Rep.* **2018**, *8*, 16866. [CrossRef]
134. Zhang, X.; Gao, F.; Wang, D.; Li, C.; Fu, Y.; He, W.; Zhang, J. Tau Pathology in Parkinson's Disease. *Front. Neurol.* **2018**, *9*, 809. [CrossRef]
135. Boman, A.; Svensson, S.; Boxer, A.; Rojas, J.C.; Seeley, W.W.; Karydas, A.; Miller, B.; Kagedal, K.; Svenningsson, P. Distinct Lysosomal Network Protein Profiles in Parkinsonian Syndrome Cerebrospinal Fluid. *J. Parkinson's Dis.* **2016**, *6*, 307–315. [CrossRef]
136. Klaver, A.C.; Coffey, M.P.; Aasly, J.O.; Loeffler, D.A. CSF lamp2 concentrations are decreased in female Parkinson's disease patients with LRRK2 mutations. *Brain Res.* **2018**, *1683*, 12–16. [CrossRef]
137. Miki, Y.; Shimoyama, S.; Kon, T.; Ueno, T.; Hayakari, R.; Tanji, K.; Matsumiya, T.; Tsushima, E.; Mori, F.; Wakabayashi, K.; et al. Alteration of autophagy-related proteins in peripheral blood mononuclear cells of patients with Parkinson's disease. *Neurobiol. Aging* **2018**, *63*, 33–43. [CrossRef]
138. Pyle, A.; Anugrha, H.; Kurzawa-Akanbi, M.; Yarnall, A.; Burn, D.; Hudson, G. Reduced mitochondrial DNA copy number is a biomarker of Parkinson's disease. *Neurobiol. Aging* **2016**, *38*, 216.e7–216.e10. [CrossRef] [PubMed]
139. Gui, Y.X.; Xu, Z.P.; Lv, W.; Zhao, J.J.; Hu, X.Y. Evidence for polymerase gamma, POLG1 variation in reduced mitochondrial DNA copy number in Parkinson's disease. *Parkinsonism Relat. Disord.* **2015**, *21*, 282–286. [CrossRef]
140. Podlesniy, P.; Vilas, D.; Taylor, P.; Shaw, L.M.; Tolosa, E.; Trullas, R. Mitochondrial DNA in CSF distinguishes LRRK2 from idiopathic Parkinson's disease. *Neurobiol. Dis.* **2016**, *94*, 10–17. [CrossRef] [PubMed]
141. Iacobazzi, V.; Castegna, A.; Infantino, V.; Andria, G. Mitochondrial DNA methylation as a next-generation biomarker and diagnostic tool. *Mol. Genet. Metab.* **2013**, *110*, 25–34. [CrossRef] [PubMed]
142. Siman, R.; Cocca, R.; Dong, Y. The mTOR Inhibitor Rapamycin Mitigates Perforant Pathway Neurodegeneration and Synapse Loss in a Mouse Model of Early-Stage Alzheimer-Type Tauopathy. *PLoS ONE* **2015**, *10*, e0142340. [CrossRef] [PubMed]
143. Berger, Z.; Ravikumar, B.; Menzies, F.M.; Oroz, L.G.; Underwood, B.R.; Pangalos, M.N.; Schmitt, I.; Wullner, U.; Evert, B.O.; O'Kane, C.J.; et al. Rapamycin alleviates toxicity of different aggregate-prone proteins. *Hum. Mol. Genet.* **2006**, *15*, 433–442. [CrossRef] [PubMed]
144. Jiang, T.; Yu, J.T.; Zhu, X.C.; Zhang, Q.Q.; Cao, L.; Wang, H.F.; Tan, M.S.; Gao, Q.; Qin, H.; Zhang, Y.D.; et al. Temsirolimus attenuates tauopathy in vitro and in vivo by targeting tau hyperphosphorylation and autophagic clearance. *Neuropharmacology* **2014**, *85*, 121–130. [CrossRef]
145. Steele, J.W.; Lachenmayer, M.L.; Ju, S.; Stock, A.; Liken, J.; Kim, S.H.; Delgado, L.M.; Alfaro, I.E.; Bernales, S.; Verdile, G.; et al. Latrepirdine improves cognition and arrests progression of neuropathology in an Alzheimer's mouse model. *Mol. Psychiatry* **2013**, *18*, 889–897. [CrossRef] [PubMed]
146. Wu, Y.; Li, X.; Zhu, J.X.; Xie, W.; Le, W.; Fan, Z.; Jankovic, J.; Pan, T. Resveratrol-activated AMPK/SIRT1/autophagy in cellular models of Parkinson's disease. *Neuro-Signals* **2011**, *19*, 163–174. [CrossRef] [PubMed]

147. Gao, J.; Perera, G.; Bhadbhade, M.; Halliday, G.M.; Dzamko, N. Autophagy activation promotes clearance of alpha-synuclein inclusions in fibril-seeded human neural cells. *J. Biol. Chem.* **2019**, *294*, 14241–14256. [CrossRef]
148. Papp, D.; Kovacs, T.; Billes, V.; Varga, M.; Tarnoci, A.; Hackler, L., Jr.; Puskas, L.G.; Liliom, H.; Tarnok, K.; Schlett, K.; et al. AUTEN-67, an autophagy-enhancing drug candidate with potent antiaging and neuroprotective effects. *Autophagy* **2016**, *12*, 273–286. [CrossRef]
149. Kovacs, T.; Billes, V.; Komlos, M.; Hotzi, B.; Manzeger, A.; Tarnoci, A.; Papp, D.; Szikszai, F.; Szinyakovics, J.; Racz, A.; et al. The small molecule AUTEN-99 (autophagy enhancer-99) prevents the progression of neurodegenerative symptoms. *Sci. Rep.* **2017**, *7*, 42014. [CrossRef]
150. Sarkar, S.; Floto, R.A.; Berger, Z.; Imarisio, S.; Cordenier, A.; Pasco, M.; Cook, L.J.; Rubinsztein, D.C. Lithium induces autophagy by inhibiting inositol monophosphatase. *J. Cell Biol.* **2005**, *170*, 1101–1111. [CrossRef]
151. Forlenza, O.V.; De-Paula, V.J.; Diniz, B.S. Neuroprotective effects of lithium: Implications for the treatment of Alzheimer's disease and related neurodegenerative disorders. *ACS Chem. Neurosci.* **2014**, *5*, 443–450. [CrossRef]
152. Forlenza, O.V.; Diniz, B.S.; Radanovic, M.; Santos, F.S.; Talib, L.L.; Gattaz, W.F. Disease-modifying properties of long-term lithium treatment for amnestic mild cognitive impairment: Randomised controlled trial. *Br. J. Psychiatry* **2011**, *198*, 351–356. [CrossRef] [PubMed]
153. Klucken, J.; Poehler, A.M.; Ebrahimi-Fakhari, D.; Schneider, J.; Nuber, S.; Rockenstein, E.; Schlotzer-Schrehardt, U.; Hyman, B.T.; McLean, P.J.; Masliah, E.; et al. Alpha-synuclein aggregation involves a bafilomycin A 1-sensitive autophagy pathway. *Autophagy* **2012**, *8*, 754–766. [CrossRef] [PubMed]
154. Zhang, J.Y.; Peng, C.; Shi, H.; Wang, S.; Wang, Q.; Wang, J.Z. Inhibition of autophagy causes tau proteolysis by activating calpain in rat brain. *J. Alzheimer's Dis.* **2009**, *16*, 39–47. [CrossRef]
155. Thome, R.; Moraes, A.S.; Bombeiro, A.L.; Farias Ados, S.; Francelin, C.; da Costa, T.A.; Di Gangi, R.; dos Santos, L.M.; de Oliveira, A.L.; Verinaud, L. Chloroquine treatment enhances regulatory T cells and reduces the severity of experimental autoimmune encephalomyelitis. *PLoS ONE* **2013**, *8*, e65913. [CrossRef]
156. Thome, R.; Issayama, L.K.; DiGangi, R.; Bombeiro, A.L.; da Costa, T.A.; Ferreira, I.T.; de Oliveira, A.L.; Verinaud, L. Dendritic cells treated with chloroquine modulate experimental autoimmune encephalomyelitis. *Immunol. Cell Biol.* **2014**, *92*, 124–132. [CrossRef] [PubMed]
157. Sachs, H.H.; Bercury, K.K.; Popescu, D.C.; Narayanan, S.P.; Macklin, W.B. A new model of cuprizone-mediated demyelination/remyelination. *ASN Neuro* **2014**, *6*. [CrossRef]
158. Yamate-Morgan, H.; Lauderdale, K.; Horeczko, J.; Merchant, U.; Tiwari-Woodruff, S.K. Functional Effects of Cuprizone-Induced Demyelination in the Presence of the mTOR-Inhibitor Rapamycin. *Neuroscience* **2019**, *406*, 667–683. [CrossRef] [PubMed]
159. Lisi, L.; Navarra, P.; Cirocchi, R.; Sharp, A.; Stigliano, E.; Feinstein, D.L.; Dello Russo, C. Rapamycin reduces clinical signs and neuropathic pain in a chronic model of experimental autoimmune encephalomyelitis. *J. Neuroimmunol.* **2012**, *243*, 43–51. [CrossRef] [PubMed]
160. Bagherpour, B.; Salehi, M.; Jafari, R.; Bagheri, A.; Kiani-Esfahani, A.; Edalati, M.; Kardi, M.T.; Shaygannejad, V. Promising effect of rapamycin on multiple sclerosis. *Mult. Scler. Relat. Disord.* **2018**, *26*, 40–45. [CrossRef] [PubMed]
161. Hertz, N.T.; Berthet, A.; Sos, M.L.; Thorn, K.S.; Burlingame, A.L.; Nakamura, K.; Shokat, K.M. A neo-substrate that amplifies catalytic activity of parkinson's-disease-related kinase PINK1. *Cell* **2013**, *154*, 737–747. [CrossRef]
162. Orr, A.L.; Rutaganira, F.U.; de Roulet, D.; Huang, E.J.; Hertz, N.T.; Shokat, K.M.; Nakamura, K. Long-term oral kinetin does not protect against alpha-synuclein-induced neurodegeneration in rodent models of Parkinson's disease. *Neurochem. Int.* **2017**, *109*, 106–116. [CrossRef] [PubMed]
163. Shiba-Fukushima, K.; Inoshita, T.; Sano, O.; Iwata, H.; Ishikawa, K.I.; Okano, H.; Akamatsu, W.; Imai, Y.; Hattori, N. A Cell-Based High-Throughput Screening Identified Two Compounds that Enhance PINK1-Parkin Signaling. *iScience* **2020**, *23*, 101048. [CrossRef]
164. Moskal, N.; Riccio, V.; Bashkurov, M.; Taddese, R.; Datti, A.; Lewis, P.N.; Angus McQuibban, G. ROCK inhibitors upregulate the neuroprotective Parkin-mediated mitophagy pathway. *Nat. Commun.* **2020**, *11*, 88. [CrossRef] [PubMed]
165. Zetterberg, H.; Burnham, S.C. Blood-based molecular biomarkers for Alzheimer's disease. *Mol. Brain* **2019**, *12*, 26. [CrossRef] [PubMed]

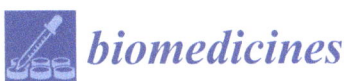

Review

News about the Role of Fluid and Imaging Biomarkers in Neurodegenerative Diseases

Jacopo Meldolesi

Division of Neuroscience, San Raffaele Institute and Vita-Salute San Raffaele University, via Olgettina 58, 20132 Milan, Italy; meldolesi.jacopo@hsr.it

Abstract: Biomarkers are molecules that are variable in their origin, nature, and mechanism of action; they are of great relevance in biology and also in medicine because of their specific connection with a single or several diseases. Biomarkers are of two types, which in some cases are operative with each other. Fluid biomarkers, started around 2000, are generated in fluid from specific proteins/peptides and miRNAs accumulated within two extracellular fluids, either the central spinal fluid or blood plasma. The switch of these proteins/peptides and miRNAs, from free to segregated within extracellular vesicles, has induced certain advantages including higher levels within fluids and lower operative expenses. Imaging biomarkers, started around 2004, are identified in vivo upon their binding by radiolabeled molecules subsequently revealed in the brain by positron emission tomography and/or other imaging techniques. A positive point for the latter approach is the quantitation of results, but expenses are much higher. At present, both types of biomarker are being extensively employed to study Alzheimer's and other neurodegenerative diseases, investigated from the presymptomatic to mature stages. In conclusion, biomarkers have revolutionized scientific and medical research and practice. Diagnosis, which is often inadequate when based on medical criteria only, has been recently improved by the multiplicity and specificity of biomarkers. Analogous results have been obtained for prognosis. In contrast, improvement of therapy has been limited or fully absent, especially for Alzheimer's in which progress has been inadequate. An urgent need at hand is therefore the progress of a new drug trial design together with patient management in clinical practice.

Keywords: neurons; astrocytes; Alzheimer's and Parkinson's diseases; fluid and imaging biomarkers; amyloid-β and tau; miRNA; extracellular vesicles; exosomes and ectosomes; PET; radiotracers; radiolabeled molecules

Citation: Meldolesi, J. News about the Role of Fluid and Imaging Biomarkers in Neurodegenerative Diseases. *Biomedicines* **2021**, *9*, 252. https://doi.org/10.3390/biomedicines9030252

Academic Editor: Arnab Ghosh

Received: 28 January 2021
Accepted: 26 February 2021
Published: 4 March 2021

Publisher's Note: MDPI stays neutral with regard to jurisdictional claims in published maps and institutional affiliations.

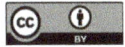

Copyright: © 2021 by the author. Licensee MDPI, Basel, Switzerland. This article is an open access article distributed under the terms and conditions of the Creative Commons Attribution (CC BY) license (https://creativecommons.org/licenses/by/4.0/).

1. Introduction

Biomarkers are molecules that are highly variable in their origin, nature, and mechanism of action, and they are connected to or are directly involved to single or various peculiar diseases. At present, biomarkers, which are addressed to cells, organs, or structures, exist for almost all diseases, including cancers. Among them, neurodegenerative diseases are receiving the greatest attention. During the last 20 years, articles about their biomarkers published in known journals have totaled over 20,000, including about 4000 reviews. Investigations of their properties, going from specificity to the mechanisms of their action, are often used to clarify various aspects of pathogenesis. Such results often play roles in processes of medical relevance, such as diagnosis, prognosis, and also therapy, and they are useful for patients and also for clinical practice. However, the relevance of biomarkers in clinical practice is variable. Some of them are well known and widely used; for others, however, knowledge is still questioned due to, for example, their limited specificity. In this review such limitations are not further illustrated. The properties of biomarkers presented here are those of general significance, identified in the last few years. Information about additional aspects can be found in other publications [1,2].

Compared to biomarkers of other organs, biomarkers of the brain exhibit distinct properties [3,4]. Initial studies about two types, the fluid and the imaging biomarkers, were developed separately. Biomarkers of the first type appeared around 2000. They are collected not in vivo but in fluid, within either of two fluids taken from patients, the central spinal fluid (CSF) and the blood plasma [5,6]. Biomarkers of the second type were developed by the use of radiolabeled molecules. Upon penetration into the living brain, these molecules are bound with high specificity as revealed by positron emission tomography (PET) imaging. A biomarker study by the latter approach, addressed to amyloid-β (Aβ) plaques of Alzheimer's disease (AD), was published in 2004 [7]. Since then, the in vivo studies of the imaging type have continued with growing success (see Section 5). Since the beginning of the two types of biomarker studies, the state of neurodegenerative diseases changed profoundly. In particular, biomarkers did recently revolutionize scientific and medical research by transforming drug trial design and also improving patient management in clinical practice [8].

So far, I have introduced the two types, i.e., fluid and imaging biomarkers. The in vivo imaging of the latter takes place upon their high affinity binding by radiolabeled specific molecules introduced in the brain. In contrast, fluid biomarkers are collected within (CSF) or away (blood) from the central nervous system. Yet, all fluid biomarkers are adequate to identify central molecules/processes, critical for patients suffering neurodegenerative diseases, not only AD but also Parkinson's disease (PD), amyotrophic lateral sclerosis (ALS), and other diseases. Initially, the disease identification was searched by the recovery in the fluids of free specific molecules. These molecules, however, are largely digested during their traffic, from the cells affected by the disease to the accumulation in the fluids. Thus, their identification was often difficult. The problem has been solved recently by changing the study from free molecules to cargo molecules segregated within extracellular vesicles (EVs). This change will be presented in detail in Section 3.

Initially, each neurodegenerative disease was considered dependent on a single specific biomarker, such as Aβ for AD and α-synuclein for PD. Now it is clear that these two, as well as many other biomarkers, are not fully specific but expressed also by patients of other neurodegenerative diseases [9]. Multispecificity of biomarkers requires caution in their operation. Caution is necessary also with another type of problem. Initially considered specific and efficient, some biomarkers have been found to be hardly reproducible, thus inappropriate for research and clinical practice [8]. A final important consideration refers to the age dependence of disease investigation/treatment. Specific biomarkers have been applied not only to mature patients, but also to patients at early stages of disease. By novel and innovated methods, it could be established whether patients at risk of long-term diseases, such as AD or dementia, can be treated only upon full development of their symptoms, or also when symptoms are absent or still at an early stage [10,11].

Summing up, I anticipate the two types of biomarker generation, and the anticipation of their properties confirms their relevance, which is demonstrated for many of them. The others, in contrast, are weak, characterized by poor specificity and limited employment. The review here includes the most important properties of the two types of biomarkers that have been identified during the last years. Following this introduction, Section 2 deals with the fluids, the environment of type one biomarker generation, followed by Section 3 about the role of EVs, and Section 4 about fluid biomarkers. Finally, Section 5 deals with the second type of biomarkers, i.e., the imaging biomarkers.

2. Fluids

In the Introduction, I already mentioned the two ways leading to the generation of neural biomarkers, i.e., the first based on the analysis of peripheral fluids containing appropriate molecules, the second in vivo, based on the imaging by PET labeling of specific brain molecules. How is it that fluids are essential for the first, very important approach? Two of their properties need to be emphasized. First, molecules of interest for their recognition as biomarkers need to be present in the biological fluids of human body;

second, the analysis of fluids, with ensuing isolation of molecules, is less expensive, much easier, and does not disrupt the body compared to the in vivo analysis of tissues. In other words, the fluids are advantageous in the development of biomarkers.

In the body of mammal animals, including humans, there are 8 types of external fluids. For our purposes, however, only two are relevant: the CSF and the blood plasma. Molecules and the small organelles EVs, released from brain cells such as neurons and astrocytes, navigate in the extracellular fluid space from which they are easily transferred to the CSF [3] (step 2 in Figure 1). At the arachnoid villi, the EVs of the CSF can move to venous blood within large vacuoles (step 4 in Figure 1). In addition, the molecules and EVs have been shown to traffic through the blood–brain barrier [12,13] (step 3 in Figure 1). The latter is the structure known to reduce/exclude the traffic of many other molecules and organelles to and from the brain.

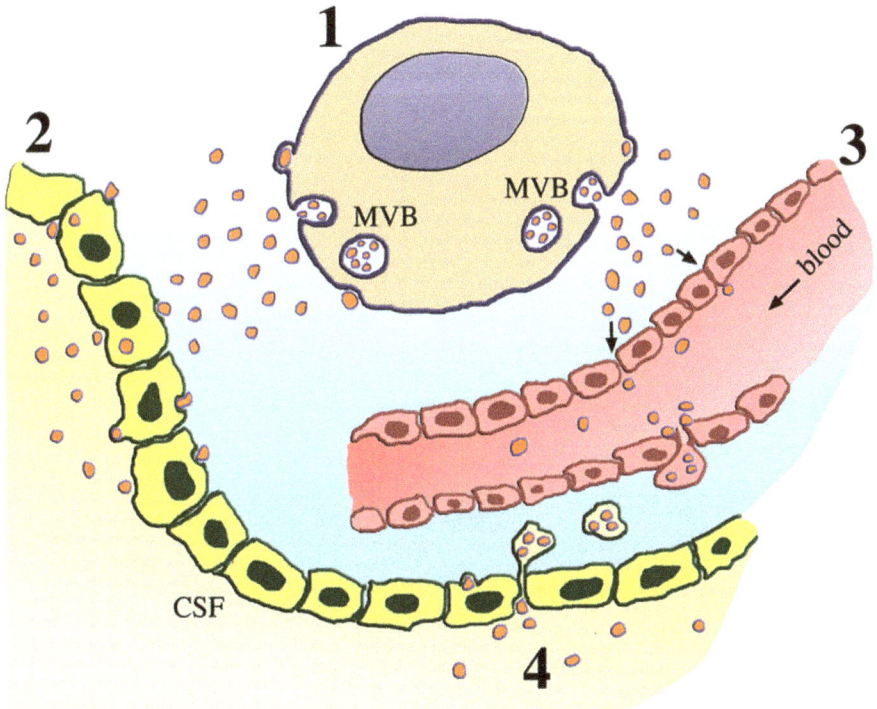

Figure 1. Traffic of extracellular vesicles (EVs) released by a neural cell. The neural cell at the top (cytoplasm of grain color, marked 1) releases the two types of EVs, the small exosomes by exocytosis of multivesicular bodies (MVB), and the larger ectosomes by shedding of plasma membrane rafts. Upon release, the vesicles navigate in the extracellular fluid (light blue). Their targeting relevant for fluid biomarker generation can be accumulate either to the central spinal fluid (CSF) of the ventricular system (left, peach color, marked 2) or as shown by the arrows to the blood (right, red-pink color, marked 3). Additional CSF-to-blood EV transfer occurs by large vacuoles operative at the arachnoid villi (bottom, marked 4). Thus, molecules and EVs can move from the extracellular space and the CSF to the blood plasma. In the case of neurodegenerative diseases, the molecules and EVs of such origin account for significant fractions of the total transferred to the fluids.

Recent studies have shown that biomarkers of the two fluids, CSF and blood plasma, are employed approximately with the same frequency. The choice of one fluid, however, is not due to a negative evaluation of the other. In recent reviews, both are reported as valid [12,14]. Rather, the choice appears to depend on advantages existing in either fluid. High levels of molecules and EVs are present in CSF (Figure 1), which is more invasive and requires more expenses than the blood for biomarker generation. Yet, the CSF fluid has made it possible to have processes of low concentrated proteins, for example, those of the COVID-19 disease reported this year in patients exhibiting neurological symptoms, evident of cerebral infection [15]. In the blood, plasma withdrawal can be large, frequently repeated, and not expensive. However the levels of molecules/EVs in this fluid are lower than in the CSF. The transfer of various EVs across the blood–brain barrier (BBB) has been shown to be different, with ensuing variability of the plasma levels [16]. In many cases, however, they have emerged in the study of neurodegenerative diseases, with enormous potential as a diagnostic, evaluation of therapeutics, and treatment tool.

Summing up, both fluids are employed for biomarker generation. However, the choices depend on their distinct properties. The processes of biomarker generation, previously defined of liquid biopsy [13], have been shown to identify not only the fluid molecules but also the brain pathologic EVs inaccessible in vivo. In addition, fluids have offered unique opportunities, as seen from recent clinical trials, to improve the quality and applicability of results. The processes involved will be developed by approaches presented in the subsequent Section 4 of this review.

3. From Molecules to Extracellular Vesicles

Neurodegenerative diseases are heterogeneous disorders characterized by a progressive and severe cognitive and functional decline leading to the progressive loss of function and death of neuronal cells. Due to the complexity of their diagnosis, early detection and treatments are difficult to recognize, and this is critical for the development of successful therapies. In addition, current diagnostic approaches are often poorly effective. Thus, their therapeutic effects are limited [16]. For several years, progress in diagnosis and therapy has been searched by molecules, such as proteins and nucleotides, via the generation of biomarkers, specific in the diagnosis and possibly in the therapy of the diseases investigated. However, during their traffic and maintenance within the fluids, the molecules were extensively digested by proteases and ribonucleases. Thus, the attempts based on free proteins and nucleotides remained with limited success. The attempt changed considerably when the search for biomarkers started to be made by the use of EVs containing the molecules of interest within their lumen (Figure 1). Now it is clear that when segregated within EVs, the molecules are protected, making them suitable candidates for noninvasive biomarkers [16–18].

EVs are small vesicles of two types released by all cells. The first, widely called exosomes, are produced and accumulated within a vacuole of endosomal nature, the multivesicular body (MVB); the second, the ectosomes, are released by shedding of rafts, directly from the plasma membrane (Figure 1). Interestingly, the two EV types share similar properties. Their membranes are different from the two membranes of origin; their cargoes, segregated within their lumen, contain peculiar molecules, namely many proteins, many nucleotides, most often the noncoding miRNAs, lipids, and others. EVs of neuronal and astrocytic origin, when harvested from blood, can be used to interrogate brain pathologic processes. Moreover, in the case of proteins involved in the development of neurodegeneration, their segregation within EVs and even more their transfer to the fluids decrease the levels within the cells and can thus alter the disease progression [17].

Isolation from CSF or blood plasma of specific brain-cell-derived EVs, confirmed by neural markers [12], is theoretically simple. Thus, the approach has been successful recently and offers great promises for the near future [17,18]. The EVs, released by neurons and astrocytes of patients affected by neurodegenerative disease, can be identified by specific biomarkers found in their cargoes, such as Aβ and phosphorylated tau in AD, α-synuclein in PD, and the transactive response DNA/RNA binding protein of 43 kDa (TDP-43) in ALS [13,19–22] (Table 1). Other biomarkers investigate the subclinical declines of the diseases, for example, the decline of middle age in AD. This can be done with tau and insulin signaling biomarkers [23,24]. A problem considered is that of multiple dementias, only some are connected to neurodegenerative diseases such as AD and PD.

Among the proteins of EVs from specific neurodegenerative diseases, some have been recently shown to concern synaptic and axon injury, inflammations, stress responses and other defects [14,25–28]. Other dementias that are independent of neurodegenerative diseases still need identification of their specific biomarkers [29].

Table 1. Gene expression and disease specificity of proteins/biomarkers.

Genes	Proteins/Biomarkers	Diseases
APP	amyloid precursor protein/Aβ *	AD
PSEN1	presenilin1 *	AD
PSEN2	presenilin2	AD
MAPT	tau *	AD, PD, DLB, FTD
C9orf72	C9orf72 *	FTD, ALS
GRN	progranulin *	FTD, ALS
VCP	valosin-containing protein *	ALS, FTD, PD
TARDBP	TDP-43 *	ALS
FUS	fused in sarcoma (FUS)	ALS
HTT	huntingtin *	HD
SNCA	α-synuclein *	PD, DLB, AD
GBA	β-glucocerebrosidase	PD, DLB
ApoE	apolipoprotein-E	AD (risk factor)
TREM2	TREM2	AD (risk factor)

Well-known fluid biomarkers related to the mentioned proteins are marked by an asterisk (*). The dependence of several diseases may explain the low specificity of some fluid biomarkers. Abbreviations not used elsewhere in this Review: C9orf72, chromosome9 open reading frame 72 gene; DLB, dementia with Lewy's bodies; FTD, frontotemporal dementia; FUS, fused in sarcoma gene; HD, Huntington disease; MAPT, gene of the microtubule-associated protein tau; SNCA, synuclein alpha gene; TARDPB, TAR DNA binding protein gene; TREM2, triggering receptor expressed on myeloid cells 2.

In addition to many proteins, EVs include in their cargo various types of nucleotides, with predominance of miRNAs. The latter are members of a noncoding family involved in various functions, the best known being translational gene expression. Within fluids, miRNAs investigated have been numerous. Whether or not they play the role of biomarkers has been discussed. Positive evidence, analogous to that of proteins, has been recently reported but without precise identification of many miRNAs involved [30–33]. Interestingly, biomarkers of miRNA origin were shown active in the ALS disease [31]. Another positive conclusion has been found, but it concerns children, healthy and patients of their diseases [33]. Additional studies have focused on a new form of noncoding RNA, namely circular RNA (circRNA), known to traffic within EVs. At present, however, the function of these RNAs is unknown. CircRNAs might be involved in age-related diseases [34,35]. RNAs of this type may also operate in neuropsychiatric disorders [35]. The next section, focused exclusively on AD, intends to reconsider in more detail the origin, the multiplicity, and the role of its biomarkers, with special attention on their heterogeneity with perspectives of innovative therapies.

4. AD and Its Multiple Fluid Biomarkers

AD is the neurodegenerative disease of greatest importance for two reasons, namely its much larger number of patients (at least 50 million worldwide) and the many scientists committed to its investigation. The choice of this disease has been made to illustrate its general properties. The task is to provide a current landscape, largely common to PD [21,29,36] but not always to other neurodegenerative diseases (see, for example, [9,17,28,31,32]).

A property common to many neurodegenerative diseases is heterogeneity. Various factors are considered as possible con-causes of its starting. Among these are oxidative stress, neural network dysfunctions, and defects in protein regulation and degradation. In the case of AD, two additional factors need to be considered, i.e., inflammation and immune dysregulation [37]. Such defects are expected to induce alterations in neurons, synapses, axons, and possibly also on glial cells. As already assumed in Section 3, some of these factors have been recognized by the identification of the corresponding biomarkers. For other defects, however, biomarkers are not available yet. Although incomplete, the present knowledge appears of interest to establish the properties of some AD heterogeneous forms, such as responses to treatments. The study of multiple biomarkers, identified during the last months, might be sufficient to characterize at clinical level various aspects of AD, including diagnosis and prognosis [38–40]. Heterogeneity exists also for tau. The fraction inducing tau biomarkers in the CSF was found to stage Alzheimer's disease, and this is potentially useful for tau-directed therapeutics [41]. Other proteins, such as mesenchymal stem cells and exosomes, appear of considerable potential for therapy. The role of some other properties, including heterogeneity, remains to be established [42,43].

An additional approach relevant for AD diagnosis and therapy has been recently reported based on two different miRNAs that are active as EV biomarkers in the blood plasma. Although not identical, the evaluation of the two miRNAs could be considered in parallel. Effects in AD patients, induced by increased miRNA levels in the blood, were revealed by neuronal viability and neuroinflammation followed by a mini-mental state examination. Additional effects were investigated also in fluid, using well-known neural cells such as SH-SY5Y cells, affected by Aβ treatment and evaluated in terms of proliferation, apoptosis, and neuroinflammation. Interestingly, significant upregulation of the first miRNA, miR-485-3p, was shown in patients and cell models, accompanied by severity of DA in vivo and in fluid [44]. The response induced by the second miRNA, miR-331-3p, appears the opposite. Both in vivo and in fluid, the increased miRNA induced significant and persistent attenuation of AD [45]. The two types of results induced by these miRNA opened the possibility of new, promising therapies based on the two biomarkers investigated [44,45].

In conclusion, the actions by EV biomarkers based on multiple properties of proteins and miRNAs have recently offered ample chances of both nature and specificity, showing enormous potential as diagnostic, evaluation and treatment tools. Their new results allow researchers to test hypotheses by proof of concept studies at the preclinical phase, with further opportunities to develop therapeutic discoveries in neurodegenerative diseases [46].

5. Imaging Biomarkers from AD and PD

As already reported in Section 1, the identification of Aβ as the key factor of AD, which was already demonstrated in fluid, was confirmed in vivo by the development and investigation of an appropriate radiolabeled molecule. Upon its penetration into the living brain, such a molecule made it possible to have a clear Aβ imaging by PET [7]. By now, such an approach of investigation plays roles much more important than its historical role. Advanced technologies of the near future are expected to further improve the present success of such studies. The biomarkers obtained by this approach are usually named imaging biomarkers.

The advantages offered by such biomarkers include properties that are different and integrative with respect to the fluid biomarkers illustrated in the previous sections. Among the results of imaging biomarkers are their demonstrations occurring in the living brain, distinct from the peripheral demonstrations of fluid biomarkers; their data obtained from larger numbers (hundreds) of patients; and the quantitation of their measurements, necessary for many assays. The relevance of these properties emerges from a recent group of papers based on the comparison between the results obtained with fluid and imaging biomarkers. In these reports, the relevance of the results obtained by the imaging techniques is emphasized [36,47,48]. Another difference between the two approaches has emerged with respect to the amyloid cascade, a concept activated by elevated levels of Aβ and tau, which is completed by severe cognition and functional impairments [49]. In this case, the data by CSF biomarkers were found to emerge before those by PET imaging, demonstrating a high sensitivity that is relevant for the study of early AD stages [50]. Further studies with CSF biomarkers, compared with those obtained by PET and resonance (MRI) imaging, confirmed the relevance of the latter approach in many preclinical AD investigations [51,52].

Among additional problems adequately investigated by brain imaging is the heterogeneity of neurodegenerative diseases. Detailed recent studies have focused not only on the various forms of AD but also on PD and its atypical syndromes. In an initial study, several PDs that were hindered by substantial clinical and pathological heterogeneities were investigated by numerous imaging techniques including PET and MRI [53]. More recently, combinations with new techniques have been established to investigate, in distinct areas and pathways of the brain, the various molecules and processes, i.e., the molecular imaging of Aβ, tau and α-synuclein, as well as neuroinflammation. This integrative "multimodal approach" was found to be superior to single modality-based methods, with expected future advancements in the field [54]. Other innovative combinations of imaging biomarkers, revealed by MRI and PET, have been employed to investigate subtypes of AD. At the level of previously established groups of patients, the average and clinical characteristics appeared similar. In subtype assignments, however, disagreements were considerable. The subtypes therefore need to be further investigated, with an establishment of their harmonization by appropriate methods [55].

Additional new studies have expanded the investigation of in vivo biomarker-driven profiles by the reinforcement of the techniques employed. In a first example, a versatile form of PET imaging was found able to quantify the molecular targets of interest. By such approach, age-related neurodegenerative diseases, inducing dysregulation of synapses, neuroinflammation, protein misfolding, and other dysfunctions, were appropriately identified. Discussion of these processes has led to the identification of novel biomarkers [56]. A second approach was based on the development of optical imaging (OPI) probes and devices, which are affordable by imaging studies but are limited by their low depth of penetration. The combination of the OPI technique with PET, which is characterized by high depth penetration, resulted in the elimination of each limitation. The affording of new radiolabeled fluorophores made the activation of the dual PET/OPI mode possible, with excellent preclinical imaging results in various pathological conditions [57].

Summing up, the imaging biomarkers presented in this section are profoundly different from the biomarkers of the fluid type. Being recognized from the analysis of brain tissue, they do not fit strictly the definition of biomarkers as distinct molecules related to pathology, given in the first lines of the Introduction. Yet, a growing class of radiotracers, addressed to specific proteins such as Aβ and tau, have recently contributed to the growing knowledge about AD. In other words, the targets of the imaging processes can now be identified as molecules based on which the identification of imaging biomarkers is established [58,59].

6. Conclusions

This review focused on the new developments of two types of biomarkers, i.e., fluid and imagining biomarkers, generated via two distinct operative pathways originated in the brain. As emphasized in Section 5, even if the structure and the mechanisms of action of the two types are largely different, at least some of their effects are similar, to the point that their results, when considered together, give rise to positive integrations [36,47,48].

How relevant is the medical work of biomarkers? The experience accumulated during the last decade appears positive and encouraging. Many of their properties, such as specificity, multiplicity, and affinity, have strengthened their use in the course of AD, PD, and other neurodegenerative diseases. The present investigation about the pathogenesis of AD and the other neurodegenerative diseases is largely due to biomarker-based data. To understand the issues underlying complex symptoms such as dementia, biomarkers often operate combined with other disciplines [60].

In basic and applied research, the impact of biomarkers has increased, sustained by the improvement of their technologies. In the fluid field, the recent experience with EVs as tools for biomarker generation has improved their success considerably. An additional development is the recent recognition of increased number of proteins and peptides in the CSF of AD patients [61]. The imaging technology has been strengthened by the development of new radiolabeled molecules, by the use of improved imaging techniques, and by their combination with different procedures. In these studies, the best successes has been obtained when working on early stages of AD, including the identification of pathological alterations and a selective cognitive decline [62].

The results obtained by the use of biomarkers are often of relevance in medical practice. This in particular is the case of diagnosis: O often inadequate when based only on medical practice, it has been recently improved by the multiplicity and specificity of biomarkers. By the use of the latter, it has been established that a disease can be diagnosed even before the appearance of symptoms [10,11,51,52]. Moreover, the intensity of the responses can contribute to the prognosis of patients [28,44]. Thus, diagnostic and prognostic results obtained by biomarkers are often analogous. In contrast, therapy is still problematic. Although open to all neurodegenerative diseases, such problem is particularly aggressive for AD and ALS, for which appropriate therapy is not available. An initial attempt to improve the present situation involves the investigation of diseases at early or even pre-symptomatic conditions. Drugs slowing down the development of the disease should delay its progress, ultimately resulting in a progressive decrease of the AD mature state. Up to now, however, the results of clinical trials to evaluate the state of the AD therapy have been disappointing. In the future, development should be based on multiple criteria, including the state of the disease, its progression, and the activity of biomarkers focused on critical processes [40].

In conclusion, the recent identification and employment of biomarkers have resulted in increased knowledge and improvement of both basic and applied research. However, as emphasized in the first and subsequent sections of this review, various aspects of their function are still not completely or even inappropriately known. In the future, it appears desirable that intense research about biomarkers will include their critical evaluation and their further improvement, especially in terms of new therapy practice.

Funding: This research received no external funding.

Institutional Review Board Statement: Not applicable.

Informed Consent Statement: Not Applicable.

Data Availability Statement: All the data reported in this review are available at the American Program PubMed.

Acknowledgments: I thank Palma Gallana for the support in the final version of this Review and Gabriella Racchetti for the preparation of Figure 1.

Conflicts of Interest: The authors declare no conflict of interest.

Abbreviations

AD	Alzheimer's disease
ALS	amyotrophic lateral sclerosis
BBB	blood-brain barrier
CSF	central spinal fluid
EV	extracellular vesicle

miRNA and circRNA	micro and circular RNAs
MVB	multivesicular body
OPI	ocular imaging
PD	Parkinson's disease
TDP-43	transactive response DNA/RNA binding protein of 43 kDa

References

1. Gromova, M.; Vaggelas, A.; Dallmann, G.; Seimtz, D. Biomarkers: Opportunities and challenges for drug development in the current regulatory landscapes. *Biomark. Insights* **2020**, *15*. [CrossRef]
2. Diray-Arce, J.; Conti, M.G.; Petrova, B.; Kanarek, N.; Angelidou, A.; Levy, O. Integrative metabolomics to identify molecular signatures of responses to vaccines and infections. *Metabolites* **2020**, *10*, 492. [CrossRef] [PubMed]
3. Rabbito, A.; Dulewicz, M.; Kulczynska-Przybik, A.; Moczko, B. Biochemical markers in Alzheimer's disease. *Int. J. Mol. Sci.* **2020**, *21*, 1989. [CrossRef]
4. Casamitjana, A.; Petrone, P.; Molinuevo, J.L.; Gispert, J.D.; Vilaplana, V. Projection to latent spaces entangles pathological effects on brain morphology in the symptomatic phase of Alzheimer's disease. *Front. Neurol.* **2020**, *11*, 648. [CrossRef]
5. Laulagnier, K.; Javalet, C.; Hemming, F.J.; Sadoul, R. Purification and analysis of exosomes released by mature cortical neurons following synaptic activation. *Methods Mol. Biol.* **2017**, *1545*, 129–138. [PubMed]
6. Maraoka, S.; Lin, W.; Chen, M.; Hersh, S.W.; Emil, A.; Xia, W.; Ikezu, T. Assessment of separation methods for extracellular vesicles from human and mouse brain tissues and human cerebrospinal fluids. *Methods* **2020**, *177*, 35–49. [CrossRef]
7. Klunk, W.E.; Engler, H.; Nordberg, A.; Wang, Y.; Blomqvist, G.; Holt, D.P.; Bergstrom, M.; Savitcheva, I.; Huang, G.F.; Es-trada, S.; et al. Imaging brain amyloid in Alzheimer's disease with Pittsburgh compound. *Ann. Neurol.* **2004**, *55*, 306–319. [CrossRef] [PubMed]
8. Mattson-Calgren, N.; Palmqvist, S.; Blennow, K.; Hansson, O. Increasing the reproducibility of fluid biomarker studies in neurodegenerative studies. *Nat. Commun.* **2020**, *11*, 6252. [CrossRef] [PubMed]
9. Torok, N.; Tanaka, M.; Vecsei, L. Searching for peripheral biomarkers in neurodegenerative diseases: The tryptophan-kynurenine metabolic pathway. *Int. J. Mol. Sci.* **2020**, *21*, 9338. [CrossRef] [PubMed]
10. Mantzavinos, V.; Alexiou, A. Biomarkers for Alzheimer's disease diagnosis. *Curr. Alzheimer Res.* **2017**, *14*, 1149–1154. [CrossRef] [PubMed]
11. Boniecki, V.; Zetterberg, H.; Aarsland, D.; Vannini, P.; Kvartsberg, H.; Winblad, B.; Blennow, K.; Freud-Levi, Y. Are neuropsychiatric symptoms in dementia linked to CSF biomarkers of synaptic and axonal degeneration? *Alzheimer's Res. Ther.* **2020**, *12*, 153. [CrossRef] [PubMed]
12. Banks, A.W.; Sharma, P.; Bullock, K.M.; Hansen, K.M.; Ludwig, N.; Whiteside, T.L. Transport of extracellular vesicles across the blood-brain barrier: Brain pharmacokinetics and effects of inflammation. *Int. J. Mol. Sci.* **2020**, *21*, 4407. [CrossRef]
13. Badhwar, A.; Haqqani, A.S. Biomarker potential of brain-secreted extracellular vesicles in blood in Alzheimer's disease. *Alzheimer's Dement.* **2020**, *12*, e12001. [CrossRef] [PubMed]
14. Gaetani, L.; Paolini Paoletti, F.; Bellomo, G.; Mancini, A.; Simoni, S.; Di Filippo, M.; Parnetti, L. CSF and blood biomarkers in neuroinflammatory and neurodegenerative diseases: Implications for treatment. *Trends Pharmacol. Sci.* **2020**, *41*, 1023–1037. [CrossRef] [PubMed]
15. Eden, A.; Kanberg, N.; Gostner, J.; Fuchs, D.; Hagberg, L.; Andersson, L.M.; Lindh, M.; Price, R.W.; Zetterberg, H.; Gisslen, M. CSF biomarkers in patients with COVID-19 and neurological symptoms: A case series. *Neurology* **2021**, *96*, e294–e300. [PubMed]
16. Lim, C.Z.J.; Natalia, A.; Sundah, N.R.; Shao, H. Biomarker organization in circulating extracellular vesicles: New applica-tions in detecting neurodegenerative diseases. *Adv. Biosyst.* **2020**, *4*, e1900309. [CrossRef] [PubMed]
17. Wang, L.; Zhang, L. Circulating exosomal miRNA as diagnostic biomarkers of neurodegenerative diseases. *Front. Mol. Neurosci.* **2020**, *13*, 53. [CrossRef]
18. Kapogiannis, D. Exosome biomarkers revolutionize preclinical diagnosis of neurodegenerative diseases and assessment of treatment responses in clinical trials. *Adv. Exp. Med. Biol.* **2020**, *1195*, 149. [CrossRef] [PubMed]
19. Hornung, S.; Dutta, S.; Bitan, G. CNS-derived blood exosomes as a promising source of biomarkers: Opportunities and challenges. *Front. Mol. Neurosci.* **2020**, *13*, 38. [CrossRef] [PubMed]
20. Yo, Y.K.; Lee, J.; Kim, H.; Hwang, K.S.; Yoon, D.S.; Lee, J.H. Toward exosome-based neuronal diagnostic devices. *Micromachines* **2018**, *9*, 634. [CrossRef]
21. Wang, H.; Wang, W.; Shi, H.; Han, L.; Pan, P. Blood neurofilament light chain in Parkinson disease and atypical parkin-sonisms, A protocol for systematic review and meta-analysis. *Medicine* **2020**, *99*, e21871. [CrossRef] [PubMed]
22. Yin, O.; Ji, X.; Ly, R.; Pei, J.J.; Du, Y.; Shen, C.; Hou, X. Targeting exosomes as a new biomarker and therapeutic approach for Alzheimer's disease. *Clin. Interv. Aging* **2020**, *15*, 195–205. [CrossRef] [PubMed]
23. Eren, E.; Hunt, J.F.; Shardell, M.; Chawla, S.; Tran, J.; Gu, J.; Vogy, N.M.; Johnson, S.C.; Bendlin, B.B.; Kapogiannis, D. Ex-tracellular vesicle biomarkers of Azheimer's disease associated with sub-clinical cognitive-decline in late middle age. *Alzheimer's Dement.* **2020**, *16*, 1293–1304. [CrossRef] [PubMed]
24. Cantero, J.; Atienza, M.; Amos-Cejudo, J.; Fossai, S.; Wisniewski, T.; Osorio, R.S. Plasma tau predicts cerebral vulnerability in aging. *Aging* **2020**, *12*, 21004–21022. [CrossRef] [PubMed]

25. Guha, D.; Lorenz, D.R.; Misra, V.; Chettimada, S.; Morgello, S.; Gabuzda, D. Proteomic analysis of cerebrospinal fluid extracellular vesicles reveals synaptic injury, inflammation, and stress response markers in HIV patients with cognitive impairment. *Neuroinflammation* **2019**, *16*, 254. [CrossRef]
26. Mazzucchi, S.; Palermo, G.; Campese, N.; Galgani, A.; Della Vecchia, A.; Vergallo, A.; Siciliano, G.; Ceravolo, R.; Hamel, H.; Baldacci, F. The role of synaptic biomarkers in the spectrum of neurodegenerative diseases. *Expert Rev. Proteom.* **2020**, *17*, 543–559. [CrossRef] [PubMed]
27. Xiang, Y.; Xin, J.; Le, W.; Yang, Y. Neurogranin, A potential biomarker of neurological and mental diseases. *Front. Aging Neurosci.* **2020**, *12*, 584743. [CrossRef] [PubMed]
28. Lin, C.H.; Li, C.H.; Yang, K.C.; Lin, F.J.; Wu, C.C.; Chieh, J.J.; Chu, M.J. Blood NfL: A biomarker for disease severity and progression in Parkinson disease. *Neurology* **2019**, *93*, e1104–e1111. [CrossRef] [PubMed]
29. Gamez-Valero, A.; Beyer, K.; Borras, F.E. Extracellular vesicles, new actors in the search for biomarkers of dementia. *Neurobiol. Aging* **2019**, *74*, 15–20. [CrossRef] [PubMed]
30. Lugli, C.; Cohen, A.M.; Bennett, D.A.; Shah, R.C.; Fields, C.J.; Hernandez, A.G.; Smalheiser, N.R. Plasma exosomal miRNAs in persons with and without Alzheimer's disease: Altered expression and prospects for biomarkers. *PLoS ONE* **2015**, *10*, e139233. [CrossRef] [PubMed]
31. Hosaka, T.; Yamashita, T.; Tamaoka, A.; Swak, S. Extracelluar RNAs as biomarkers of sporadic amyotrophic lateral sclerosis and other neurodegenerative disease. *Int. J. Mol. Sci.* **2019**, *20*, 3148. [CrossRef]
32. Jimenez-Avalos, J.A.; Ferandez-Macias, J.C.; Galez-Palomo, A.K. Circulating exosomal microRNAs: New non-invasive biomarkers of non-communicable disease. *Mol. Biol. Rep.* 2020. [CrossRef]
33. Prieto-Fernandez, E.; Lopez-Lopez, E.; Martin-Guerrero, I.; Barcen, L.; Gonzalez-Lopez, M.; Aransay, A.M.; Lozano, J.J.; Benito, J.; Falcon-Perez, J.M.; Garcia-Orad, A. Variability in cerebrospinal fluid microRNA through life. *Mol. Neurobiol.* **2020**, *57*, 4134–4142. [CrossRef] [PubMed]
34. Pan, W.H.; Wu, W.P.; Xiong, X.D. Circular RNAs: Promising biomarkers for age related diseases. *Aging Dis.* **2020**, *11*, 1585–1593. [CrossRef] [PubMed]
35. Zhuo, C.J.; Hou, W.H.; Jiang, D.G.; Tian, H.J.; Wang, L.N.; Jia, F.; Zhou, C.H.; Zhu, J.J. Circular RNAs in early brain development and their influence and clinical significance in neuropsychiatric disorders. *Neural Regen. Res.* **2020**, *15*, 817–823. [CrossRef] [PubMed]
36. Compta, Y.; Revesz, T. Neuropathological and biomarker findings in Parkinson's disease and Alzheimer's disease from protein aggregates to synaptic dysfunction. *J. Parkinsons Dis.* **2020**, *11*, 102–121.
37. Kim, J.; Kim, Y.K. Inflammatory biomarkers in AD: Implications for diagnosis. *Curr. Alzheimer's Res.* **2020**, *17*, 962–971. [CrossRef]
38. Vasileff, N.; Cheng, L.; Hill, A.F. Extracellular vesicles-propagators of neuropathology and sources of potential biomarkers and therapeutics for neurodegenerative diseases. *J. Cell Sci.* **2020**, *133*, jcs243139. [CrossRef] [PubMed]
39. Nguyen, T.T.; Ta, Q.T.H.; Nguyen, T.K.O.; Nguyen, T.T.D.; Vo, V.G. Role of body-fluid biomarkers in Alzheimer's disease diagnosis. *Diagnostics* **2020**, *10*, 326. [CrossRef] [PubMed]
40. Tarawsneh, R. Biomarkers, Our path towards a cure for Alzheimer's disease. *Biomark. Insights* **2020**, *15*, 1177271920976367. [CrossRef]
41. Horie, K.; Barthlemy, N.R.; Sato, C.; Bateman, R.J. CSF tau microtubule binding region identifies tau tangle and clinical stages of Alzheimer's disease. *Brain* **2020**, awaa373. [CrossRef]
42. Guo, M.; Yin, Z.; Chen, F.; Ping, L. Mesenchymal stem cell-derived exosome: A promising alternative in the therapy of Alzheimer's disease. *Alzheimer's Res. Ther.* **2020**, *12*, 109. [CrossRef]
43. Martins, T.S.; Trindade, D.; Vaz, M.; Campelo, I.; Almeida, M.; Trigo, G.; da Cruz E Silva, O.A.B.; Henriques, A.G. Diagnostic and therapeutic potential of exosomes in Alzheimer's disease. *J. Neurochem.* **2020**, *156*, 162–181. [CrossRef] [PubMed]
44. Yu, L.; Haiting, L.I.; Liu, W.; Zhang, L.; Tia, O.; Li, H.; Li, M. MiR-485-3p serves as a biomarker and therapeutic target of Alzheimer's disease via regulating neuronal cell viability and neurofiammation by target AKT3. *Mol. Genet. Genom. Med.* **2020**, e1548. [CrossRef]
45. Liu, Q.; Lei, C. Neuroprotective effects of miR-331-3p through improved cell viability and inflammatory marker expression, Correlation of serum miR-331-3p levels with diagnosis and severity of Alzheimer's disease. *Exp. Gerontol.* **2020**, *144*, 111187. [CrossRef] [PubMed]
46. Cummings, J. Drug development for psychotropic, cognitive-enhancing and disease-modifying treatments for Alzheimer's disease. *J. Neuropsychiatry Clin. Neurosci.* **2020**, *33*, 3–13. [CrossRef]
47. Clifford, R.J.; Bennett, D.A.; Blennow, K.; Carillo, M.C.; Feldman, H.H.; Frisono, G.B.; Hampel, H.; Jagust, W.J.; Johnson, K.A.; Knopman, D.S.; et al. A/T/N, An unbiased descriptive classification scheme for Alzheimer's disease biomarkers. *Neurology* **2016**, *87*, 539–547.
48. Lashley, T.; Shott, J.M.; Weston, P.; Murray, C.E.; Wellington, H.; Keshavan, A.; Foti, S.C.; Foinani, M.; Toombs, J.; Rohrer, J.D.; et al. Molecular biomarkers of Alzheimer's disease: Progress and prospects. *Dis. Model. Mech.* **2018**, *11*, dmm031781. [CrossRef] [PubMed]
49. Hardy, J.; Selkoe, D.J. The amyloid hypothesis of the Alzheimer's disease: Progress and problems on the road to therapeutics. *Science* **2002**, *297*, 229–240. [CrossRef] [PubMed]

50. Insel, P.; Donohue, M.C.; Berron, D.; Hansson, O.; Mattson-Calgren, N. Time between milestone events in the Alzheimer's disease amyloid cascade. *Neuroimage* **2020**, *22*, 117676. [CrossRef]
51. Babulal, G.M.; Johnson, A.; Fagan, A.M.; Morris, J.C.; Roe, C.M. Identifying preclinical Alzheimer's disease using everyday driving behavior: Proof of concepts. *J. Alzheimer's Dis.* **2021**, *79*, 1009–1014. [CrossRef]
52. Li, T.R.; Wu, Y.; Jiang, J.J.; Lin, H.; Han, C.L.; Jang, J.H.; Han, Y. Radiomic analysis of magnetic resonance imaging facili-tates the identification of preclinical Alzheimer's disease: An exploratory study. *Cell Dev. Biol.* **2020**, *8*, 605734. [CrossRef]
53. Saed, U.; Compagnone, J.; Aviv, R.; Strafella, A.P.; Black, S.E.; Lang, A.E.; Masellis, M. Imaging biomarkers in Parkinson's disease and parkinsonin syndromes: Current and emergins concepts. *Transl. Neurodegener.* **2017**, *6*, 8. [CrossRef] [PubMed]
54. Saeed, U.; Lang, A.E.; Masellis, M. Neuroimaging advances in Parkinson's disease and atypical parkinsonian syndromes. *Front. Neurol.* **2020**, *11*, 572976. [CrossRef] [PubMed]
55. Mohanty, R.; Martensson, G.; Poulakis, K.; Muelboueck, J.S.; Rodriguez-Vieitez, E.; Chotis, K.; Grothe, M.J.; Nordberg, A.; Ferreira, D.; Westman, E. Comparison of subtyping methods for neuroimaging studies in Alzheimer's disease, A call for harmonization. *Brain Commun.* **2020**, *2*, fcaa192. [CrossRef] [PubMed]
56. Wilson, H.; Politis, M.; Rabiner, E.A.; Middleton, L.T. Novel PET biomarkers to disentangle molecular pathways across age-related neurodegenerative diseases. *Cells* **2020**, *9*, 2581. [CrossRef] [PubMed]
57. Munch, M.; Rotstein, B.H.; Ulrich, G. Florine-18-labeled fluorescent dyes for dual-mode molecular imaging. *Molecules* **2020**, *25*, 6042. [CrossRef] [PubMed]
58. Rowley, P.A.; Samsonov, A.A.; Betthauser, T.J.; Pirasteh, A.; Johnson, S.C.; Eisenmenger, L.B. Amyloid and tau PET imaging of Alzheimer's disease and other neurodegenerative conditions. *Semin. Ultrasound CT MR* **2020**, *41*, 572–583. [CrossRef] [PubMed]
59. Knopman, D.S.; Jagust, W.J. Alzheimer's disease spectrum: Syndrome and etiology from clinical and PET imaging per-spectives. *Neurology* 2020. [CrossRef]
60. Ehremberg, A.J.; Khatun, A.; Coomans, E.; Betts, M.J.; Capraro, F.; Thijssen, E.H.; Senkevich, K.; Bharucha, T.; Jafarpour, M.; Young, P.N.E.; et al. Relevance of biomarkers across different neurodegenerative diseases. *Alzheimer's Res. Ther.* **2020**, *12*, 56. [CrossRef]
61. Pedrero-Prieto, C.M.; Garcia-Capitero, S.; Frontinan-Rubio, J.; Llanos-Gonzalez, E.; Aguilera-Garcia, C.; Alcan, F.C.; Lind-berg, I.; Duran-Prado, M.; Peinado, J.R.; Rabanal-Luiz, Y. A comprehensive systematic review of CSF proteins and peptides to define Alzheimer's disease. *Clin. Proteom.* **2020**, *17*, 21. [CrossRef] [PubMed]
62. Wang, X.; Huang, W.; Su, L.; Xing, Y.; Fessen, F.; Sun, Y.; Shu, N.; Han, Y. Neuroimaging advances regarding subjective cognitive decline in preclinical Alzheimer's disease. *Mol. Neurodegener.* **2020**, *15*, 55. [CrossRef] [PubMed]

MDPI
St. Alban-Anlage 66
4052 Basel
Switzerland
Tel. +41 61 683 77 34
Fax +41 61 302 89 18
www.mdpi.com

Biomedicines Editorial Office
E-mail: biomedicines@mdpi.com
www.mdpi.com/journal/biomedicines

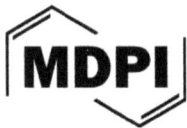

www.ingramcontent.com/pod-product-compliance
Lightning Source LLC
LaVergne TN
LVHW070707100526
838202LV00013B/1044